Insights into Antibiotics in Human, Animal, and Agriculture: Resistance, Determinant, and Treatment

Insights into Antibiotics in Human, Animal, and Agriculture: Resistance, Determinant, and Treatment

Editors

Anusak Kerdsin
Jinquan Li
Jonathan Frye

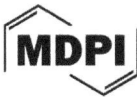

Basel • Beijing • Wuhan • Barcelona • Belgrade • Novi Sad • Cluj • Manchester

Editors

Anusak Kerdsin
Faculty of Public Health
Kasetsart University,
Chalermphrakiat Sakon
Nakhon Province Campus
Sakon Nakhon
Thailand

Jinquan Li
College of Food Science and
Technology
Huazhong Agricultural
University
Wuhan
China

Jonathan Frye
Poultry Microbiological
Safety and Processing
Research Unit
USDA ARS Russell Research
Center (RRC)
Athens
United States

Editorial Office
MDPI
St. Alban-Anlage 66
4052 Basel, Switzerland

This is a reprint of articles from the Special Issue published online in the open access journal *Antibiotics* (ISSN 2079-6382) (available at: www.mdpi.com/journal/antibiotics/special_issues/ insights_antibiotics).

For citation purposes, cite each article independently as indicated on the article page online and as indicated below:

Lastname, A.A.; Lastname, B.B. Article Title. *Journal Name* **Year**, *Volume Number*, Page Range.

ISBN 978-3-7258-1392-6 (Hbk)
ISBN 978-3-7258-1391-9 (PDF)
doi.org/10.3390/books978-3-7258-1391-9

Contents

Preface

The overuse and inappropriate use of antibiotics in medicine, agriculture, fishery, and food animal production is an under-appreciated problem. This problem is considered to have potential public health implications. The agricultural, food animal, and aquatic environments have been regarded as vital reservoirs and sources of antibiotic residues, antibiotic-resistant bacteria, and resistance genes. Antibiotic residues have been reported to have a negative impact on public health and food safety with regard to drug toxicity, immunopathological diseases, carcinogenicity, allergic reactions, etc., whereas antibiotic-resistant bacteria lead to treatment failure in humans and animals, increasing the number and spread of infections worldwide.

This Special Issue assembles a set of fifteen articles, consisting of one review and fourteen research articles. The review by Liang S. and colleagues covers the application of bacteriophage therapy. The 14 research articles included (1) methodologies and techniques to detect AMR organisms, such as VRE by Saenhom N et al. and carbapenemase-producing Eterobacterales by Hatrongjit R. et al.; (2) characterization of AMR from patients, foods, and the environment, such as by Yinsai et al., Li R. et al., Kamal Hossain M., et al., Kansaen R., et al., Tabut et al., Lopes E.S. et al., and Kumar Rout A. et al., respectively; (3) antibiotics residue management approached, such as by Chokejaroenrat et al. and Sakulthaew et al., and (4) medical care of AMR patients and carriage, such as by Ngamprasertchai T et al. and Miranda-Novales et al.

Finally, on behalf of the guest editors of the Special Issue, we wish to thank the authors for their contributions and for their commitment to improving their work, the reviewers for investing time and effort into analysing and providing valuable comments and corrections, and the editorial staff for managing the review and publication process efficiently and thoroughly. We hope that these articles will provide in-depth research results, advance knowledge, impact the scientific community, and motivate researchers to pursue their scientific goals.

Anusak Kerdsin, Jinquan Li, and Jonathan Frye
Editors

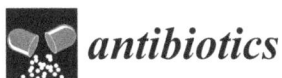

antibiotics

MDPI

Review

Bacteriophage Therapy as an Application for Bacterial Infection in China

Shuang Liang[1], Yanling Qi[1], Huabo Yu[1], Wuwen Sun[1,2], Sayed Haidar Abbas Raza[3], Nada Alkhorayef[4], Samia S. Alkhalil[5], Essam Eldin Abdelhady Salama[6] and Lei Zhang[1,2,*]

1 College of Animal Science and Technology, Jilin Agricultural University, Changchun 130000, China
2 Borui Technology Co., Ltd., Changchun 130000, China
3 College of Animal Science and Technology, Northwest A&F University, Yangling 712100, China
4 Department of Clinical Laboratory Science, College of Applied Medical Sciences, Al-Quway'iyah, Shaqra University, Riyadh 19257, Saudi Arabia
5 Department of Clinical Laboratory Sciences, Faculty of Applied Medical Sciences, Shaqra University, Shaqra 11961, Saudi Arabia
6 Anatomy Department College of Medicine, King Saud University, Riyadh 11495, Saudi Arabia
* Correspondence: zhanglei0221@jlau.edu.cn

Abstract: Antibiotic resistance has emerged as a significant issue to be resolved around the world. Bacteriophage (phage), in contrast to antibiotics, can only kill the target bacteria with no adverse effect on the normal bacterial flora. In this review, we described the biological characteristics of phage, and summarized the phage application in China, including in mammals, ovipara, aquatilia, and human clinical treatment. The data showed that phage had a good therapeutic effect on drug-resistant bacteria in veterinary fields, as well as in the clinical treatment of humans. However, we need to take more consideration of the narrow lysis spectrum, the immune response, the issues of storage, and the pharmacokinetics of phages. Due to the particularity of bacteriophage as a bacterial virus, there is no unified standard or regulation for the use of bacteriophage in the world at present, which hinders the application of bacteriophage as a substitute for antibiotic biological products. We aimed to highlight the rapidly advancing field of phage therapy as well as the challenges that China faces in reducing its reliance on antibiotics.

Keywords: phage therapy; animal models; clinical application; anti-infection; bacterial resistance

Citation: Liang, S.; Qi, Y.; Yu, H.; Sun, W.; Raza, S.H.A.; Alkhorayef, N.; Alkhalil, S.S.; Salama, E.E.A.; Zhang, L. Bacteriophage Therapy as an Application for Bacterial Infection in China. *Antibiotics* **2023**, *12*, 417. https://doi.org/10.3390/antibiotics12020417

Academic Editors: Anusak Kerdsin, Jinquan Li and Jonathan Frye

Received: 25 December 2022
Revised: 31 January 2023
Accepted: 5 February 2023
Published: 20 February 2023

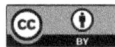

1. Introduction

At present, the main treatment for bacterial infection is antibiotics. Due to the extensive use of antibiotics, there have been numerous problems, such as the emergence of drug-resistant bacteria, immunosuppression, drug residues in animal products, environmental pollution, and so on. According to statistics, 75% of bacteria in the United States are resistant to at least one kind of antibiotic, and nearly 2 million people's health is at risk each year due to drug-resistant bacteria [1]. In addition, more than half of the clinical *Staphylococcus* isolated in Japan have multidrug resistances to antibiotics [2]. A report from the British government in 2016 showed that the deaths caused by drug-resistant bacteria could reach about 700,000 each year [3]. It is estimated that by the year 2050, upwards of 10 million people will die each year due to antimicrobial resistance. In 2017, the World Health Organization (WHO) published a list of global priority pathogens comprising 12 species of bacteria which were categorized into critical, high, and medium priority based on their level of resistance and available therapeutics (Table 1). It is crucial to discover, design, and develop new and alternative antimicrobial therapies. The current rate of resistance development far exceeds the level of antibiotic discovery and development and represents a global public health challenge.

Table 1. WHO pathogen priority list, 2017.

Priority	Pathogen Name	Resistance
Critical	*Acinetobacter baumannii*	Carbapenem
	Pseudomonas aeruginosa	Carbapenem
	Enterobacteriaceae	Carbapenem and produces extended-spectrum lactamase (ESBL)
High	*Enterococcus faecalis*	Vancomycin
	Staphylococcus aureus	Methicillin and Vancomycin intermediary
	Helicobacterpylori	Clarithromycin
	Campylobacter	Fluoroquinolones
	Salmonella	Fluoroquinolones
	Neisseria gonorrhoeae	Cephalosporin and Fluoroquinolones
Medium	*Streptococcus pneumoniae*	Penicillin
	Haemophilus influenzae	Ampicillin
	Shigella	Fluoroquinolones

Note: Critical priority pathogens are bacteria that cause severe infection and high mortality in hospitalized patients; High priority pathogens are bacteria that cause a large number of infections in healthy people; Medium priority pathogens are three types of bacteria that are developing more resistance to available drugs.

The Chinese government placed a high priority on bacterial drug resistance and included it on the agenda of the G20 Hangzhou Summit. In order to control the development of bacterial resistance, the Ministry of Agriculture and Rural Affairs of the People's Republic of China issued *the National Action Plan for Reducing the Use of Veterinary Antimicrobials (2021–2025)* and *the List of Banned Drugs and Other Compounds for Food Animals.* In addition, the Chinese government encourages large-scale animal husbandry to cut off pathogen infection at the source. Companies have tried to develop new antibiotics, but few are available in terms of their commercial value [4]. Faced with the problem of increasing bacterial resistance year by year, it is urgent to find a new treatment that can replace antibiotics. Antimicrobial peptides and biological enzymes are also popular alternatives to antibiotic therapy. However, the utilization of these medications is constrained due to their lengthy research cycles and limited antibacterial properties [5].

Bacteriophage(phage) is a virus that can infect microorganisms such as bacteria, fungi, actinomycetes, and spirochetes. Phages have been used as antibacterial agents since their discovery in the 1920s. However, with the discovery of antibiotics and their widespread use, people gradually ignored the in-depth study of phage therapy. Since the 1980s, due to the continuous emergence of drug-resistant bacteria worldwide, antibiotic therapy has been facing great challenges, and bacteriophage as a traditional antimicrobial therapy has attracted attention again. Phage has the characteristics of strong specificity, little toxicity, good bactericidal effect, good biological safety, and great potential in the prevention and control of bacterial infection. Recently, some scholars from western countries have published special papers on bacteriophage antibacterial technology, sharing positive comments on the basic research and development of bacteriophage. They believed that the natural targeting effect, specificity, and high efficiency of bacteriophages had opened up a new field for the control and prevention of bacterial diseases [6–8]. Haddad et al. collated the literature on phage therapy published from 1985 to 2018, and the results showed that phage therapy was effective in reducing bacterial concentration, degrading biofilms, healing wounds, and improving outcomes in most studies (87%, 26/30) [9].

In this review, we summarized the research and application of phage in the prevention and control of bacterial infections in China, and discussed the limitations and challenges of phage therapy, hoping to provide a reference for promoting the clinical application of phage therapy.

2. Overview of Phages

Bacteriophages (phages) are highly abundant in the environment and may be the source of low-cost antimicrobials. Bacteriophages coexist with their bacterial hosts and play an important role in many biological processes such as bacterial evolution and microorganism diversity [10–15]. In general, the biological characteristics of a phage include its optimum pH, temperature, one-step growth curve, morphology, etc. Like other viruses, phages are simple in structure, consisting of a protein capsid and core. According to their morphological and structural characteristics, there are three types of phages: *Caudovirales* (which are divided into *Siphoviridae*, *Podoviridae*, and *Myoviridae*), *Ballabactivirus*, and *Inoviridae* [16]. Ling Chen et al. described the biological characteristics of phage ValSw3-3, which belonged to the *Siphoviridae* [17]. ValSw3-3 had a latent period of about 15 min and a burst size of 95 ± 2 PFU/cell. Its infectivity remained above 80% at pH 6–10. Meanwhile, this phage was able to exist stably at 4–50 °C. Because of their tail fiber proteins, which can specifically recognize receptors on the surface of bacteria, phages can form a strict specificity with the host bacteria. Although the life cycle of phages is well understood, we will discuss it briefly based on the article of Zhang (Figure 1) [18]. According to the life cycle of phages, they can be divided into lytic phages and temperate phages. Lytic phages, also known as virulent phages, have the ability to inject their genomes into the bacteria, hijack the metabolic function of the host, and lyse the host cells to produce new progeny phages [19]. Temperate phages live a different life cycle and infect their hosts by initiating a lysogenic cycle. In the lysogenic cycle, the phage genome remains dormant as a prophage, replicates alongside its host, and occasionally bursts into a lytic cycle in response to a specific trigger [20].

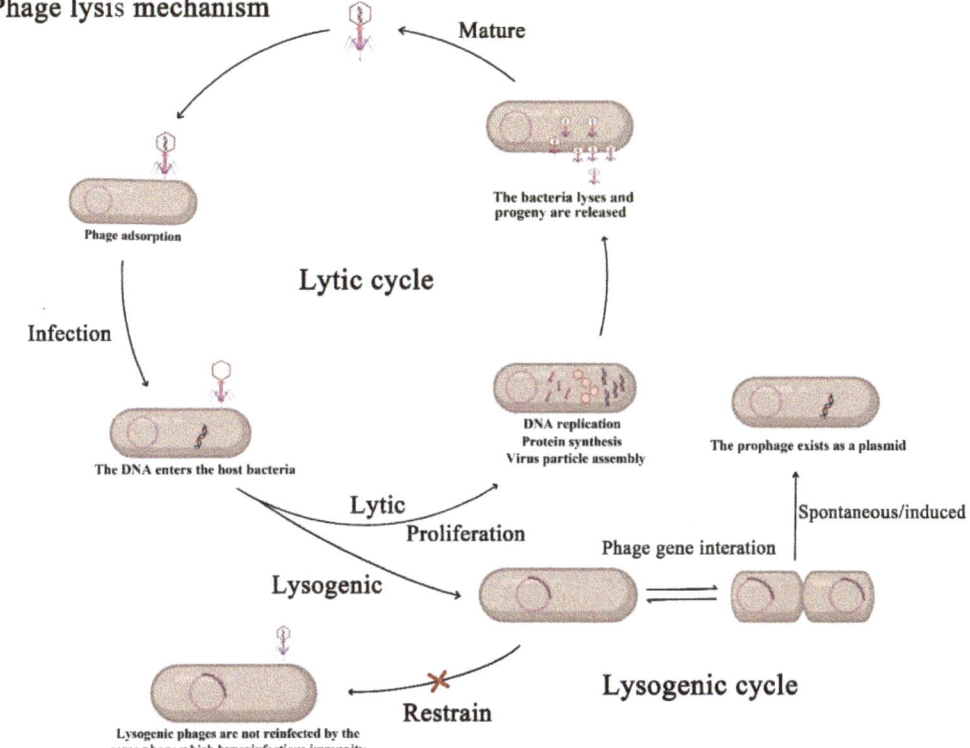

Figure 1. Mechanisms of action of lytic phage and lysogenic phage.

3. Phage Therapy in Animal Models

By 2022, we have found more than 95,400 articles about phage research on the National Center for Biotechnology Information (NCBI) database (URL: https://www.ncbi.nlm.nih.gov/, accessed on 27 July 2022), of which more than 4500 were published by Chinese researchers, accounting for 4.72% (Figure 2). Along with the gradual deepening of phage research, scientists have assessed the value of phages in animal models through more rigorous and detailed experiments. We are attempting to explore the possible clinical application of phage therapy based on the animal experiments. We summarized the progress of phage application in mammals, oviparous animals, and aquatic animals by Chinese researchers (Table 2).

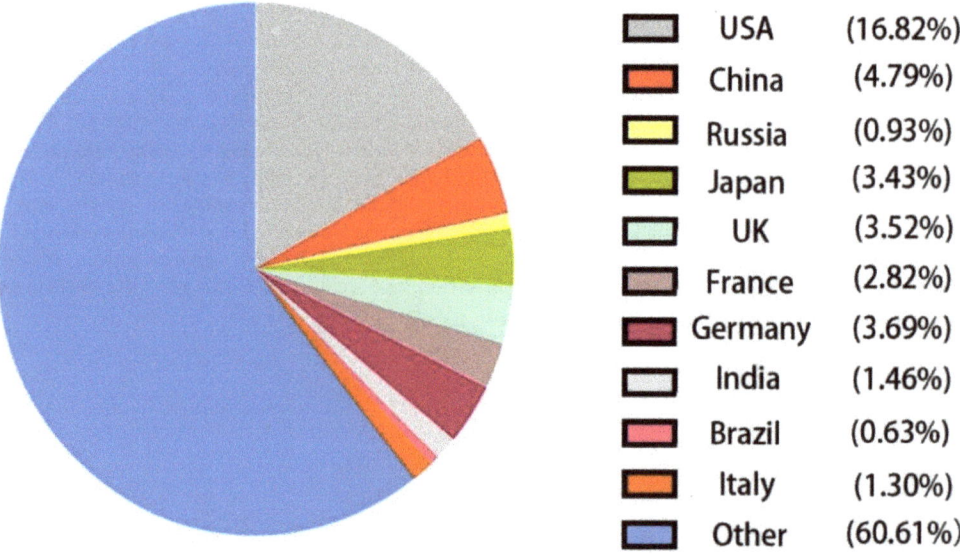

Figure 2. Percentage of articles published on the National Center for Biotechnology Information (NCBI) database.

Table 2. Summary of Bacteriophage Therapy for Bacterial Infection in Animal Models in China.

Reference	Host Organism	Animal	Infection	Delivery (b-Bacterial, p-Phage, bp-Bacterial and Phage)	Phage Log (CFU)	Phage Log (CFU)	Phage Species	Reduce Bacterial Concentration	Clear Infection	Effect of Delay in Treatment	Dose Related Studies	Continuous Injection of Phage
[21]	Escherichia coli	Calve	Colibacillosis	Take Orally: bp	10.0	11.0	4	B	B			
[22]	Escherichia coli	Calve	Mastitis	Intraperitoneal Injection: bp	1.8	8.7	3	A	A			
[23]	Aeromonas salmonicida	Turbot	Inflammation	Intraperitoneal Injection: bp	4–6	2.9–6.9	1	A	B		A	
[24]	Pseudomonas aeruginosa	Mouse	Mastitis / Colibacillosis	Intraperitoneal Injection: bp	5.3	6.3	1	B	B			
[25]	Escherichia coli	Mouse	Colibacillosis	Take Orally: b; Intraperitoneal Injection: p	8.0	5–7	1	A	B		A	
[26]	Klebsiella pneumoniae	Mouse	Bacteremia	Intraperitoneal Injection: bp	7.3	6–7	1	A	B		A	
[27]	Highly pathogenic Salmonella	Chicken	Pullorum disease	Take Orally: bp	6.3	7.0	1	B	B			
[28]	Acinetobacter baumannii	Duck	Colibacillosis	Intramuscular Injection: bp	5.3	8.5	1	B	B			A
[29]	Acinetobacter baumannii	Mouse	Sepsis	Transnasal Entry: bp	8.3	9.3	1	A	A	A		
[30]		Mouse	Pneumonia	Intraperitoneal Injection: bp	7.7	8.0	1	A	A	A		
[31]	Pseudomonas aeruginosa			Intraperitoneal Injection: bp	10.0	5–7	1	A	A		A	

Table 2. Cont.

Phage Therapy Outcome legend: A Remarkable Effect; B Medium Effect; C No Effect.
Delivery legend: b-Bacterial; p-Phage; bp-Bacterial and Phage.

Reference	Host Organism	Animal	Infection	Delivery	Phage Log (CFU)	Phage Log (CFU)	Phage Species	Reduce Bacterial Concentration	Clear Infection	Effect of Delay in Treatment	Dose Related Studies	Continuous Infection of Phage
[32]	Salmonella	Chicken		Take Orally (bp)	7.7	4.9–8.9	1	A	A		A	
[33]	Salmonella, Pasteurella	Mouse	Salmonellosis	Intraperitoneal Injection (bp)	9.3	10.3	1	B	B			A
[34]	Staphylococcus aureus, Klebsiella pneumoniae	Rabbit	Pneumonia	Transnasal Entry (bp)	8.5	6.5–9.5	1	B	B		A	A
[35]	Staphylococcus aureus	Mouse	Systemic	Intraperitoneal Injection (bp)	1.9	8.0	1	B	B		A	A
[36]		Mouse	Mastitis	Breast Injection (bp)	4.8	7.3	2	B	A			A
[37]		Mouse	Pneumonia	Transnasal Entry (bp)	8.3	7.3–9.3	1	B	A		A	
[38]	Escherichia coli	Mouse	Bacteremia	Intraperitoneal Injection (bp)	8.0	5.0	2	A	A			
[39]	Escherichia coli	Rabbit	Intestine	Take Orally (bp)	10.0	11.0	1	A	A			
[40]	Streptococcus agalactiae	Tilapia mossambica	Nephritis	Intestinal Injection (bp)	5.1	9.8	1	A	B			
[41]	Pasteurella	Mouse	Pneumonia	Intraperitoneal Injection (bp)	4.5	8.0	1	B	B			
[42]	Pseudomonas aeruginosa, Citrobacter freundii	Mouse	Bacteremia	Breast Injection (bp)	7.5	9.8	1	A	A	A		
[43]			Crap, Bacteremia	Intestinal Injection (bp)	9.3	7.0	1	C	B		A	A

Table 2. *Cont.*

Host Organism													Animal									Infection													Delivery (b-Bacterial, p-Phage, bp-Bacterial and Phage)						Phage Log (CFU)	Phage Log (CFU)	Phage Species	Phage Therapy Outcome (A Remarkable Effect, B Medium Effect, C No Effect)					Reference
Escherichia coli	*Pseudomonas aeruginosa*	*Aeromonas salmonicida*	*Klebsiella pneumoniae*	Highly pathogenic *Salmonella*	*Acinetobacter baumanii*	*Salmonella*	*Staphylococcus aureus*	*Pasteurella*	*Streptococcus agalactiae*	*Citrobacter freundii*	*Yersinia*	*Enterococcus faecalis*	Mouse	Bird	Chicken	Calve	Mink	Turbot	Duck	Rabbit	*Tilapia mossambica*	Crap	Colibacillosis	Mastitis	Pneumonia	Inflammation	Bacteremia	Pullorum disease	Sepsis	Placenta and endometritis	Salmonellosis	Systemic	Intestine	Nephritis	Take Orally	Transnasal Entry	Intraperitoneal Injection	Intramuscular Injection	Breast Injection	Intestinal Injection				Reduce Bacterial Concentration	Clear Infection	Effect of Delay in Treatment	Dose Related Studies	Continuous Infection of Phage	
			◆										◆														◆											bp			8.4	3.5–4.5	3	A	A	A	A		[44]
						◆							◆																				◆					bp			8.7	9.5	1	B	B				[45]
						◆					◆		◆																	◆			◆					bp			3.3	5.0	1	A	A	A			[46]
												◆	◆														◆									bp				9.4	9.3	1	A	A	C	A		[47]
																																						bp			9.3	5.6	1	A	A	A	A		[48]

Note: The site where ◆ appeared is indicated as that Host Organism/Animal/Infection.

3.1. Mammals

Many studies have shown that bacteriophages have a good therapeutic effect in mammals. Mice models are widely used in the treatment of diseases such as pneumonia, sepsis, and intestinal infection with phage therapy. As a result of a study conducted by Cao, after mice were infected with multiple drug-resistant *Klebsiella pneumoniae* bacteria for 2 h, the survival rate could reach about 80% by nasally inhaling phage 1513 (2×10^9 PFU/mouse) [37]. Moreover, the injury of the lung was effectively improved in the treatment group, while the mice in the untreated control group all died, indicating that phage had a good effect on lung infection caused by drug-resistant bacteria. Wang infected mice with imipenem-resistant *Pseudomonas aeruginosa* [42]. In this experiment, all the animals died within 24 h after the minimal lethal dose of bacteria (3×10^7 CFU/mL) injected. If phage was injected 15 and 30 min after the bacteria infection (MOI > 0.1), the survival rate could reach 100%. In contrast, the survival rate decreased to 50% and 20% respectively, when phage treatment was administered at 3 h and 6 h. Thus, phages should be used as early as possible to treat bacterial infections. Bacteriophages are also effective in treating *Escherichia coli*, *Acinetobacter baumannii,* and *Yersinia enterocolitica* infections [49–51]. *Yersinia enterocolitica* is generally considered an important food-borne pathogen, particularly in the European Union. Xue established a mouse enteritis model caused by a *Yersinia enterocolitica* infection with serotype O:3, and evaluated the therapeutic effect of the instillation of phage X1 [47]. The result showed that a single oral administration of phage X1 (1.95×10^8 PFU/mouse) at 6 h post infection was sufficient to eliminate *Yersinia enterocolitica* in 33.3% of mice (15/45). In addition, the number of *Yersinia enterocolitica* strains in the mice was also dramatically reduced to approximately 10^3 CFU/g after 18 h, compared to 10^7 CFU/g in the mice without phage treatment. Phage X1 treatment significantly improved of intestinal tissue, and the level of pro-inflammatory cytokines (IL-6, TNF-α and IL-1β) was significantly reduced ($p < 0.05$). These results indicated that phage was a promising candidate to control infection by bacteria in mice. In mice models, Prof. Hongping Wei and Prof. Hang Yang from the Laboratory of Diagnostic Microbiology, CAS Key Laboratory of Special Pathogens and Biosafety, Center for Biosafety Mega-Science, Wuhan Institute of Virology, Chinese Academy of Sciences also contributed to the application of phage and lysin therapy in the treatment of drug-resistant bacterial infections [52,53].

Phage therapy is also widely used in large mammals such as pigs, cattle, and sheep. For weaned piglets, *Escherichia coli* is the main pathogen causing diarrhea. In 2019, Zeng YD et al. found that adding phage in diets can improve growth performance and reduce the diarrhea index of weaned piglets [54]. Moreover, the phage supplement can improve the morphological structure and function of intestines, regulate the activity of intestinal digestive enzymes, improve the structure of intestinal microorganisms, and promote the intestinal health of piglets [55]. Foot-and-mouth disease (FMD) is a highly contagious disease in cloven-hoofed animals, which causes severe economic losses. To prevent this disease, Hai demonstrated the potential of T7 bacteriophage, based on nanoparticles displaying a genetically fused G-H loop peptide (T7-GH) as a FMDV vaccine candidate [56]. They found that the T7-GH phage nanoparticles were effective in eliciting antigen-specific immune responses in pigs. Qu YG invented a bacteriophage cocktail (six species of *Escherichia coli* phages of bovine mastitis; two species of cow mastitis source *Streptococcus* phages; two dairy cow mastitis, source *Staphylococcus aureus* bacteriophage; 1×10^9 PFU of each phage) in 2021 for clinical dairy cow mastitis and recessive mastitis, of which the effect was superior to antibiotic treatment and antimicrobial peptide treatment [57,58]. There were many other experiments on the successful treatment of bacterial infection in mammals by phage, but we have not provided any more examples.

3.2. Ovipara

Phage can be used as a prophylactic agent to protect chickens from lethal *Escherichia coli* infestation. Inoculation of the phage (BP16, 1.5×10^8 PFU) suspension prior to infection with *Escherichia coli* (O2 serotype, 1.5×10^8 CFU) enabled a 100% protection rate [59]. When the chicken were injected with phage after the bacteria infected them, the survival rate could reach around 80%, compared with 70% in the antibiotic-treated group. The results showed that phage was effective in preventing and treating poultry infection caused by lethal *Escherichia coli*. *Salmonella pullorum* is the major pathogen that is harmful to the poultry industry in developing countries, and the treatment of chicken diarrhea caused by drug-resistant *Salmonella pullorum* has become increasingly difficult. A lytic bacteriophage of YSP2 was used, which was able to specifically infect *Salmonella* [32]. Experiments in vivo demonstrated that a single oral administration of YSP2 (1×10^{10} PFU/mL, 80 µL/chicken) 2 h after *Salmonella pullorum* administration at a double median lethal dose was sufficient to protect chickens against diarrhea. Bacteriophages and their phage cocktails are also widely used as disinfectants specifically to eliminate pathogens in poultry [60,61].

3.3. Aquatilia

People often use antibiotics and water disinfectants in aquaculture to treat bacterial infections. However, the entry of residual drugs into the natural environment affects the composition and activity of microorganisms, disrupting the balance of microbiome. Phage therapy is used in aquaculture, which can effectively control pathogenic bacteria including *Citrobacter freundii*, *Aeromonas hydrophila*, *Vibrio parahaemolyticus*, *Vibrio harveyi*, etc. Zhang Lei et al. from Jilin Agricultural University, committed to the research of phage therapy, found that bacteriophage had good therapeutic effects in the treatment of aquatic drug-resistant bacteria. They isolated a phage, IME-JL18, which had strong activity against *Citrobacter freundii*, and applied it to the treatment of carp enteritis models [43]. In this study, a dose of IME-JL18 at 1×10^7 PFU effectively counteracted the lethal dose of *Citrobacter freundii* (1×10^9 CFU/carp), inhibiting the formation of the host bacterial biofilms. To treat an *Aeromonas hydrophila* infection, a phage mixture therapy was established based on the analysis of the genomic sequences and biological characteristics of vB_AHAp_PZL-AH8 and vB_AHAp_PZL-AH1 [62]. The results also showed that phage therapy was a good method to inhibit the production of phage-resistant strains. This team recently found a bacteriophage named PZL-Ah152, which had good efficacy in reducing the pathogenic *Aeromonas hydrophila* strain 152 in vivo and in vitro [63]. Furthermore, a 12-day consecutive injection of PZL-Ah152 (2×10^9 PFU) did not cause significant adverse effects on the main organs of the treated fish, such as liver, spleen, kidney, gut, and gill. They also found that members of the genus *Aeromonas* can enter and colonize the gut. The phage PZL-Ah152 reduced the number of colonies of the genus *Aeromonas*. However, no significant changes were observed in α-diversity and β-diversity parameters, which suggested that the consumed phage had little effect on the gut microbiota. Other researchers have also studied the application of bacteriophages in aquatic products. A study found that vB_VpaS_PG07 (7.6×10^9 PFU/mL) significantly reduced the mortality of shrimps challenged with *Vibrio parahaemolyticus* (2.27×10^6 CFU/shrimp), a bacterium causing acute hepatopancreatic necrosis disease (AHPND). The findings highlighted the potential of PG07 as an effective antibacterial agent for phage prophylaxis and phage therapy in aquaculture [64]. Another study found that phage qdvp001 (1.0×10^7 PFU/mL) could purify *Vibrio parahaemolyticus* (1.0×10^8 CFU/mL) in both oyster cultured environment and oyster bodies [65]. Simultaneously, this phage could inhibit the expression of pro-inflammatory factors including IL-1β, IL-6, and CD-14, and regulate the immune response caused by the bacteria. In addition, *Vibrio harveyi* can cause infections and diseases in a variety of marine vertebrates and invertebrates, which is very harmful to the aquaculture industry. Cui et al. isolated two bacteriophages [66], vB_VhaP_Vh-5 and vB_VhaM_VH-8, and discussed the practicability of feeding phages as a route of administration to protect turbot from *Vibrio harveyi* infection. When the MOI was 10 and 100, the phages could enhance the resistance of turbot to *Vibrio harveyi* VH5 infection, indicating feeding phage cocktails may be another optimal therapeutic agent against *Vibrio harveyi* infection in turbot culture.

4. Application of Bacteriophages in Clinics

In the 1940s, with the discovery of Penicillin, rapid and effective sterilization became the most effective treatment for bacterial diseases, heralding the golden age of antibiotics. Scientists have largely abandoned in-depth research on phage therapy ever since [67]. However, scientists in the former Soviet Union and some eastern European countries were not affected by the abandonment of phage therapy by western European countries and the United States, and still carried out in-depth research on the anti-infection effect of phages [68,69]. Currently, phage preparations have been approved for commercial use in many countries, including Georgia, Poland, and Russia. In China, the application of phage therapy to treat clinical diseases also has a long history. The former Dalian Institute of Biological Products was the first to develop phage research and related production (used for the prevention and treatment of dysentery) in China [70]. The Wuhan Institute of Biological Products also carried out a period of trial production around 1958. In 2017, the Shanghai Institute of Phage was established, which was the first institution to obtain the qualification for clinical treatment of bacteriophages in China. The institute launched the first ethically approved clinical trial of phage therapy in 2018 in China. Since then, teams such as the Chinese Academy of Sciences have also been working on the development of engineered phages to treat drug-resistant bacterial infections. In 2020, the Chinese team published a paper on the clinical practice of bacteriophages and proposed a new protocol of "non-sensitive antibiotic-phage combination," providing a new strategy for the treatment of "super-bacteria" that was resistant to both antibiotics and bacteriophages [71]. The leading enterprises of phage industrialization in China also include Qingdao Nuoan Baxter Biotechnology Co., Ltd. and Phagelux Inc. These companies applied bacteriophage formulations to animals, aquatic products, agriculture, and human health. Here, we summarize some successful cases of phage application in clinical therapy in China (Figure 3), hoping to promote the wider application of phage in clinical practice (Table 3).

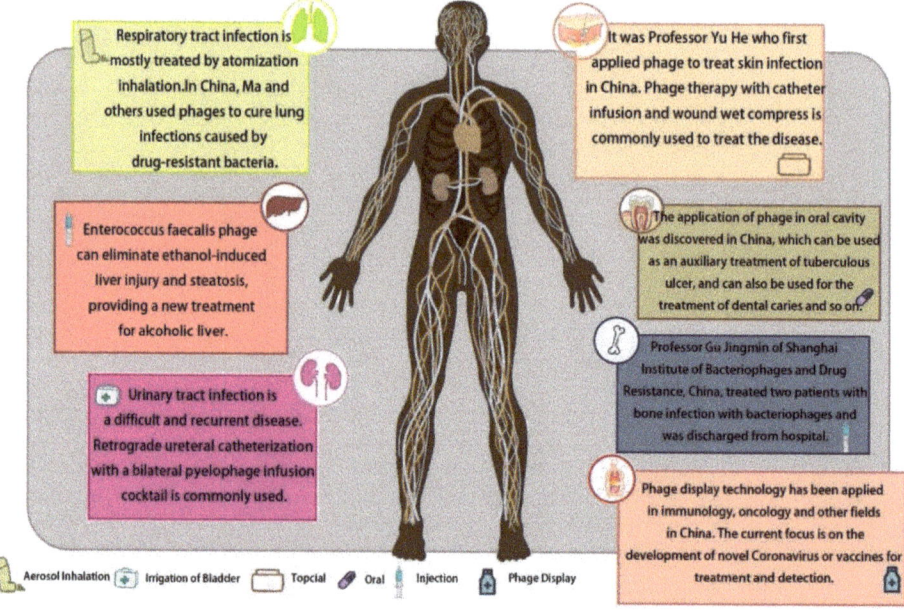

Figure 3. Summary of the clinical application of bacteriophage in China. Includes respiratory [72], skin [73], mouth [74], liver [75], urinary tract [76], bones, and phage display [77].

Table 3. Summary of the clinical treatment of bacterial infections by bacteriophages in China.

No.	Age–Year	Host Organism	Type of Infection	Delivery	Phage(s) Used	Outcome
[1]	66	MDR *Klebsiella pneumoniae*	Urinary tract infections	Irrigated simultaneously via the kidney and bladder	A two-phage cocktail (ΦJD902 + ΦJD905) and a three-phage cocktail (ΦJD905 + ΦJD907 + ΦJD908), combined with antibiotic treatment	Discharged and did not recur after two months of follow-up
[2]	65	Complex pan-resistant *Klebsiella pneumoniae*	Urinary tract infections	Bladder infusion	A four-phage cocktail (117, 135, 178, and GD168 phage) and a three-phage cocktail (130, 131, and 909 phage)	Pan-resistant *Klebsiella pneumoniae* was cleared and bladder infection was significantly improved.
[3]	Patient 1: 62 Patient 2: 64 Patient 3: 81 Patient 4: 78	Carbapenem-resistant *Acinetobacter baumannii* (CRAB)	Pulmonary infection	Via nebulization	A phage cocktail (2Φ)	Patient 1 and Patient 2: Discharged Patient 3: CRAB was eliminated but an un-subdued Carbapenem-resistant CRKP infection was followed and died on day 10 Patient 4: Discharged from ICU Day 7, however died of respiratory failure a month.
[4]	54	*Klebsiella pneumoniae*	Pulmonary infection	Via nebulization	Single-phage preparation (Φ59)	The symptoms of cough and expectoration were improved, and the inflammatory reaction was reduced
[5]	82	Carbapenem-resistant *Acinetobacter baumannii* (CRAB) and Carbapenem-resistant *Pseudomon asaeruginosa* (CRPA)	Pulmonary infection	Via nebulization	A two-phage cocktail (ΦPA3 + ΦPA39) and single-phage preparation (ΦAB3), combined with antibiotic treatment	The pulmonary infection was significantly improved
[6]	88	Carbapenem-resistant *Acinetobacter baumannii* (CRAB)	Pulmonary infection	Via nebulization	Single-phage preparation (Ab_SZ3), combined with antibiotic treatment	CRAB was cleared and the pulmonary infection was significantly improved

4.1. Skin Infection

Gram-negative bacilli, including *Escherichia coli, Klebsiella pneumoniae, Pseudomonas aeruginosa,* and *Acinetobacter baumannii,* are important pathogens of nosocomial infections. The majority of patients who suffered from chronic wounds/ulcers (86.1%, n = 310) and skin infections (94.9%, n = 734) experienced remission or improvement after phage therapy [78]. In 1958, Professor Yu He successfully cured patients infected with *Pseudomonas aeruginosa* using phage therapy [73]. This was the first successful clinical application of phage in

China. In 2021, a patient in Shanghai Public Health Clinical Center was infected with drug-resistant *Pseudomonas aeruginosa* after surgery. Following expert consultation, phage therapy with catheter perfusion and wound wet compress was implemented. After the treatment, the patient was cured.

4.2. Respiratory Tract Infection

Clinically, aerosol inhalation techniques enable accurate delivery of bacteriophages to the site of infection [79]. In the treatment of lung infection caused by drug-resistant *Klebsiella pneumoniae*, clinical symptoms were effectively relieved after two inhalations of phage aerosol preparations [80]. The team led by Ma also used the aerosol method of bacteriophage to treat patients and, after two weeks of treatment, successfully cleared the lung infection caused by *Acinetobacter baumannii* [72]. This was the first case in Shenzhen (China) using phage to treat drug-resistant bacteria infections. Furthermore, Wu assessed the efficacy and safety of compassionate phage therapy on secondary carbapenem-resistant *Acinetobacter baumannii* (CRAB) infections in patients hospitalized with critical COVID-19. They suggested the potential of phages on rapid responses to secondary CRAB outbreak in COVID-19 patients [81,82]. For the patient who suffered from chronic obstructive pulmonary disease (caused by carbapenem-resistant *Acinetobacter baumannii*), Tan used a specific lysing pathogen-specific phage (phage Ab_SZ3, 5×10^6 PFU-5×10^{10} PFU) in combination with tigecycline and colistin for a 16-day treatment [83]. The patient's pathogen clearance rate and lung function were clinically improved.

4.3. Urinary Tract Infection

Urinary tract infection (UTI) with extensively drug-resistant *Klebsiella pneumoniae* (XDRKp) is a challenging infection complication to immunocompromised patients, such as transplant recipients and patients with cancer and diabetes. In the context of increasing antibiotic resistance, phage therapy is effective in treating urinary tract infections. In 2018, Zhu successfully cured the first urinary tract infection caused by multidrug-resistant *Klebsiella pneumoniae* in China. In 2019, another patient infected with complex pan-drug-resistant *Klebsiella pneumoniae* recovered by using a 3-strain phage mixture through continuous bladder perfusion and retrograde ureteral intubation in both renal–pelvis [76]. The following year, Bao reported a case of a 63-year-old female patient who developed a recurrent urinary tract infection with extensively drug-resistant *Klebsiella pneumoniae* (ERKp) [71]. The combination of antibiotic (Trimethoprim-sulfamethoxazole, SMZ-TMP, 800mg-100mg) with a phage mixture (Kp152, Kp154, Kp155, Kp164, Kp6377, and HD001, 5×10^8 PFU/mL for each phage) inhibited the appearance of phage-resistant mutants in vitro and successfully cured the patient. There is a possibility that, instead of replacing antibiotics with phages, a combination of these two types of antibacterial agents may be more effective compared with use of either independently [84]. Qin et al. used a cocktail phage therapy to treat a man with multifocal urinary tract infection caused by MDR *Klebsiella pneumoniae* in 2021 [85]. Finally, the patient recovered. These successful cases provided valuable treatment ideas and solutions for phage treatment of complex infections.

4.4. Others

In addition to the above aspects, Chinese researchers are also attempting to apply phages in the treatment of chronic rhinosinusitis, dental ulcers, and alcoholic hepatitis. In 2018, Zhang identified bacteriophages (Sa83 and Sa87, 1×10^5 PFU) that could effectively kill multidrug-resistant *Staphylococcus aureus* in the nasal passages of patients with chronic sinusitis [86]. Moreover, Li used phage topical application to treat the tuberculous oral ulcer, and the patient soon recovered [74]. Meng found that using *Enterobacter faecalis* phage can significantly reduce liver cytolytic level and fecal enterococcus quantity [75], which can eliminate ethanol-induced liver injury and steatosis. Phages can target specific bacteria, providing a new treatment for alcoholic hepatitis.

5. Limitation of Phage Therapy

There is no doubt that phage therapy is an attractive solution to combat escalating antibiotic resistance. Numerous studies have highlighted the potential of therapeutic phages in vitro and in vivo, and many clinical trials have been conducted over the past decade [87]. Despite the promise of phage therapy, many issues must be addressed before it can be used as a treatment: ① The immune response. As a foreign substance, phage can stimulate the immune response of the body, and the antibodies produced may inhibit the ability of phage to eliminate bacteria, thereby reducing phage efficacy [88]. Moreover, the reticuloendothelial system can quickly eliminate phages. Optimizing the dose of phage can reduce the production of specific antibodies. In addition to reducing the dose of phage application, phage packaging can also alleviate specific antibodies [89]. Similarly, an encapsulation approach for standard phage therapy can also provide effective and targeted delivery of phages to the site of infection to protect the phages from immune system clearance [90]. ② The host spectrum of phages is relatively narrow; a certain type of phage can only infect and lyse the corresponding species or type of bacteria [91]. Phage cocktail therapy can combine species–specific phages to improve the efficacy of phage therapy and also reduce the production of phage-resistant mutants [92]. ③ Phage therapy has limitations in dose and duration. According to the pharmacokinetics, phages can only proliferate when the bacteria reach a certain density [93]. Therefore, early or inappropriate bacteriophage inoculation may be cleared by the immune system before proliferation. Optimal inoculation time and dose will be the key to phage therapy. ④ When bacteriophages are stored for a long time, there will be a certain inactivation or reduced titers. Bacteriophages as viruses have protein structures, so they are susceptible to known protein denaturation factors. These factors include exposure to organic solvents, high temperatures, pH, ionic strength, and interface effects [94]. Therefore, when choosing a storage method, careful consideration of its physical and chemical properties is required. The current preservation methods are: a. Broth lysate; b. 50% glycerol dilution; c. Saturating filter paper with lysate and then drying; d. Phage lyophilization [95]. ⑤ Safety of phage application. Some toxin genes carried by phages may have adverse effects on the body. Therefore, phages should be sequenced before they are used to ensure that they do not have virulence genes or integrase genes. The important step in the process of isolation and purification of phage is to remove endotoxin. Bacterial endotoxin, as an important part of Gram-negative bacteria, is released when bacteriophage lyses bacteria, which is toxic to the human body and has potential safety hazards. At present, bacteriophage preparation can be purified by affinity chromatography, commercial kits, and other methods to remove endotoxin from bacteriophage particles. ⑥ Criteria for clinical use of phages. It is necessary to ensure the activity of phages and remove contaminants from bacteria as much as possible. Information critical to the success of clinical trials includes: a. The adequate characterization and selection of phages as well as of subjects (humans) and the target bacteria. b. The formulations, dosing, and efficacy of the phage [96]. c. The sterility and purity of the phage preparation [97].

6. Regulation of Phage Application in China and Western Countries

Phage therapy has made great achievements both in animals and clinically. When it comes to the clinical treatment of phages, we definitely mention Hirszfeld Institute in Wroclaw, Poland and the Eliava Institute in Tbilisi, Georgia. The Eliava Institute focuses on the production and therapeutic use of phage cocktails for specific pathogenic bacteria. The Hirszfeld Institute supports the development of a more personalized phage therapeutic approach [98]. Both institutions have demonstrated convincing success rates in the use of phage therapy. Data from clinical trials at the Eliava Institute showed that phage therapy was approximately 70% and 55% effective in the treatment of *Staphylococcal* infection and *Staphylococcal* sepsis, respectively [69]. The Hirszfeld Institute pointed out that the good response rate to phage therapy was about 40% [97]. However, only a few phage therapies currently have completed phase I and phase II clinical trials, both of which lacked strict criteria and did not have evidence of properly controlled clinical trials [99]. The reports from Poland, Georgia, and other former Soviet Union countries have provided good experiences, but this form of treatment still lacks modern, properly controlled, double-blind clinical trials, and an appropriate framework is needed to make phage therapy a reality. Although phage-based clinical products have been commercialized in some eastern European countries, in western Europe and the United States, phage products for clinical applications have not yet reached the commercialization stage [7]. Currently, sporadic applications of bacteriophage therapy are carried out in western countries, where it is allowed to be used as a placebo in clinical treatment when antibiotic therapy is ineffective. Its research process and application are supervised by the Ethics Review Board and are generally protected by Article 37 of the New Helsinki Declaration [100]. The Declaration, although not a document with the force of law, became the standard for medical research ethics and serves as the basis for the development of other international guidelines. In fact, an increasing number of patients have been treated on an emergency IND (eIND) basis with the approval of the U.S. Food and Drug Administration (FDA) or the European Medicines Agency [101]. Belgium is currently implementing a pragmatic framework for phage therapy that centers on the magistral preparation (compounding pharmacy in the US) of tailor-made phage medicines [102]. This made Belgium the only western country that routinely produced phage drugs under prescription.

D'Herelle successfully treated four patients using phage injection in 1919. The earliest clinical use of phages in China can be traced back to 1958. As phage research develops in China, the cooperation between China and western countries in this field is closer. In 2022, Professor Martha Clokie from the University of Leicester, UK, in collaboration with the Institute of Animal Husbandry and Veterinary Medicine of Shandong Academy of Agricultural Sciences, published a book named *Phage Pharmacology and Experimental Methods* [103]. The book focused on pharmacology and had a strong practical application of phages. Since 2018, the Shanghai Institute of Phage and Drug Resistance (China) has conducted clinical trials on phage therapy. As far as we know, the patients receiving phage therapy must meet the following conditions:

(1) The patients were between 14 and 90 years of age who suffered from multi-drug resistant bacterial infections.
(2) The pathogenic bacteria that the patient is infected with should meet the following conditions:
    a. The patient is infected with pathogenic bacteria that are fully resistant to antibiotics.
    b. Pathogenic bacteria are resistant to key antibiotics (WHO has published a list of 12 superbug categories for 2017, as seen in Figure 1).
    c. The pathogen is sensitive to the key antibiotic but this antibiotic treatment is ineffective.
(3) To receive at least one or more phages capable of lysing drug-resistant bacteria.
(4) Be able to administer the phage by topical application, focal spraying of infection, nebulized inhalation, perfusion, local injection, or infusion tube.

7. The Direction of Phage Application

Due to the emergence of drug-resistant bacteria, researchers reattached importance to the study of bacteriophages as biological antibacterial agents. At present, the research and development directions of phage are as follows: strong lysis ability, good environmental adaptability and stability, no virulence genes on the genome, easy isolation and purification, no negative effect on the human immune system, and establishment of scientific pharmaceutical standards for phage preparations. Phage cocktail preparations are commonly used in clinical settings to respond to infections with different bacteria. Phage cocktails can broaden the host spectrum and reduce the frequency with which bacteria develop resistance to phages [104]. Phage cocktail therapy was approved by the U.S. government and its regulators as the first phage product for agriculture in 2005. The Shanghai Institute of Phage and Drug Resistance in China has also used phage cocktail therapy to cure patients with multi-drug resistant bacterial infections. The genetic modification of phages can broaden the host spectrum of phages, reduce cytotoxicity, and prolong the cycle time of phages in vivo. The genetic modification of phages is full of infinite possibilities to overcome some limitations of natural phage applications and improve the performance and therapeutic efficacy of phages. In addition, appropriate genetic modification strategies were used to extract lytic enzymes. Phage lysozyme is also one of the directions. The advantages of lysin lie in its easy purification, easy directional operation, high specificity, no damage to normal bacteria, and good antibacterial activity. Phages and antibiotics have different bactericidal mechanisms. The combination of the two could also improve antibacterial efficacy and produce synergistic therapeutic effects on bacteria. Genetically modified phages were used to increase or inhibit bacterial susceptibility to antibiotics. The introduction of *rpsL* and *gyrA* genes into the genome of drug-resistant *E. coli* using bacteriophage λ restored the susceptibility of the host bacteria to streptomycin [105]. Particularly, the combination of genetically modified phages and antibiotics can broaden the host lytic spectrum, which is one of the important directions for the development of phage therapy in the future. Phage has been properly investigated for its clinical potential for a long time. The upcoming years could be seen as a major milestone for phage and endolysin in terms of clinical recognition as viable alternatives to antibiotics. In order to bridge the gap and increase the packing of antibacterial drugs, researchers and clinicians must explore improved delivery strategies and creative approaches to designing phage and endolysin, as well as advancements in clinical trials [106].

8. Conclusions

Due to the widespread prevalence of multidrug-resistant bacteria and the slow development of antibiotics, the application of bacteriophages in the prevention, control, and treatment of bacterial infections has attracted people's attention again. The existing research showed that phage therapy had considerable prospects and effects in clinic trials, veterinary medicine, food, and other fields. An ideal phage for clinical trials should have strong lysis ability, no toxin gene, easy separation and purification, good environmental adaptability and stability, and be harmless to the body. However, phage has some limitations, such as immune response, narrow host spectrum, dosage of administration, and preservation conditions. These problems need to be solved urgently. We can use molecular biology technology to modify the phage genome, expanding the host spectrum, improving the lytic ability and modifying the lysin. Additionally, global criteria for clinical use of phage need to be developed as soon as possible so that phages can be used more widely. It is hoped that on the basis of the existing research, we can break through the current limitations and make bacteriophages safe, green, and effective products for drug-resistant bacteria.

Author Contributions: Conceptualization, L.Z. and S.L.; validation, L.Z.; formal analysis, S.L. and H.Y.; investigation, S.L. and Y.Q.; data curation, S.L.; writing—original draft preparation, S.L.; writing—review and editing, S.L., L.Z., S.H.A.R., N.A., S.S.A. and E.E.A.S.; supervision, L.Z. and W.S. All authors have read and agreed to the published version of the manuscript.

Funding: This work was founded by the Jilin Province Science and technology development plan project, grant No. 20210508006R Q.

Institutional Review Board Statement: Not applicable.

Informed Consent Statement: Not applicable.

Data Availability Statement: No new data were created or analyzed in this study. Data sharing is not applicable to this article.

Acknowledgments: Shuang Liang and Yanling Qi contributed equally to this work. The authors thank Jilin Agricultural University and Borui Technology Co for their support for this project.

Conflicts of Interest: The authors declare that the research was conducted in the absence of any commercial or financial relationships that could be construed as a potential conflict of interest.

Antibiotics **2023**, *12*, 417

References

1. Perry, J.; Waglechner, N.; Wright, G. The Prehistory of Antibiotic Resistance. *Cold Spring Harb. Perspect. Med.* **2016**, *6*, a025197. [CrossRef]
2. Merril, C.R.; Scholl, D.; Adhya, S.L. The prospect for bacteriophage therapy in Western medicine. *Nat. Rev. Drug Discov.* **2003**, *2*, 489–497. [CrossRef] [PubMed]
3. Górski, A.; Międzybrodzki, R.; Weber-Dąbrowska, B.; Fortuna, W.; Letkiewicz, S.; Rogóż, P.; Jończyk-Matysiak, E.; Dąbrowska, K.; Majewska, J.; Borysowski, J. Phage Therapy: Combating Infections with Potential for Evolving from Merely a Treatment for Complications to Targeting Diseases. *Front. Microbiol.* **2016**, *7*, 1515. [CrossRef] [PubMed]
4. Rex, J.H.; Outterson, K. Antibiotic reimbursement in a model delinked from sales: A benchmark-based worldwide approach. *Lancet. Infect. Dis.* **2016**, *16*, 500–505. [CrossRef] [PubMed]
5. Waglechner, N.; Wright, G.D. Antibiotic resistance: It's bad, but why isn't it worse? *BMC Biol.* **2017**, *15*, 84. [CrossRef]
6. Khalid, A.; Lin, R.C.Y.; Iredell, J.R. A Phage Therapy Guide for Clinicians and Basic Scientists: Background and Highlighting Applications for Developing Countries. *Front. Microbiol.* **2020**, *11*, 599906. [CrossRef]
7. Royer, S.; Morais, A.P.; da Fonseca Batistão, D.W. Phage therapy as strategy to face post-antibiotic era: A guide to beginners and experts. *Arch. Microbiol.* **2021**, *203*, 1271–1279. [CrossRef]
8. Caflisch, K.M.; Suh, G.A.; Patel, R. Biological challenges of phage therapy and proposed solutions: A literature review. *Expert. Rev. Anti-Infect. Ther.* **2019**, *17*, 1011–1041. [CrossRef]
9. El Haddad, L.; Harb, C.P.; Gebara, M.A.; Stibich, M.A.; Chemaly, R.F. A Systematic and Critical Review of Bacteriophage Therapy Against Multidrug-resistant ESKAPE Organisms in Humans. *Clin. Infect. Dis.* **2019**, *69*, 167–178. [CrossRef]
10. Wendling, C.C.; Goehlich, H.; Roth, O. The structure of temperate phage–bacteria infection networks changes with the phylogenetic distance of the host bacteria. *Biol. Lett.* **2018**, *14*, 20180320. [CrossRef]
11. Fineran, P.; Petty, N.; Salmond, G. Transduction: Host DNA transfer by bacteriophages. In *Encyclopedia of Microbiology*; Elsevier: Oxford, UK, 2009; pp. 666–679. [CrossRef]
12. Engelhardt, T.; Kallmeyer, J.; Cypionka, H.; Engelen, B. High virus-to-cell ratios indicate ongoing production of viruses in deep subsurface sediments. *ISME J.* **2014**, *8*, 1503–1509. [CrossRef] [PubMed]
13. Suttle, C.A. Viruses in the sea. *Nature* **2005**, *437*, 356–361. [CrossRef] [PubMed]
14. Suttle, C.A. Marine viruses–major players in the global ecosystem. *Nat. Rev. Microbiol.* **2007**, *5*, 801–812. [CrossRef]
15. Williamson, K.E.; Corzo, K.A.; Drissi, C.L.; Buckingham, J.M.; Thompson, C.P.; Helton, R.R. Estimates of viral abundance in soils are strongly influenced by extraction and enumeration methods. *Biol. Fertil. Soils* **2013**, *49*, 857–869. [CrossRef]
16. Letarov, A.V.; Kulikov, E.E. Adsorption of Bacteriophages on Bacterial Cells. *Biochemistry* **2017**, *82*, 1632–1658. [CrossRef]
17. Chen, L.; Liu, Q.; Fan, J.; Yan, T.; Zhang, H.; Yang, J.; Deng, D.; Liu, C.; Wei, T.; Ma, Y. Characterization and Genomic Analysis of ValSw3-3, a New Siphoviridae Bacteriophage Infecting Vibrio alginolyticus. *J. Virol.* **2020**, *94*, e00066-20. [CrossRef]
18. Zhang, M.; Zhang, T.; Yu, M.; Chen, Y.L.; Jin, M. The Life Cycle Transitions of Temperate Phages: Regulating Factors and Potential Ecological Implications. *Viruses* **2022**, *14*, 1904. [CrossRef]
19. Casjens, S.R.; Hendrix, R.W. Bacteriophage lambda: Early pioneer and still relevant. *Virology* **2015**, *479*, 310–330. [CrossRef]
20. Shen, J.; Zhou, J.; Fu, H.; Mu, Y.; Sun, Y.; Xu, Y.; Xiu, Z. A Klebsiella pneumoniae bacteriophage and its effect on 1, 3-propanediol fermentation. *Process Biochem.* **2016**, *51*, 1323–1330. [CrossRef]
21. Niu, Y.D.; Xu, Y.; McAllister, T.A.; Rozema, E.A.; Stephens, T.P.; Bach, S.J.; Johnson, R.P.; Stanford, K. Comparison of fecal versus rectoanal mucosal swab sampling for detecting Escherichia coli O157:H7 in experimentally inoculated cattle used in assessing bacteriophage as a mitigation strategy. *J. Food Prot.* **2008**, *71*, 691–698. [CrossRef]
22. Guo, M.; Gao, Y.; Xue, Y.; Liu, Y.; Zeng, X.; Cheng, Y.; Ma, J.; Wang, H.; Sun, J.; Wang, Z.; et al. Bacteriophage Cocktails Protect Dairy Cows Against Mastitis Caused By Drug Resistant Escherichia coli Infection. *Front. Cell. Infect. Microbiol.* **2021**, *11*, 690377. [CrossRef] [PubMed]
23. Xu, Z.; Jin, P.; Zhou, X.; Zhang, Y.; Wang, Q.; Liu, X.; Shao, S.; Liu, Q. Isolation of a Virulent Aeromonas salmonicida subsp. masoucida Bacteriophage and Its Application in Phage Therapy in Turbot (*Scophthalmus maximus*). *Appl. Environ. Microbiol.* **2021**, *87*, e0146821. [CrossRef] [PubMed]
24. Wang, Z.; Xue, Y.; Gao, Y.; Guo, M.; Liu, Y.; Zou, X.; Cheng, Y.; Ma, J.; Wang, H.; Sun, J.; et al. Phage vB_PaeS-PAJD-1 Rescues Murine Mastitis Infected With Multidrug-Resistant Pseudomonas aeruginosa. *Front. Cell. Infect. Microbiol.* **2021**, *11*, 689770. [CrossRef] [PubMed]
25. Sui, B.; Han, L.; Ren, H.; Liu, W.; Zhang, C. A Novel Polyvalent Bacteriophage vB_EcoM_swi3 Infects Pathogenic Escherichia coli and Salmonella enteritidis. *Front. Microbiol.* **2021**, *12*, 649673. [CrossRef]
26. Shi, Y.; Peng, Y.; Zhang, Y.; Chen, Y.; Zhang, C.; Luo, X.; Chen, Y.; Yuan, Z.; Chen, J.; Gong, Y. Safety and Efficacy of a Phage, kpssk3, in an in vivo Model of Carbapenem-Resistant Hypermucoviscous Klebsiella pneumoniae Bacteremia. *Front. Microbiol.* **2021**, *12*, 613356. [CrossRef]
27. Huang, J.; Liang, L.; Cui, K.; Li, P.; Hao, G.; Sun, S. Salmonella phage CKT1 significantly relieves the body weight loss of chicks by normalizing the abnormal intestinal microbiome caused by hypervirulent Salmonella Pullorum. *Poult. Sci.* **2022**, *101*, 101668. [CrossRef]
28. Xu, J.; Chen, M.; He, L.; Zhang, S.; Ding, T.; Yao, H.; Lu, C.; Zhang, W. Isolation and characterization of a T4-like phage with a relatively wide host range within Escherichia coli. *J. Basic. Microbiol.* **2016**, *56*, 405–421. [CrossRef]

29. Wang, Y.; Mi, Z.; Niu, W.; An, X.; Yuan, X.; Liu, H.; Li, P.; Liu, Y.; Feng, Y.; Huang, Y.; et al. Intranasal treatment with bacteriophage rescues mice from Acinetobacter baumannii-mediated pneumonia. *Future. Microbiol.* **2016**, *11*, 631–641. [CrossRef]

30. Deng, L.Y.; Yang, Z.C.; Gong, Y.L.; Huang, G.T.; Yin, S.P.; Jiang, B.; Peng, Y.Z. Therapeutic effect of phages on extensively drug-resistant Acinetobacter baumannii-induced sepsis in mice. *Zhonghua Shao Shang Za Zhi* **2016**, *32*, 523–528. [CrossRef]

31. Gu, J.; Li, X.; Yang, M.; Du, C.; Cui, Z.; Gong, P.; Xia, F.; Song, J.; Zhang, L.; Li, J.; et al. Therapeutic effect of Pseudomonas aeruginosa phage YH30 on mink hemorrhagic pneumonia. *Vet. Microbiol.* **2016**, *190*, 5–11. [CrossRef]

32. Tie, K.; Yuan, Y.; Yan, S.; Yu, X.; Zhang, Q.; Xu, H.; Zhang, Y.; Gu, J.; Sun, C.; Lei, L.; et al. Isolation and identification of Salmonella pullorum bacteriophage YSP2 and its use as a therapy for chicken diarrhea. *Virus Genes* **2018**, *54*, 446–456. [CrossRef] [PubMed]

33. Tang, F.; Zhang, P.; Zhang, Q.; Xue, F.; Ren, J.; Sun, J.; Qu, Z.; Zhuge, X.; Li, D.; Wang, J.; et al. Isolation and characterization of a broad-spectrum phage of multiple drug resistant Salmonella and its therapeutic utility in mice. *Microb. Pathog.* **2019**, *126*, 193–198. [CrossRef] [PubMed]

34. Ji, Y.; Cheng, M.; Zhai, S.; Xi, H.; Cai, R.; Wang, Z.; Zhang, H.; Wang, X.; Xue, Y.; Li, X.; et al. Preventive effect of the phage VB-SavM-JYL01 on rabbit necrotizing pneumonia caused by Staphylococcus aureus. *Vet. Microbiol.* **2019**, *229*, 72–80. [CrossRef] [PubMed]

35. Chen, Y.; Sun, E.; Yang, L.; Song, J.; Wu, B. Therapeutic Application of Bacteriophage PHB02 and Its Putative Depolymerase Against Pasteurella multocida Capsular Type A in Mice. *Front. Microbiol.* **2018**, *9*, 1678. [CrossRef] [PubMed]

36. Geng, H.; Zou, W.; Zhang, M.; Xu, L.; Liu, F.; Li, X.; Wang, L.; Xu, Y. Evaluation of phage therapy in the treatment of Staphylococcus aureus-induced mastitis in mice. *Folia Microbiol.* **2020**, *65*, 339–351. [CrossRef]

37. Cao, F.; Wang, X.; Wang, L.; Li, Z.; Che, J.; Wang, L.; Li, X.; Cao, Z.; Zhang, J.; Jin, L.; et al. Evaluation of the efficacy of a bacteriophage in the treatment of pneumonia induced by multidrug resistance Klebsiella pneumoniae in mice. *Biomed. Res. Int.* **2015**, *2015*, 752930. [CrossRef]

38. Yu, L.; Wang, S.; Guo, Z.; Liu, H.; Sun, D.; Yan, G.; Hu, D.; Du, C.; Feng, X.; Han, W.; et al. A guard-killer phage cocktail effectively lyses the host and inhibits the development of phage-resistant strains of Escherichia coli. *Appl. Microbiol. Biotechnol.* **2018**, *102*, 971–983. [CrossRef]

39. Zhao, J.; Liu, Y.; Xiao, C.; He, S.; Yao, H.; Bao, G. Efficacy of Phage Therapy in Controlling Rabbit Colibacillosis and Changes in Cecal Microbiota. *Front. Microbiol.* **2017**, *8*, 957. [CrossRef]

40. Luo, X.; Liao, G.; Liu, C.; Jiang, X.; Lin, M.; Zhao, C.; Tao, J.; Huang, Z. Characterization of bacteriophage HN48 and its protective effects in Nile tilapia Oreochromis niloticus against Streptococcus agalactiae infections. *J. Fish Dis.* **2018**, *41*, 1477–1484. [CrossRef]

41. Chen, Y.; Guo, G.; Sun, E.; Song, J.; Yang, L.; Zhu, L.; Liang, W.; Hua, L.; Peng, Z.; Tang, X.; et al. Isolation of a T7-Like Lytic Pasteurella Bacteriophage vB_PmuP_PHB01 and Its Potential Use in Therapy against Pasteurella multocida Infections. *Viruses* **2019**, *11*, 86. [CrossRef]

42. Wang, J.; Hu, B.; Xu, M.; Yan, Q.; Liu, S.; Zhu, X.; Sun, Z.; Reed, E.; Ding, L.; Gong, J.; et al. Use of bacteriophage in the treatment of experimental animal bacteremia from imipenem-resistant Pseudomonas aeruginosa. *Int. J. Mol. Med.* **2006**, *17*, 309–317. [CrossRef]

43. Jia, K.; Yang, N.; Zhang, X.; Cai, R.; Zhang, Y.; Tian, J.; Raza, S.H.A.; Kang, Y.; Qian, A.; Li, Y.; et al. Genomic, Morphological and Functional Characterization of Virulent Bacteriophage IME-JL8 Targeting Citrobacter freundii. *Front. Microbiol.* **2020**, *11*, 585261. [CrossRef]

44. Gu, J.; Liu, X.; Li, Y.; Han, W.; Lei, L.; Yang, Y.; Zhao, H.; Gao, Y.; Song, J.; Lu, R.; et al. A method for generation phage cocktail with great therapeutic potential. *PLoS ONE* **2012**, *7*, e31698. [CrossRef]

45. Bao, H.; Zhou, Y.; Shahin, K.; Zhang, H.; Cao, F.; Pang, M.; Zhang, X.; Zhu, S.; Olaniran, A.; Schmidt, S.; et al. The complete genome of lytic Salmonella phage vB_SenM-PA13076 and therapeutic potency in the treatment of lethal Salmonella Enteritidis infections in mice. *Microbiol. Res.* **2020**, *237*, 126471. [CrossRef]

46. Wang, X.; Ji, Y.; Su, J.; Xue, Y.; Xi, H.; Wang, Z.; Bi, L.; Zhao, R.; Zhang, H.; Yang, L.; et al. Therapeutic Efficacy of Phage P(IZ) SAE-01E2 against Abortion Caused by Salmonella enterica Serovar Abortusequi in Mice. *Appl. Environ. Microbiol.* **2020**, *86*, e01366-20. [CrossRef] [PubMed]

47. Xue, Y.; Zhai, S.; Wang, Z.; Ji, Y.; Wang, G.; Wang, T.; Wang, X.; Xi, H.; Cai, R.; Zhao, R.; et al. The Yersinia Phage X1 Administered Orally Efficiently Protects a Murine Chronic Enteritis Model Against Yersinia enterocolitica Infection. *Front. Microbiol.* **2020**, *11*, 351. [CrossRef] [PubMed]

48. Cheng, M.; Liang, J.; Zhang, Y.; Hu, L.; Gong, P.; Cai, R.; Zhang, L.; Zhang, H.; Ge, J.; Ji, Y.; et al. The Bacteriophage EF-P29 Efficiently Protects against Lethal Vancomycin-Resistant Enterococcus faecalis and Alleviates Gut Microbiota Imbalance in a Murine Bacteremia Model. *Front. Microbiol.* **2017**, *8*, 837. [CrossRef]

49. Salazar, K.C.; Ma, L.; Green, S.I.; Zulk, J.J.; Trautner, B.W.; Ramig, R.F.; Clark, J.R.; Terwilliger, A.L.; Maresso, A.W. Antiviral Resistance and Phage Counter Adaptation to Antibiotic-Resistant Extraintestinal Pathogenic Escherichia coli. *mBio* **2021**, *12*, e00211-21. [CrossRef] [PubMed]

50. Easwaran, M.; De Zoysa, M.; Shin, H.J. Application of phage therapy: Synergistic effect of phage EcSw (ΦEcSw) and antibiotic combination towards antibiotic-resistant Escherichia coli. *Transbound. Emerg. Dis.* **2020**, *67*, 2809–2817. [CrossRef]

51. Rouse, M.D.; Stanbro, J.; Roman, J.A.; Lipinski, M.A.; Jacobs, A.; Biswas, B.; Regeimbal, J.; Henry, M.; Stockelman, M.G.; Simons, M.P. Impact of Frequent Administration of Bacteriophage on Therapeutic Efficacy in an A. baumannii Mouse Wound Infection Model. *Front. Microbiol.* **2020**, *11*, 414. [CrossRef]

52. Yang, H.; Zhang, H.; Wang, J.; Yu, J.; Wei, H. A novel chimeric lysin with robust antibacterial activity against planktonic and biofilm methicillin-resistant Staphylococcus aureus. *Sci. Rep.* **2017**, *7*, 40182. [CrossRef]

53. Li, C.; Jiang, M.; Khan, F.M.; Zhao, X.; Wang, G.; Zhou, W.; Li, J.; Yu, J.; Li, Y.; Wei, H.; et al. Intrinsic Antimicrobial Peptide Facilitates a New Broad-Spectrum Lysin LysP53 to Kill Acinetobacter baumannii In Vitro and in a Mouse Burn Infection Model. *ACS Infect. Dis.* **2021**, *7*, 3336–3344. [CrossRef] [PubMed]

54. Zeng, Y.; Wang, Z.; Zou, T.; Zheng, L.; Li, S.; You, J. Effects of Bacteriophage on Growth Performance, Intestinal pH, Volatile Fatty Acid Contents and Disaccharase Activity of Weaned Piglets. *Chin. J. Anim. Nutr.* **2020**, *32*, 682–690. (In Chinese)

55. Lin, Y.; Zhou, B.; Zhu, W. Pathogenic Escherichia coli-Specific Bacteriophages and Polyvalent Bacteriophages in Piglet Guts with Increasing Coliphage Numbers after Weaning. *Appl. Environ. Microbiol.* **2021**, *87*, e0096621. [CrossRef] [PubMed]

56. Xu, H.; Bao, X.; Lu, Y.; Liu, Y.; Deng, B.; Wang, Y.; Xu, Y.; Hou, J. Immunogenicity of T7 bacteriophage nanoparticles displaying G-H loop of foot-and-mouth disease virus (FMDV). *Vet. Microbiol.* **2017**, *205*, 46–52. [CrossRef] [PubMed]

57. Qu, Y.; Liang, Y.; Yang, R.; Chang, J.; Liu, G.; Wang, L.; Zhang, Q. Preparation and application of phage cocktail preparation for dairy cow mastitis. CN113082060A, 9 July 2021. Available online: https://www.patentguru.com/search?q=CN113082060A (accessed on 25 November 2022).

58. Zeng, Y.; Wang, Z.; Zou, T.; Chen, J.; Li, G.; Zheng, L.; Li, S.; You, J. Bacteriophage as an Alternative to Antibiotics Promotes Growth Performance by Regulating Intestinal Inflammation, Intestinal Barrier Function and Gut Microbiota in Weaned Piglets. *Front. Vet. Sci.* **2021**, *8*, 623899. [CrossRef]

59. Li, M.; Zhao, Z.; Yang, T.; Zhang, H. Prevention and Treatment Effect of Escherichia coli Phage BP16 on Chicken Colibacillosis. *China Anim. Husb. Vet. Med.* **2022**, *49*, 776–782. (In Chinese) [CrossRef]

60. Yu, X.; Yan, C.; Ren, J.; Zhang, C.; Ren, H. The effect of *E. coli* bacteriophage Bp7 on the disinfection of the chicken coop environment. *Heilongjiang Anim. Sci. Vet. Med.* **2016**, *56*, 107–109. (In Chinese) [CrossRef]

61. Bao, H.; Zhang, H.; Li, G.; Zhou, Y.; Wang, R. Sterilization of Foodborne Pathogens by Aerosol Spray Treatments with Phages and Their Cocktails. *Food Sci.* **2013**, *34*, 10–13. (In Chinese)

62. Yu, H.; Zhang, L.; Feng, C.; Chi, T.; Qi, Y.; Abbas Raza, S.H.; Gao, N.; Jia, K.; Zhang, Y.; Fan, R.; et al. A phage cocktail in controlling phage resistance development in multidrug resistant Aeromonas hydrophila with great therapeutic potential. *Microb. Pathog.* **2022**, *162*, 105374. [CrossRef]

63. Feng, C.; Jia, K.; Chi, T.; Chen, S.; Yu, H.; Zhang, L.; Haidar Abbas Raza, S.; Alshammari, A.M.; Liang, S.; Zhu, Z.; et al. Lytic Bacteriophage PZL-Ah152 as Biocontrol Measures Against Lethal Aeromonas hydrophila Without Distorting Gut Microbiota. *Front. Microbiol.* **2022**, *13*, 898961. [CrossRef]

64. Ding, T.; Sun, H.; Pan, Q.; Zhao, F.; Zhang, Z.; Ren, H. Isolation and characterization of Vibrio parahaemolyticus bacteriophage vB_VpaS_PG07. *Virus Res.* **2020**, *286*, 198080. [CrossRef] [PubMed]

65. Ding, Y. Isolation, Identification and Preliminary Application of Bacteriophage qdvp001 Host Vibrio Para-Haemolyticus in Oyster Purification. Master's Thesis, Ocean University of China, Qingdao, China, 2012.

66. Cui, H.; Cong, C.; Wang, L.; Li, X.; Li, J.; Yang, H.; Li, S.; Xu, Y. Protective effectiveness of feeding phage cocktails in controlling Vibrio harveyi infection of turbot Scophthalmus maximus. *Aquaculture* **2021**, *535*, 736390. [CrossRef]

67. Sulakvelidze, A.; Alavidze, Z.; Morris, J.G., Jr. Bacteriophage therapy. *Antimicrob. Agents Chemother.* **2001**, *45*, 649–659. [CrossRef] [PubMed]

68. Lu, T.K.; Koeris, M.S. The next generation of bacteriophage therapy. *Curr. Opin. Microbiol.* **2011**, *14*, 524–531. [CrossRef] [PubMed]

69. Kutateladze, M.; Adamia, R. Phage therapy experience at the Eliava Institute. *Med. Mal. Infect.* **2008**, *38*, 426–430. [CrossRef]

70. Chen, T. Trial phages to stop superbug infection–recall a long-forgotten place in the original 'Dalian Institute'. *Prog. Microbiol. Immunol.* **2010**, *38*, 57–61. (In Chinese) [CrossRef]

71. Bao, J.; Wu, N.; Zeng, Y.; Chen, L.; Li, L.; Yang, L.; Zhang, Y.; Guo, M.; Li, L.; Li, J.; et al. Non-active antibiotic and bacteriophage synergism to successfully treat recurrent urinary tract infection caused by extensively drug-resistant Klebsiella pneumoniae. *Emerg. Microbes. Infect.* **2020**, *9*, 771–774. [CrossRef]

72. Chen, P.; Kong, Y.; Wen, S.; Gu, X.; Zhou, Y.; Tan, X.; Ma, Y.; Lu, H. A case report of phage therapy against lung infection caused by Carbapenem-resistant *Acinetobacter baumannii* and Carbapenem-resistant *Pseudomonas aeruginosa*. *Electron. J. Emerg. Infect. Dis.* **2022**, *7*, 71–75. (In Chinese) [CrossRef]

73. Qing, N. China's first doctor of bacteriology–Yu He. *Acta Microbiol. Sin.* **2007**, 949–950. (In Chinese) [CrossRef]

74. Li, H.; Wan, X.; Li, W. Bacteriophages in the treatment of tuberculosis uicers. *J. Oral Maxillofac. Surg.* **2009**, *19*, 151–152. (In Chinese)

75. Meng, F.; Sun, Y.; Yuan, G.; Gao, Y. Progress in the application of phage in the treatment of alcoholic liver disease. *Chin. Hepatol.* **2021**, *26*, 956–957. (In Chinese) [CrossRef]

76. Zeng, Y.; Bao, J.; Tan, D.; Zhang, Y.; Guo, M.; Zhu, Z.; Shao, E.; Zhu, T. Application of phage in patients with pan-drug resistant Klebsiella pneumoniae infection in urinary tract. *Chin. J. Urol.* **2020**, *41*, 677–680. (In Chinese)

77. Zhang, X.; Zhang, X.; Gao, H.; Qing, G. Phage display derived peptides for Alzheimer's disease therapy and diagnosis. *Theranostics* **2022**, *12*, 2041–2062. [CrossRef]

78. Qin, J.; Wu, N.; Bao, J.; Shi, X.; Ou, H.; Ye, S.; Zhao, W.; Wei, Z.; Cai, J.; Li, L.; et al. Heterogeneous Klebsiella pneumoniae Co-infections Complicate Personalized Bacteriophage Therapy. *Front. Cell. Infect. Microbiol.* **2020**, *10*, 608402. [CrossRef] [PubMed]

79. Wu, N.; Dai, J.; Guo, M.; Li, J.; Zhou, X.; Li, F.; Gao, Y.; Qu, H.; Lu, H.; Jin, J.; et al. Pre-optimized phage therapy on secondary Acinetobacter baumannii infection in four critical COVID-19 patients. *Emerg. Microbes. Infect.* **2021**, *10*, 612–618. [CrossRef] [PubMed]

80. Li, L.; Li, J.; He, B.; Wu, N.; Zhu, T.; Guo, X.; Chen, Z. Clinical application and effect of phage on the treatment of pulmonary infection by pan-drug resistant Klebsiella pneumoniae. *J. Shanghai Jiao Tong Univ.* **2021**, *41*, 1272–1276. (In Chinese)

81. Tan, X.; Chen, H.; Zhang, M.; Zhao, Y.; Jiang, Y.; Liu, X.; Huang, W.; Ma, Y. Clinical Experience of Personalized Phage Therapy Against Carbapenem-Resistant Acinetobacter baumannii Lung Infection in a Patient With Chronic Obstructive Pulmonary Disease. *Front. Cell. Infect. Microbiol.* **2021**, *11*, 631585. [CrossRef] [PubMed]

82. Steele, A.; Stacey, H.J.; de Soir, S.; Jones, J.D. The Safety and Efficacy of Phage Therapy for Superficial Bacterial Infections: A Systematic Review. *Antibiotics* **2020**, *9*, 754. [CrossRef] [PubMed]

83. Wang, X.; Xie, Z.; Zhao, J.; Zhu, Z.; Yang, C.; Liu, Y. Prospects of Inhaled Phage Therapy for Combatting Pulmonary Infections. *Front. Cell. Infect. Microbiol.* **2021**, *11*, 758392. [CrossRef]

84. Wu, N.; Chen, L.K.; Zhu, T. Phage therapy for secondary bacterial infections with COVID-19. *Curr. Opin. Virol.* **2022**, *52*, 9–14. [CrossRef]

85. Li, X.; He, Y.; Wang, Z.; Wei, J.; Hu, T.; Si, J.; Tao, G.; Zhang, L.; Xie, L.; Abdalla, A.E.; et al. A combination therapy of Phages and Antibiotics: Two is better than one. *Int. J. Biol. Sci.* **2021**, *17*, 3573–3582. [CrossRef] [PubMed]

86. Zhang, G.; Zhao, Y.; Paramasivan, S.; Richter, K.; Morales, S.; Wormald, P.J.; Vreugde, S. Bacteriophage effectively kills multidrug resistant Staphylococcus aureus clinical isolates from chronic rhinosinusitis patients. *Int. Forum. Allergy Rhinol.* **2018**, *8*, 406–414. [CrossRef] [PubMed]

87. Furfaro, L.L.; Payne, M.S.; Chang, B.J. Bacteriophage Therapy: Clinical Trials and Regulatory Hurdles. *Front. Cell. Infect. Microbiol.* **2018**, *8*, 376. [CrossRef]

88. Gembara, K.; Dąbrowska, K. Phage-specific antibodies. *Curr. Opin. Biotechnol.* **2021**, *68*, 186–192. [CrossRef]

89. Singla, S.; Harjai, K.; Katare, O.P.; Chhibber, S. Encapsulation of Bacteriophage in Liposome Accentuates Its Entry in to Macrophage and Shields It from Neutralizing Antibodies. *PLoS ONE* **2016**, *11*, e0153777. [CrossRef] [PubMed]

90. Loh, B.; Gondil, V.S.; Manohar, P.; Khan, F.M.; Yang, H.; Leptihn, S. Encapsulation and Delivery of Therapeutic Phages. *Appl. Environ. Microbiol.* **2020**, *87*, e01979-20. [CrossRef] [PubMed]

91. Hyman, P.; Abedon, S.T. Bacteriophage host range and bacterial resistance. *Adv. Appl. Microbiol.* **2010**, *70*, 217–248. [CrossRef] [PubMed]

92. Malik, S.; Sidhu, P.K.; Rana, J.S.; Nehra, K. Managing urinary tract infections through phage therapy: A novel approach. *Folia. Microbiol.* **2020**, *65*, 217–231. [CrossRef]

93. Nilsson, A.S. Pharmacological limitations of phage therapy. *Upsala J. Med. Sci.* **2019**, *124*, 218–227. [CrossRef]

94. Malik, D.J.; Sokolov, I.J.; Vinner, G.K.; Mancuso, F.; Cinquerrui, S.; Vladisavljevic, G.T.; Clokie, M.R.J.; Garton, N.J.; Stapley, A.G.F.; Kirpichnikova, A. Formulation, stabilisation and encapsulation of bacteriophage for phage therapy. *Adv. Colloid. Interface Sci.* **2017**, *249*, 100–133. [CrossRef] [PubMed]

95. Clark, W.A. Comparison of several methods for preserving bacteriophages. *Appl. Microbiol.* **1962**, *10*, 466–471. [CrossRef] [PubMed]

96. Loganathan, A.; Manohar, P.; Eniyan, K.; VinodKumar, C.S.; Leptihn, S.; Nachimuthu, R. Phage therapy as a revolutionary medicine against Gram-positive bacterial infections. *Beni-Suef Univ. J. Basic Appl. Sci.* **2021**, *10*, 49. [CrossRef]

97. Międzybrodzki, R.; Borysowski, J.; Weber-Dąbrowska, B.; Fortuna, W.; Letkiewicz, S.; Szufnarowski, K.; Pawełczyk, Z.; Rogóż, P.; Kłak, M.; Wojtasik, E.; et al. Clinical aspects of phage therapy. *Adv. Virus Res.* **2012**, *83*, 73–121. [CrossRef] [PubMed]

98. Kakasis, A.; Panitsa, G. Bacteriophage therapy as an alternative treatment for human infections. A comprehensive review. *Int. J. Antimicrob. Agents* **2019**, *53*, 16–21. [CrossRef] [PubMed]

99. Kutter, E.; De Vos, D.; Gvasalia, G.; Alavidze, Z.; Gogokhia, L.; Kuhl, S.; Abedon, S.T. Phage therapy in clinical practice: Treatment of human infections. *Curr. Pharm. Biotechnol.* **2010**, *11*, 69–86. [CrossRef]

100. Onsea, J.; Soentjens, P.; Djebara, S.; Merabishvili, M.; Depypere, M.; Spriet, I.; De Munter, P.; Debaveye, Y.; Nijs, S.; Vanderschot, P.; et al. Bacteriophage Application for Difficult-to-treat Musculoskeletal Infections: Development of a Standardized Multidisciplinary Treatment Protocol. *Viruses* **2019**, *11*, 891. [CrossRef] [PubMed]

101. Luong, T.; Salabarria, A.C.; Edwards, R.A.; Roach, D.R. Standardized bacteriophage purification for personalized phage therapy. *Nat. Protoc.* **2020**, *15*, 2867–2890. [CrossRef]

102. Pirnay, J.P.; Verbeken, G.; Ceyssens, P.J.; Huys, I.; De Vos, D.; Ameloot, C.; Fauconnier, A. The Magistral Phage. *Viruses* **2018**, *10*, 64. [CrossRef]

103. Clokie, R.J.M. *Phage Pharmacology and Experimental Methods*; Chemical Industry Press: Beijing, China, 2022.

104. Chan, B.K.; Abedon, S.T.; Loc-Carrillo, C. Phage cocktails and the future of phage therapy. *Future. Microbiol.* **2013**, *8*, 769–783. [CrossRef]

105. Li, G.; Hu, F. History and development of phage therapy. *Chin. J. Antibiot.* **2017**, *42*, 807–813. (In Chinese) [CrossRef]
106. Gondil, V.S.; Khan, F.M.; Mehra, N.; Kumar, D.; Khullar, A.; Sharma, T.; Sharma, A.; Mehta, R.; Yang, H. Clinical Potential of Bacteriophage and Endolysin Based Therapeutics: A Futuristic Approach. In *Microbial Products for Health, Environment and Agriculture*; Springer: Berlin/Heidelberg, Germany, 2021; pp. 39–58.

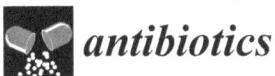

Article

Mortality in Thai Nursing Homes Based on Antimicrobial-Resistant *Enterobacterales* Carriage and COVID-19 Lockdown Timing: A Prospective Cohort Study

Thundon Ngamprasertchai [1,*,†], Muthita Vanaporn [2,†], Sant Muangnoicharoen [1,‡], Wirichada Pan-ngum [3], Narisa Ruenroengbun [4], Pittaya Piroonamornpun [5], Thitiya Ponam [5], Chatnapa Duangdee [5], Phanita Chankete [2], Anupop Jitmuang [6] and Visanu Thamlikitkul [6]

[1] Department of Clinical Tropical Medicine, Faculty of Tropical Medicine, Mahidol University, Bangkok 10400, Thailand; sant.mua@mahidol.ac.th
[2] Department of Microbiology and Immunology, Faculty of Tropical Medicine, Mahidol University, Bangkok 10400, Thailand; muthita.van@mahidol.ac.th (M.V.); teerarut.cha@mahidol.ac.th (P.C.)
[3] Department of Tropical Hygiene, Faculty of Tropical Medicine, Mahidol University, Bangkok 10400, Thailand; wirichada.pan@mahidol.ac.th
[4] Department of Pharmaceutics (Clinical Pharmacy), Faculty of Pharmacy, Slipakorn University, Nakornprathom 73000, Thailand; polladew@gmail.com
[5] Hospital for Tropical Diseases, Faculty of Tropical Medicine, Mahidol University, Bangkok 10400, Thailand; pittaya.pir@mahidol.ac.th (P.P.); thitiya.pon@mahidol.ac.th (T.P.); chatnapa.dua@mahidol.ac.th (C.D.)
[6] Department of Medicine, Faculty of Medicine Siriraj Hospital, Mahidol University, Bangkok 10700, Thailand; anupopmix@yahoo.co.th (A.J.); visanu.tha@mahidol.ac.th (V.T.)
* Correspondence: thundon.ngm@mahidol.ac.th
† These authors contributed equally to this work.
‡ Essentially intellectual contributor.

Citation: Ngamprasertchai, T.; Vanaporn, M.; Muangnoicharoen, S.; Pan-ngum, W.; Ruenroengbun, N.; Piroonamornpun, P.; Ponam, T.; Duangdee, C.; Chankete, P.; Jitmuang, A.; et al. Mortality in Thai Nursing Homes Based on Antimicrobial-Resistant *Enterobacterales* Carriage and COVID-19 Lockdown Timing: A Prospective Cohort Study. *Antibiotics* **2022**, *11*, 762. https://doi.org/10.3390/antibiotics11060762

Academic Editors: Anusak Kerdsin, Jinquan Li and Jonathan Frye

Received: 7 May 2022
Accepted: 30 May 2022
Published: 2 June 2022

Publisher's Note: MDPI stays neutral with regard to jurisdictional claims in published maps and institutional affiliations.

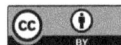

Abstract: Antimicrobial-resistant *Enterobacterales* carriage and the coronavirus disease 2019 (COVID-19) lockdown measures may impact the incidence all-cause mortality rate among nursing home residents. To determine the all-cause mortality rate in the presence/absence of antimicrobial-resistant *Enterobacterales* carriage and the incidence all-cause mortality rate before and during COVID-19 pandemic lockdown, this prospective closed-cohort study was conducted at various types of nursing homes in Bangkok, Thailand, from June 2020 to December 2021. The elderly residents included 142 participants (aged ≥60 years) living in nursing homes ≥3 months, who did not have terminal illnesses. Time-to-event analyses with Cox proportional hazards models and stratified log-rank tests were used. The all-cause mortality rate was 18%, and the incidence all-cause mortality rate was 0.59/1000 person-days in residents who had antimicrobial-resistant *Enterobacterales* carriage at baseline. Meanwhile, the incidence all-cause mortality rate among noncarriage was 0.17/1000 person-days. The mortality incidence rate of carriage was three times higher than residents who were noncarriage without statistical significance (HR 3.2; 95% CI 0.74, 13.83). Residents in nonprofit nursing homes had a higher mortality rate than those in for-profit nursing homes (OR 9.24; 95% CI 2.14, 39.86). The incidence mortality rate during and before lockdown were 0.62 and 0.30, respectively. Effective infection-control policies akin to hospital-based systems should be endorsed in all types of nursing homes. To limit the interruption of long-term chronic care, COVID-19 prevention should be individualized to nursing homes.

Keywords: *Enterobacterales*; colonization; nursing home; COVID-19; lockdown

1. Introduction

Residents in nursing homes are favorable carriers of microbes [1] and spread antibiotic-resistant microbes, leading to antimicrobial resistance (AMR) [2]. Previous studies have shown that 4.7–64% of the residents of nursing homes had multidrug-resistant Gram-negative bacteria [3–6] that were subsequently transmitted to and infected [7] other patients or healthcare workers [8]. Although nursing homes provide limited healthcare services and have fewer beds than healthcare facilities, the probability of transmission of antimicrobial-resistant pathogens remains high [2]. Overuse and prolonged empirical administration of antimicrobial agents accompanied by poor infection-control policies increase AMR burden. [9] Furthermore, ineffective infection-control procedures resulted in the outbreak of the COVID-19 pandemic in nursing homes [10]. Therefore, nursing homes must improve their infection-control policies.

Thailand is experiencing a rapid increase in its aging population. One report estimated that the number of elderly persons aged ≥ 80 years would increase from 1.9 to 3 million persons in the from 2020 to 2040 [11]. Consequently, there has been an expansion of long-term care services (also known as nursing homes) in Thailand [12]. However, there are suboptimal standards of care offered, staff competencies, and ineffective systems within long-term care services [13]. Additionally, research regarding AMR bacteria situations in Thai nursing homes are limited. In community settings, 52.1–58.2% of Thai healthy volunteers had CTX-M beta-lactamase-producing *Enterobacterales* (EC) carriage [14,15]. We postulate that carriage rates in nursing homes have been described as a proxy composite indicator of AMR in the community [16]. The mortality rate of nursing home residents is determined by several factors, including advanced age, the presence of comorbidities, and having impaired cognitive or physical function or sarcopenia [17–19]. The outcomes resulting from AMR carriage or infection in nursing homes are diverse. Some studies showed lower mortality rates among residents without AMR carriage when compared with residents with AMR carriage; other studies showed similar mortality outcomes in the two groups [20,21]. However, Aliyu S et al. illustrated worse outcomes among residents infected with multidrug-resistant organisms [22]. We hypothesize that nursing home residents with AMR carriage are likely to develop an infection from their antimicrobial-resistant colonies for which they may receive inappropriate empirical antimicrobial agents. We also hypothesize that residents with AMR carriage would have a higher mortality rate than those with AMR noncarriage.

The COVID-19 pandemic not only affected nursing home residents but also impacted on the healthcare delivery system. In western countries, more than one-fourth of the documented deaths due to COVID-19 were reported among nursing home residents [23]. At the end of 2020, the number of COVID-19 cases in Thailand gradually increased but were successfully controlled. Nursing home policies were changed to limit the influx of residents and visiting family members. Henceforth, until April 2021, the number of community COVID-19 cases increased, resulting in the imposition of travel restrictions and social distancing measures in May 2021. Subsequently, all nursing homes were in full lockdown; thus, residents were unable to see their families or visit doctors in charge of their chronic illnesses. Although healthcare delivery was moved to telehealth platforms, the impact of the pandemic-related transition and patient outcomes has not yet been established.

We set out to compare the all-cause mortality rate among Thai nursing home residents with and without AMR-EC carriage. We also compared the all-cause mortality rate before and after the countrywide COVID-19 pandemic lockdown measures were imposed among Thai nursing home residents. Additionally, we described the risk factors for AMR-EC carriage and all-cause mortality among nursing home residents.

2. Results

Table 1 demonstrates the baseline characteristics of nursing home residents. We included 142 residents in total, with minimal loss to follow-up (5; 3.5%). Residents with multiple comorbidities or retaining catheter or having incontinence or pressure ulcer were frequently found AMR-EC carriage. The definitions of study variables were available in material and method part.

Table 1. Baseline and characteristics of antimicrobial-resistant *Enterobacterales* carriage of Thai nursing home residents at study enrolment.

Characteristics	Residents $N = 142$, N. (%)	*Enterobacterales* Carriage * ($N = 136$)		*p* Value
		Antimicrobial-Resistant Carriage ($N = 101$; 74.3%), No. (%)	No Antimicrobial-Resistant Carriage ($N = 35$; 25.8%) No. (%)	
Sex				
Male	57 (40.1)	37 (36.6)	19 (54.3)	0.067
Female	85 (59.9)	64 (63.4)	16 (45.7)	
Age, year				
<80	67 (47.2)	49 (48.5)	14 (40.0)	0.384
≥80	75 (52.8)	52 (51.5)	21 (60.0)	
Comorbidities				
None	5 (3.5)	1 (1)	4 (11.4)	0.014 +
Single	33 (23.2)	26 (25.7)	6 (17.1)	
Multiple	104 (73.2)	74 (73.3)	25 (71.4)	
Duration of living, year				
<1	46 (32.4)	33 (32.7)	11 (31.4)	0.892
≥1	96 (67.6)	68 (67.3)	24 (68.6)	
Types of nursing home				
Nonprofit	73 (51.4)	56 (55.5)	15 (42.9)	0.199
Profit	69 (48.6)	45 (44.6)	20 (57.1)	
Activities of Daily Living (ADLs)				
Dependence	53 (37.6)	39 (39.0)	12 (34.3)	0.078
Partial dependence	76 (53.9)	56 (56.0)	17 (48.6)	
Independence	12 (8.5)	5 (5.0)	6 (17.1)	
Incontinence or pressure ulcer existing				0.016 +
Yes	62 (43.7)	51 (50.5)	8 (22.9)	
No	80 (56.3)	50 (49.5)	27 (77.1)	
Catheter or foreign material retaining				0.016+
Yes	59 (41.6)	48 (47.6)	7 (20.0)	
No	83 (58.5)	53 (52.5)	28 (80.0)	
Recent antimicrobial agents use				0.156
Yes	50 (38.2)	39 (41.1)	8 (26.7)	
No	81 (61.8)	56 (59.0)	22 (73.3)	
Need regular follow-up				0.189
Yes	60 (72.2)	41 (68.3)	14 (70.0)	
No	23 (27.7)	18 (30.0)	4 (20.0)	
Recent in hospital admission				0.829
Yes	41 (49.3)	28 (46.7)	9 (45.0)	
No	42 (50.6)	31 (51.7)	11 (55.0)	
Recent ICU admission				
Yes	8 (22.2)	6 (25.0)	1 (11.1)	0.385
No	28 (77.8)	18 (75.0)	8 (88.9)	

+ statistical significance; * Carriage/noncarriage was defined as the presence/absence of AMR-EC was in rectal swabs, respectively.

2.1. Characteristics and Factors Associated EC Carriage

Nearly 74% of residents had AMR-EC carriage at enrollment (Table 1). Almost 38% of residents had 3GCR-EC carriage, and 70% had QREC carriage. *E. coli* was the most isolated EC (68.6%) (Supplementary Materials Table S1). No carbapenem-resistant EC was found in our study population. Factors associated with AMR-EC carriage at enrollment and QREC carriage were incontinence or pressure ulcer (OR 3.44; 95% CI 1.43, 8.30), foreign materials or retained catheters (OR 3.62; 95% CI 1.45, 9.05), and multiple comorbidities (OR 17.33; 95% CI 1.63, 184.36). Elderly residents who had been living in nursing homes for more than 1 year developed 3GCR-EC less than those who had been living in nursing homes for less than 1 year (OR 0.46; 95% CI 0.22, 0.96). After confounding adjustment, elderly residents who had incontinence or existing pressure ulcers (OR 2.15; 95% CI 0.75, 6.18) and a catheter or retained foreign material (OR 2.30; 95% CI 0.77, 6.90) were more likely to have AMR-EC carriage (Table 2).

Table 2. Factors associated with antimicrobial-resistant *Enterobacterales* carriage of Thai nursing home residents at study enrolment.

Characteristics	Quinolone-Resistant EC * Carriage		Third-Generation Cephalosporin-Resistant EC ** Carriage		Antimicrobial Resistant EC *** Carriage	
	Crude OR (95% CI)	Adjusted OR (95%CI)	Crude OR (95% CI)	Adjusted (OR 95% CI)	Crude OR (95% CI)	Adjusted OR (95%CI)
Comorbidities						
None	-				-	
Single	1				1	
Multiple	12 (1.16,123.68)				17.33 (1.63,184.36)	
Duration of living, year						
<1			1			
≥1			0.46 (0.22,0.96)			
Activities of Daily Living (ADLs)						
Dependence	4.63 (1.17,18.27)	0.96 (0.19,4.91)				
Partial dependence	4.64 (1.22, 17.57)	3.52 (0.92,13.45)				
Independence	1	1				
Incontinence or pressure ulcer existing						
Yes	3.95 (1.70, 9.17)				3.44 (1.43, 8.30)	2.15 (0.75, 6.18)
No	1				1	1
Catheter or foreign material retaining						
Yes	4.96 (2.00, 12.29)	9.52 (2.74,33.11)			3.62 (1.45, 9.05)	2.30 (0.77, 6.90)
No	1	1			1	1
Recent antimicrobial agents use						
Yes	2.437 (1.00, 5.96)					
No	1					

* Quinolone resistant *Enterobacterales* (EC) defined as EC resistant to either ciprofloxacin or levofloxacin or both; ** third-generation cephalosporin-resistant EC (3GCR-EC) defined as EC were resistant to either ceftazidime or cefotaxime or both; *** antimicrobial resistant (AMR) EC defined as EC were either QREC or 3GC-EC or both.

2.2. Mortality Rate of EC Carriage

The all-cause mortality rate in residents who had AMR-EC carriage at baseline was approximately 18%; similar rates were seen in residents with 3GCR-EC and QREC carriage (Supplementary Materials Table S2). The incidence all-cause mortality rate among residents with AMR-EC carriage was 0.59 per 1000 person-days (95% CI 0.37, 0.93). The mortality incidence rate among residents with AMR-EC carriage was thrice that of those with AMR-EC noncarriage without statistical significance (HR 3.2; 95% CI 0.74, 13.83). The Kaplan–Meier curve (Figure 1) represented survival probability between residents who were carriage at enrollment and those who were noncarriage showed that noncarriage had higher survival probability than carriage by all types of resistance without statistical significance. The hazard ratios of AMR carriage have a similar trend in residents with 3GCR-EC (HR 1.57; 95% CI 0.64, 3.87) and QREC (HR 2.45, 95% CI 0.71, 8.42) without statistical significance.

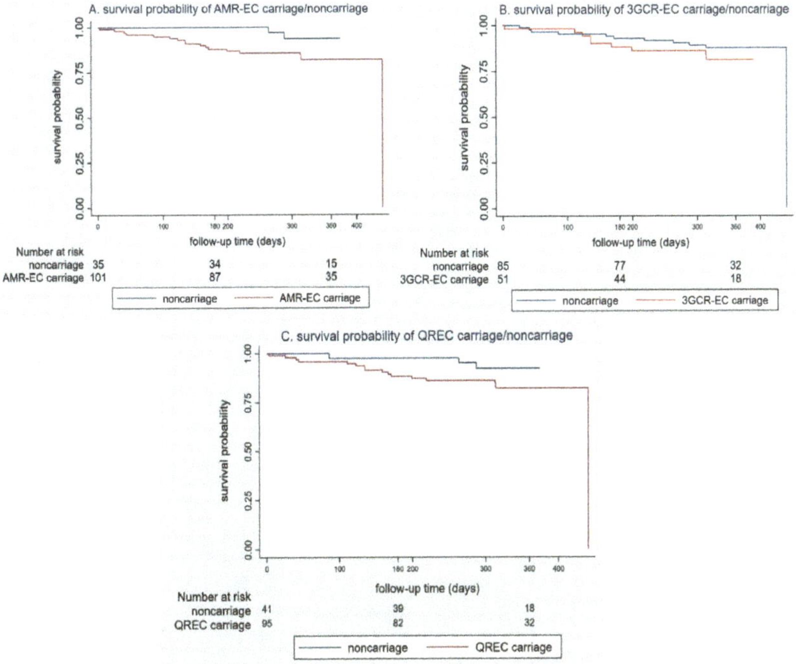

Figure 1. The survival probability between carriage (red line) and noncarriage (blue line) antimicrobial-resistant *Enterobacterales* stratified by types of resistance: (**A**) AMR-EC (*p* value log-rank 0.10); (**B**) 3GCR-EC (*p* value log-rank 0.32); (**C**) QREC (*p* value log-rank 0.14).

2.3. Associated Factors and Incidence Mortality Rate among Residents

The overall mortality rate among residents who had been living in nursing homes at the 1-year follow-up date was 14.8%. The mortality rate before and during the lockdown was approximately 4% and 11%, respectively (Supplementary Materials Table S3). The incidence mortality rate during the lockdown period (0.62; 95% CI 0.37, 1.02) was double that before the lockdown period (0.30; 95% CI 0.14, 0.67). The Kaplan–Meier curve (Supplementary Materials Figure S1) shows mortality probability before and during the COVID-19 pandemic lockdown. Only one case was mortality reported because of COVID-19 infection during the lockdown period. After confounding adjustments, the factors of nonprofit nursing home, incontinence, pressure ulcer existing, and catheter or foreign material retaining were poor prognostic factors for nursing home residents (Figure 2). Supplementary Materials Figure S2 showed that residents in nonprofit homes had the lowest survival probability when compared with residents in for-profit nursing homes (*p* < 0.001). Dependent residents had the worst survival outcome when compared with more able residents (Supplementary Materials Figure S3) (*p* = 0.004) and had a mortality rate that was triple that of partially dependent residents (OR 3.71; 95% CI 1.43, 9.67). We performed a global test to check the constant of the coefficient over time; *p* value was 0.326, which was represented the validity of the assumption.

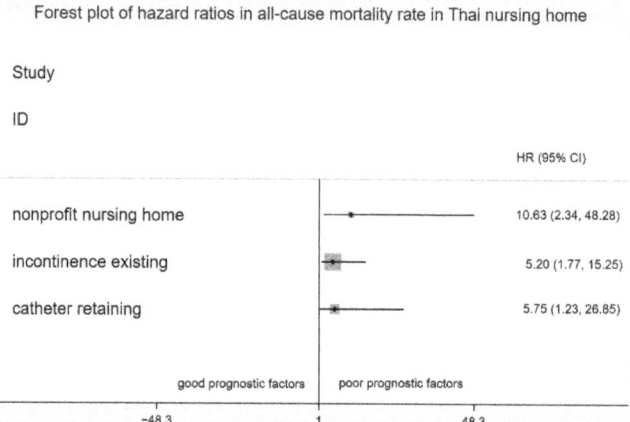

Figure 2. Forest plot of adjusted hazard ratios in all-cause mortality rate in Thai nursing homes.

3. Discussion

In this cohort of 142 nursing home residents, the all-cause mortality rate in 1 year follow-up was 14.8%, which was relatively lower than that in the literature, which was approximately 28–30% [17,19]. Only one death was caused by COVID-19. Residents with AMR-EC, 3GCR-EC, and QREC had a mortality rate of approximately 17.8%, which was also lower than in previous studies which approximately was 25–50% [8,20,24]; meanwhile, the mortality rate among noncarriage was approximately 5.7–13%. Our results concurred with the results in the literature regarding the incidence all-cause mortality rate among persons with drug-resistant carriage that is usually higher than in persons with noncarriage without statistical significance, i.e., almost triple, as they developed infection from their antimicrobial-resistant colonies. These may result from infection after the carriage and inappropriate empirical antimicrobial use; however, previous reports have demonstrated controversial results regarding the clinical significance of carriage [8,20,24,25]. Effective infection-control strategies such as hand hygiene or the use of standard personal protective equipment similar to that practiced in hospitals should be enforced in nursing homes. Residents who are likely to be carriers, for example, of poor ADLs status or with the presence of risk factors for AMR-EC, should be isolated in a cohort ward. Only trained staff should perform standard nursing care. We found that residents who had been living in a nursing home for more than 1 year were less likely to develop 3GCR-EC carriage. This implies that carriage would be substituted by noncarriage over time if there was no antimicrobial pressure effect [26]. We therefore recommend antimicrobial stewardship programs in nursing homes to reduce AMR-EC carriage. The 3GCR-EC carriage rate was less than that found in the community [14,15], since most of the residents have lived in nursing homes for more than 1 year. Overall, AMR-EC carriage in Thai nursing homes was higher than in the previous studies [8,27,28], which were either conducted in high-income countries or had different AMR pathogens other than EC.

The COVID-19 pandemic has had a devastating effect on nursing home residents in many countries, but our study illustrated favorable results. Although there was no COVID-19 outbreak in our cohort, the incidence all-cause mortality rate during the COVID-19 pandemic was double that before the lockdown. All their family members and their doctors' meetings were transposed to a virtual platform. Nearly 70% of our cohort residents who needed regular follow-up had their care interrupted during the COVID-19 pandemic lockdowns. With telehealth, essential physical examinations cannot be done by a doctor, which may lead to an incorrect or a missed diagnosis. It is possible that the aggravation of their underlying chronic illnesses or missed diagnoses were the main causes of death during the lockdown period. Though telehealth will not solve this situation all, it is appropriate in settings which infrastructure remains intact and doctors are able to see patients [29]. Flexible and appropriate COVID-19 prevention policies should be individualized in diverse settings. There was an unequal mortality rate in different nursing homes; an attribute related to nursing home quality ratings. Highly rated nursing homes had lower death rates, as well as fewer cases of COVID-19 [30–32]. Nonprofit nursing homes had the worst survival probability among nursing homes since they did not offer doctor-provided care, which the hospital-based and private nursing homes did. Although residents in hospital-based nursing homes tend to develop drug-resistant carriage and are more likely to have severe chronic diseases, hospital settings implement standardized nursing care and appropriate antimicrobial use. We recommend that the Ministry of Public Health endorse standardized nursing care akin to that in hospital-based nursing homes to improve the quality of life and the survival outcomes of residents in nonprofit nursing homes. Furthermore, the COVID-19 pandemic has also affected the health service, controlling AMR at both the hospital level and the community level [33]. Increasing antimicrobial usage and infection-control system interruption might impact on AMR situation in near future.

Our study had several strengths. First, we included residents from different types of nursing homes to enhance the generalizability of our results. Additionally, we prospectively followed up our participants and had a minimal loss to follow-up. Lastly, we were able to establish the impact of moving to telehealth, strict infection-control policies, and the inequality experienced by residents of different types of nursing homes. However, some study limitations must be addressed. First, our results regarding the association between AMR-EC carriage and mortality did not attain statistical significance. This could be due to our limited sample size. Second, we assessed for AMR-EC carriage only at one point during enrollment; our results may have been more robust if we had prospectively measured AMR-EC carriage over the whole study period. Longitudinal AMR-EC surveillance study may be needed to understand natural progression of carriage/noncarriage. Lastly, we performed COVID-19 testing in participants who were symptomatic when they first arrived at a nursing home; thus, asymptomatic residents who may have had COVID-19 were not be captured by our study.

4. Materials and Methods

4.1. Study Design and Setting

This prospective closed-cohort study was conducted from June 2020 to December 2021. The enrolment date began on 1st June 2020 and followed up till 30th April 2021, which was the beginning of COVID-19 lockdown. Then, we followed up with participants 6 months afterward. Our cohort nursing home limited new members of residents before COVID-19 lockdown. However, during lockdown, all residents who went outside nursing homes for any reason were tested and isolated. All their family members and their doctors' meetings were transposed to a virtual platform. We recruited residents living in six different types of nursing homes in Bangkok. We collected data from three for-profit nursing homes: one hospital-based nursing home located in and run by the Hospital for Tropical Diseases, Faculty of Tropical Medicine, Mahidol University; and two private centers run by the private sector. We also collected data from three nonprofit nursing homes.

4.2. Study Populations

We enrolled residents, aged $\geq$60 years without a terminal illness or illnesses, who had been living in nursing homes for at least 3 months preceding the interview date. Exclusion criteria included residents who developed end-of-life conditions or there was tendency to be lost to follow-up within 1 year after enrollment. Participants for whom rectal sampling also was contraindicated were excluded.

4.3. Study Procedure and Data Collection

4.3.1. Rectal Sampling and Microbiological Outcome Measurement

We assessed EC carriage using rectal swabs since they are easier to collect than stool samples, and results obtained from rectal swabs are highly correlated with those obtained from stool samples [34]. Rectal sampling was at enrollment performed by trained investigators. Swabs were placed on BBL™ CultureSwab™ EZ II (COPAN ITALIA SpA, Brescia, Italy) at 25 °C. Samples were then sent to the microbiology laboratory for identification and drug-susceptible testing at the Hospital for Tropical Diseases and Department of Microbiology and Immunology at the Faculty of Tropical Medicine, Mahidol University, the same day they were collected. The target bacteria, EC, were identified using different media and standard biochemical conventional methods. Antimicrobial susceptibility testing (AST) was performed via disk diffusion method and interpreted according to the standard recommendation of the Clinical Laboratory Standard Institute 2021-2.

4.3.2. Study Endpoints

The primary endpoint was the incidence all-cause mortality rate in nursing home residents with or without AMR-EC. The secondary endpoint was the incidence all-cause mortality rate in nursing home residents before and during the COVID-19 pandemic lockdown. All-cause mortality was defined as death due to any cause during the entire duration of the study. Factors associated with all-cause mortality and AMR-EC carriage were also described. Prevalence, type, and pattern of carriage among residents were also defined. This study was registered in the Thai Clinical Trials Registry on 2 June 2019, with ID number (TCTR20190602003). In this study, we follow the Strengthening the Reporting of Observational Studies in Epidemiology reporting guidelines.

4.3.3. Study Variables Definition

Definition of targeted isolated bacteria were EC-categorized based on the type of drug resistance as follows: quinolone resistant EC (QREC) defined as EC resistant to either ciprofloxacin or levofloxacin or both, third-generation cephalosporin-resistant EC (3GCR-EC) were resistant to either ceftazidime or cefotaxime or both, and AMR-EC defined as EC that were either QREC or 3GC-EC or both. Carriage/noncarriage was defined as the presence/absence of AMR-EC was in rectal swabs, respectively.

We selected factors that were clinically meaningful to determine mortality rate and AMR-EC carriage. List of factors [8,17–19,27,35] were as follows; The age group was classified to be less than 80 years, or equal to and more than 80 years, based on the mean age of our study population; this age was also referred to when determining the mortality risk [36]. Comorbidities were categorized into single or multiple comorbidities; the duration of living in a nursing home was classified into two: <1 or $\geq$1 year. Physical function was measured using activities of daily living (ADLs) measures, which were grouped into dependence, partial independence, and independence. We defined dependence as being unable to perform basic ADLs, an ability to do instrumental ADLs without any assistance as independence, and the need for a caregiver to assist in instrumental ADLs as partial dependence. Incontinence was categorized as urinary or fecal incontinence. Information about the presence or absence of pressure ulcers was also collected. The use of catheters or internally retained foreign materials, such as urinary catheters, nasogastric tubes, venous or arterial catheters, and pacemakers, and having a tracheostomy were considered risk factors for AMR-EC carriage and mortality in our analyses. Some residents had to regularly visit a hospital for follow-up of a diagnosed chronic health condition and to receive their long-term medications.

4.4. Statistical Method

4.4.1. Sample Size Calculation

From previous literature, the mortality rate in noncarriage and carriage AMR-EC nursing home residents was 12–30% and 25–50%, respectively [8,20,24]. We estimated that the mortality rate among noncarriage and carriage AMR-EC would be 15% and 35%, respectively. The prevalence of the CTX-M beta-lactamase-producing EC in healthy volunteers in Thailand is 50% [14,15]; therefore, the ratio of the population with carriage and noncarriage is 1:1. From this, we aimed to recruit 73 participants in each group with a power of 80% and an α error of 0.05%.

4.4.2. Statistical Analysis

To identify risk factors for AMR-EC carriage, odds ratios (OR) and 95% confidence interval (CI) were computed using logistic regression analysis. All predictors with a p value of <0.10 in univariate analysis were included in multiple logistic regression models with stepwise forward selection. We used the time-to-events analyses (Kaplan–Meier) and stratified log-rank tests to compare time to death between the carriage and noncarriage groups. We used Cox proportional hazards models to describe factors associated with mortality, which were reported as HRs with 95% confidence intervals (CIs). The date of censoring was 30 April 2021 as COVID-19 lockdown and 6 months afterward. The incidence mortality rate was computed as the number of deaths per population per 1000 days living in a nursing home. The person-days used for AMR-EC mortality were calculated using the duration between the date of enrollment and the date of follow-up. Person-days before the COVID-19 pandemic lockdown were taken as the duration between the date of enrollment and the date of lockdown, 1 April 2021; conversely, person-days after the lockdown were taken as the duration between the date of lockdown and date of follow-up. The global test was used to check the constant of the coefficient over time. The data were analyzed using StataBE v17.0 software (StataCorp, College Station, TX, USA); p values of <0.05 were considered two-sided and statistically significant.

5. Conclusions

The incidence all-cause mortality rate among nursing home residents with AMR-EC carriage was higher than that in residents with noncarriage without statistical significance. Standard nursing care and effective infection-control policies similar to those in hospital-based systems should be endorsed in all types of nursing homes. Nursing home residents with chronic diseases whose mandatory long-term follow-up was interrupted during the COVID-19 pandemic had a higher mortality rate. The COVID-19 pandemic also affected health service's control of AMR at both the hospital level and the community level. Increasing antimicrobial usage and infection-control system interruption might impact on AMR situation in near future. Eventually, COVID-19 prevention policies should be individualized based on the type of nursing home.

Supplementary Materials: The following supporting information can be downloaded at: https://www.mdpi.com/article/10.3390/antibiotics11060762/s1, Table S1: Microbiology results at enrollment (isolations), Table S2: Incidence all-cause mortality rate among antimicrobial-resistant *Enterobacterales* carriage, Table S3: Comparison of incidence all-cause mortality rate by COVID-19 pandemic lockdown, Figure S1: The mortality probability before COVID-19 lockdown (A) and during COVID-19 lockdown (B), Figure S2: The survival probability between types of nursing home (blueline: hospital based (profit) nursing home; red line: private (profit) nursing home; green line: non-profit nursing home) (p value log-rank <0.001), Figure S3: The survival probability between types of Activities Daily Living (ADLs) (blue line: dependence; red line: partial dependence; green line: independence) (p value log-rank 0.004).

Author Contributions: M.V. and S.M., intellectual contributions; T.N., S.M., A.J. and V.T., participated in the study conception and design; T.N., P.P. and T.P., collected study factors and outcomes; M.V., P.C. and C.D., microbiological culture and antimicrobial susceptibility testing; T.N., N.R. and W.P.-n., statistical analysis plan, analyzed data, and interpretation of data; T.N., M.V. and A.J., manuscript writing. All authors contributed to reviewing, editing, and approving the manuscript before submission. All authors have read and agreed to the published version of the manuscript.

Funding: This research was funded by Faculty of Tropical Medicine, Mahidol University, Fiscal Year 2019 (grant number: 0401/2562) and The APC was funded by Faculty of Tropical Medicine, Mahidol University and Mahidol University.

Institutional Review Board Statement: The study was conducted in accordance with the Declaration of Helsinki, and approved by the Institutional Review Board (or Ethics Committee) of the Faculty of Tropical Medicine, Mahidol University (submission number TMEC 19-077 (MUTM 2020-011)).

Informed Consent Statement: Informed consent was obtained from all subjects involved in the study. Written informed consent has been obtained from the patient(s) to publish this paper.

Data Availability Statement: Not applicable.

Acknowledgments: We gratefully acknowledge the contributions of Santi Maneewatchararangsri, Jiraporn Sujjanunt, Gengpong Tangaroonsanti, Wilaiwan Pattalik, Siripun Srivilairit, Pannalin Tangpiboonwatana, Jantawan Satayarak, Amporn Rungruengkitkun, and all patients in this study. The authors also would like to thank Enago™ (http://www.enago.com/ (accessed on 20 March 2022)) for the manuscript review and editing support.

Conflicts of Interest: The authors declare no conflict of interest. The funders had no role in the design of the study; in the collection, analyses, or interpretation of data; in the writing of the manuscript, or in the decision to publish the results.

References

1. Aschbacher, R.; Pagani, E.; Confalonieri, M.; Farina, C.; Fazii, P.; Luzzaro, F.; Montanera, P.G.; Piazza, A.; Pagani, L. Review on colonization of residents and staff in Italian long-term care facilities by multidrug-resistant bacteria compared with other European countries. *Antimicrob. Resist. Infect. Control* **2016**, *5*, 33. [CrossRef] [PubMed]
2. van den Dool, C.; Haenen, A.; Leenstra, T.; Wallinga, J. The Role of Nursing Homes in the Spread of Antimicrobial Resistance over the Healthcare Network. *Infect. Control Hosp. Epidemiol.* **2016**, *37*, 761–767. [CrossRef] [PubMed]
3. Ruscher, C.; Pfeifer, Y.; Layer, F.; Schaumann, R.; Levin, K.; Mielke, M. Inguinal skin colonization with multidrug-resistant bacteria among residents of elderly care facilities: Frequency, persistence, molecular analysis and clinical impact. *Int. J. Med Microbiol.* **2014**, *304*, 1123–1134. [CrossRef] [PubMed]
4. March, A.; Aschbacher, R.; Dhanji, H.; Livermore, D.M.; Böttcher, A.; Sleghel, F.; Maggi, S.; Noale, M.; Larcher, C.; Woodford, N. Colonization of residents and staff of a long-term-care facility and adjacent acute-care hospital geriatric unit by multiresistant bacteria. *Clin. Microbiol. Infect.* **2010**, *16*, 934–944. [CrossRef] [PubMed]
5. Rooney, P.J.; O'Leary, M.C.; Loughrey, A.C.; McCalmont, M.; Smyth, B.; Donaghy, P.; Badri, M.; Woodford, N.; Karisik, E.; Livermore, D.M. Nursing homes as a reservoir of extended-spectrum β-lactamase (ESBL)-producing ciprofloxacin-resistant *Escherichia coli*. *J. Antimicrob. Chemother.* **2009**, *64*, 635–641. [CrossRef] [PubMed]
6. Cochard, H.; Aubier, B.; Quentin, R.; van der Mee-Marquet, N.; du Centre, R.D.H. Extended-Spectrumβ-Lactamase–Producing Enterobacteriaceae in French Nursing Homes: An Association between High Carriage Rate among Residents, Environmental Contamination, Poor Conformity with Good Hygiene Practice, and Putative Resident-to-Resident Transmission. *Infect. Control Hosp. Epidemiol.* **2014**, *35*, 384–389. [CrossRef]
7. Reddy, P.; Malczynski, M.; Obias, A.; Reiner, S.; Jin, N.; Huang, J.; Noskin, G.A.; Zembower, T. Screening for Extended-Spectrum -Lactamase-Producing Enterobacteriaceae among High-Risk Patients and Rates of Subsequent Bacteremia. *Clin. Infect. Dis.* **2007**, *45*, 846–852. [CrossRef]
8. Leitner, E.; Zechner, E.; Ullrich, E.; Zarfel, G.; Luxner, J.; Pux, C.; Pichler, G.; Schippinger, W.; Krause, R.; Zollner-Schwetz, I. Low prevalence of colonization with multidrug-resistant gram-negative bacteria in long-term care facilities in Graz, Austria. *Am. J. Infect. Control* **2018**, *46*, 76–80. [CrossRef]
9. Nicolle, L.E. Infection Control in Long-Term Care Facilities. *Clin. Infect. Dis.* **2000**, *31*, 752–756. [CrossRef]
10. Baker, N.R.; Dunn, D.; Greenberg, S.A.; Shaughnessy, M. Infection Control in Long-Term Care: An Old Problem and New Priority. *J. Am. Med. Dir. Assoc.* **2021**, *23*, 321–322. [CrossRef]
11. Peae, P. *Situation of the Thai Elderly 2019*; Mahidol University and Foundation of Thai Gerontology Research and Development Institute (TGRI), Institute for Population and Social Research: Nakhon Pathom, Thailand, 2020.
12. Lloyd-Sherlock, P.G.; Sasat, S.; Sanee, A.; Miyoshi, Y.; Lee, S. The rapid expansion of residential long-term care services in Bangkok: A challenge for regulation. *J. Public Health Dev.* **2021**, *19*, 89–101. Available online: https://he01.tci-thaijo.org/index.php/AIHD-MU/article/view/246485 (accessed on 20 March 2022).
13. Sasat, S.; Choowattanapakorn, T.; Pukdeeprom, T.; Lertrat, P.; Aroonsang, P. Long-Term Care Institutions in Thailand. *J. Health Res.* **2017**, *27*, 413–418. Available online: https://he01.tci-thaijo.org/index.php/jhealthres/article/view/88736 (accessed on 20 March 2022).

14. Niumsup, P.R.; Tansawai, U.; Na-Udom, A.; Jantapalaboon, D.; Assawatheptawee, K.; Kiddee, A.; Romgaew, T.; Lamlertthon, S.; Walsh, T.R. Prevalence and risk factors for intestinal carriage of CTX-M-type ESBLs in Enterobacteriaceae from a Thai community. *Eur. J. Clin. Microbiol.* **2017**, *37*, 69–75. [CrossRef] [PubMed]

15. Sasaki, T.; Hirai, I.; Niki, M.; Nakamura, T.; Komalamisra, C.; Maipanich, W.; Kusolsuk, T.; Sa-Nguankiat, S.; Pubampen, S.; Yamamoto, Y. High prevalence of CTX-M -lactamase-producing Enterobacteriaceae in stool specimens obtained from healthy individuals in Thailand. *J. Antimicrob. Chemother.* **2010**, *65*, 666–668. [CrossRef] [PubMed]

16. Thamlikitkul, V.; Tangkoskul, T.; Seenama, C. Fecal Carriage Rate of Extended-Spectrum Beta-Lactamase-Producing Enterobacteriaceae as a Proxy Composite Indicator of Antimicrobial Resistance in a Community in Thailand. *Open Forum Infect. Dis.* **2019**, *6*, ofz425. [CrossRef]

17. Hjaltadóttir, I.; Hallberg, I.R.; Ekwall, A.K.; Nyberg, P. Predicting mortality of residents at admission to nursing home: A longitudinal cohort study. *BMC Health Serv. Res.* **2011**, *11*, 86. [CrossRef]

18. Saka, B.; Ozkaya, H.; Karisik, E.; Akin, S.; Akpinar, T.; Tufan, F.; Bahat, G.; Dogan, H.; Horasan, Z.; Cesur, K.; et al. Malnutrition and sarcopenia are associated with increased mortality rate in nursing home residents: A prospective study. *Eur. Geriatr. Med.* **2016**, *7*, 232–238. [CrossRef]

19. Vossius, C.; Selbæk, G.; Benth, J.; Bergh, S. Mortality in nursing home residents: A longitudinal study over three years. *PLoS ONE* **2018**, *13*, e0203480. [CrossRef]

20. Schoevaerdts, D.; Agelas, J.-P.; Ingels, M.-G.; Jamart, J.; Frennet, M.; Huang, T.-D.; Swine, C.; Glupczynski, Y. Health outcomes of older patients colonized by multi-drug resistant bacteria (MDRB): A one-year follow-up study. *Arch. Gerontol. Geriatr.* **2013**, *56*, 231–236. [CrossRef]

21. Igbinosa, O.; Dogho, P.; Osadiaye, N. Carbapenem-resistant Enterobacteriaceae: A retrospective review of treatment and outcomes in a long-term acute care hospital. *Am. J. Infect. Control* **2019**, *48*, 7–12. [CrossRef]

22. Aliyu, S.; McGowan, K.; Hussain, D.; Kanawati, L.; Ruiz, M.; Yohannes, S. Prevalence and Outcomes of Multi-Drug Resistant Blood Stream Infections among Nursing Home Residents Admitted to an Acute Care Hospital. *J. Intensiv. Care Med.* **2021**, *37*, 565–571. [CrossRef] [PubMed]

23. Grabowski, D.C.; Mor, V. Nursing Home Care in Crisis in the Wake of COVID-19. *JAMA* **2020**, *324*, 23. [CrossRef]

24. Choi, J.-P.; Cho, E.H.; Lee, S.J.; Koo, M.S.; Song, Y.G. Influx of multidrug resistant, Gram-negative bacteria (MDRGNB) in a public hospital among elderly patients from long-term care facilities: A single-center pilot study. *Arch. Gerontol. Geriatr.* **2012**, *54*, e19–e22. [CrossRef] [PubMed]

25. Ramphal, R.; Ambrose, P.G. Extended-Spectrum β-Lactamases and Clinical Outcomes: Current Data. *Clin. Infect. Dis.* **2006**, *42*, S164–S172. [CrossRef] [PubMed]

26. Östholmbalkhed, Å.; Tärnberg, M.; Nilsson, M.; Nilsson, L.E.; Hanberger, H.; Hällgren, A.; for the Southeast Sweden Travel Study Group. Duration of travel-associated faecal colonisation with ESBL-producing Enterobacteriaceae—A one year follow-up study. *PLoS ONE* **2018**, *13*, e0205504. [CrossRef]

27. Latour, K.; Huang, T.-D.; Jans, B.; Berhin, C.; Bogaerts, P.; Noel, A.; Nonhoff, C.; Dodémont, M.; Denis, O.; Ieven, M.; et al. Prevalence of multidrug-resistant organisms in nursing homes in Belgium in 2015. *PLoS ONE* **2019**, *14*, e0214327. [CrossRef]

28. Lee, C.-M.; Lai, C.-C.; Chiang, H.-T.; Lu, M.-C.; Wang, L.-F.; Tsai, T.-L.; Kang, M.-Y.; Jan, Y.-N.; Lo, Y.-T.; Ko, W.-C.; et al. Presence of multidrug-resistant organisms in the residents and environments of long-term care facilities in Taiwan. *J. Microbiol. Immunol. Infect.* **2017**, *50*, 133–144. [CrossRef]

29. Hollander, J.E.; Carr, B.G. Virtually Perfect? Telemedicine for COVID-19. *N. Engl. J. Med.* **2020**, *382*, 1679–1681. [CrossRef]

30. Williams, C.S.; Zheng, Q.; White, A.J.; Bengtsson, A.I.; Shulman, E.T.; Herzer, K.R.; Fleisher, L.A. The association of nursing home quality ratings and spread of COVID-19. *J. Am. Geriatr. Soc.* **2021**, *69*, 2070–2078. [CrossRef]

31. Li, Y.; Temkin-Greener, H.; Shan, G.; Cai, X. COVID-19 Infections and Deaths among Connecticut Nursing Home Residents: Facility Correlates. *J. Am. Geriatr. Soc.* **2020**, *68*, 1899–1906. [CrossRef]

32. He, M.; Li, Y.; Fang, F. Is There a Link between Nursing Home Reported Quality and COVID-19 Cases? Evidence from California Skilled Nursing Facilities. *J. Am. Med. Dir. Assoc.* **2020**, *21*, 905–908. [CrossRef] [PubMed]

33. Rawson, T.M.; Ming, D.; Ahmad, R.; Moore, L.S.P.; Holmes, A.H. Antimicrobial use, drug-resistant infections and COVID-19. *Nat. Rev. Microbiol.* **2020**, *18*, 409–410. [CrossRef] [PubMed]

34. Lerner, A.; Romano, J.; Chmelnitsky, I.; Navon-Venezia, S.; Edgar, R.; Carmeli, Y. Rectal Swabs Are Suitable for Quantifying the Carriage Load of KPC-Producing Carbapenem-Resistant Enterobacteriaceae. *Antimicrob. Agents Chemother.* **2013**, *57*, 1474–1479. [CrossRef] [PubMed]

35. Suñer, C.; Ouchi, D.; Mas, M.; Alarcon, R.L.; Mesquida, M.M.; Prat, N.; Bonet-Simó, J.M.; Izquierdo, M.E.; Sánchez, I.G.; Noguerola, S.R.; et al. A retrospective cohort study of risk factors for mortality among nursing homes exposed to COVID-19 in Spain. *Nat. Aging* **2021**, *1*, 579–584. [CrossRef]

36. Panagiotou, O.A.; Kosar, C.M.; White, E.M.; Bantis, L.E.; Yang, X.; Santostefano, C.M.; Feifer, R.A.; Blackman, C.; Rudolph, J.L.; Gravenstein, S.; et al. Risk Factors Associated with All-Cause 30-Day Mortality in Nursing Home Residents with COVID-19. *JAMA Intern. Med.* **2021**, *181*, 439. [CrossRef] [PubMed]

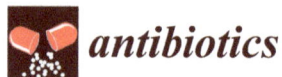 *antibiotics*

 MDPI

Article

The Real Practice Prescribing Antibiotics in Outpatients: A Failed Control Case Assessed through the Simulated Patient Method

María Guadalupe Miranda-Novales [1], Karen Flores-Moreno [2], Mauricio Rodríguez-Álvarez [3,*], Yolanda López-Vidal [3], José Luis Soto-Hernández [4], Fortino Solórzano Santos [5] and Samuel Ponce-de-León-Rosales [6]

1   Unidad de Investigación en Análisis y Síntesis de la Evidencia, Instituto Mexicano del Seguro Social, Centro Médico Nacional Siglo XXI, Mexico City 06720, Mexico
2   Laboratorio de Microbioma, Facultad de Medicina, Universidad Nacional Autónoma de México, Mexico City 04510, Mexico
3   Departamento de Microbiología y Parasitología, Facultad de Medicina, Universidad Nacional Autónoma de México, Mexico City 04510, Mexico
4   Instituto Nacional de Neurología y Neurocirugía Manuel Velasco Suárez, Mexico City 14269, Mexico; joseluis_sotohernandez@yahoo.com
5   Unidad de Investigación en Enfermedades Infecciosas, Hospital Infantil de México Federico Gómez, Secretaría de Salud, Mexico City 06720, Mexico
6   Programa Universitario de Investigación Sobre Riesgos Epidemiológicos y Emergentes, Universidad Nacional Autónoma de México, Mexico City 04510, Mexico
*   Correspondence: maurodriguez@unam.mx; Tel.: +52-55-5622-5220

Citation: Miranda-Novales, M.G.; Flores-Moreno, K.; Rodríguez-Álvarez, M.; López-Vidal, Y.; Soto-Hernández, J.L.; Solórzano Santos, F.; Ponce-de-León-Rosales, S. The Real Practice Prescribing Antibiotics in Outpatients: A Failed Control Case Assessed through the Simulated Patient Method. *Antibiotics* 2023, 12, 915. https://doi.org/10.3390/antibiotics12050915

Academic Editors: Anusak Kerdsin, Jinquan Li and Jonathan Frye

Received: 19 April 2023
Revised: 5 May 2023
Accepted: 11 May 2023
Published: 16 May 2023

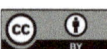
Abstract: The first level of medical care provides the largest number of consultations for the most frequent diseases at the community level, including acute pharyngitis (AP), acute diarrhoea (AD) and uncomplicated acute urinary tract infections (UAUTIs). The inappropriate use of antibiotics in these diseases represents a high risk for the generation of antimicrobial resistance (AMR) in bacteria causing community infections. To evaluate the patterns of medical prescription for these diseases in medical offices adjacent to pharmacies, we used an adult simulated patient (SP) method representing the three diseases, AP, AD and UAUTI. Each person played a role in one of the three diseases, with the signs and symptoms described in the national clinical practice guidelines (CPGs). Diagnostic accuracy and therapeutic management were assessed. Information from 280 consultations in the Mexico City area was obtained. For the 101 AP consultations, in 90 cases (89.1%), one or more antibiotics or antivirals were prescribed; for the 127 AD, in 104 cases (81.8%), one or more antiparasitic drugs or intestinal antiseptics were prescribed; for the scenarios involving UAUTIs in adult women, in 51 of 52 cases (98.1%) one antibiotic was prescribed. The antibiotic group with the highest prescription pattern for AP, AD and UAUTIs was aminopenicillins and benzylpenicillins [27/90 (30%)], co-trimoxazole [35/104 (27.6%)] and quinolones [38/51 (73.1%)], respectively. Our findings reveal the highly inappropriate use of antibiotics for AP and AD in a sector of the first level of health care, which could be a widespread phenomenon at the regional and national level and highlights the urgent need to update antibiotic prescriptions for UAUTIs according to local resistance patterns. Supervision of adherence to the CPGs is needed, as well as raising awareness about the rational use of antibiotics and the threat posed by AMR at the first level of care.

Keywords: antibiotic management; primary care; health services research

1. Introduction

Mexico's health system is made up of public and private services. The former serves the majority of the country's population, including formal workers and their families, as well as those who do not have any type of social security and cannot pay for private services, while the latter serves individuals through private insurance policies and those who can cover the costs of care with their own financial resources [1]. In recent decades, the use of private services has grown considerably. While in the year 2000, the number of visits to private medical doctors (MDs) represented 31% of the total number, this proportion increased to 37.6% and 38.9% in 2006 and 2012, respectively [2–4]

For health services, almost two decades ago, medical offices adjacent to chain pharmacies (MOAPs) began operating, mainly oriented to the sale of generic drugs for the low- and middle-income populations. These MOAPs can be classified according to the type of pharmacy to which they are linked: medical offices adjacent to independent pharmacies (MOAIPs) or to business chain pharmacies (MOABCPs) [5].

In 2013 it was estimated that nearly 13,000 MOABCPs treated 10 million patients per month and employed 32,500 physicians [6]. In 2016, the number of medical offices increased to 16,000, and according to the 2012 National Survey of Health and Nutrition (ENSANUT 2012), the visits to MOABCPs represented 41.5% of all private medical consultations in the country [4].

Until August 2010, the public sale of antibiotics in Mexico had no restrictions, and any person could buy them in pharmacies [7]; after that date, the obligation to obtain a medical prescription in order to purchase antibiotics came into force, contributing to an increase in the number of MOAPs. The main objective of the MOAP business model is to increase pharmacy sales, so the professionals who work in them are also called 'point of sale doctors' [8–10]. There is some concern regarding the quality of care at MOAPs, but most users report that it is good or even very good, with several advantages: low cost, convenience and short waiting times [11]. There is also uncertainty about the working conditions (obligations, rights and benefits) [9] which have been indicated as key elements directly related to patient care and safety [12].

The Federal Commission for Protection against Sanitary Risk (*Comisión Federal para la Protección contra Riesgos Sanitarios*, COFEPRIS) is the national regulatory authority in matters of health and is responsible for monitoring compliance with regulations regarding health risks for health service providers, as well as manufacturers and all those involved in the distribution and sale of medicines and medical devices, among other functions. From November 2013 to December 2017, COFEPRIS made 11,941 verification visits to MOAPs, resulting in 480 suspensions, equivalent to 4% of the verified establishments. At these verification visits, there was no mention of supervision of antimicrobial prescription according to clinical diagnoses [13].

The simulated patient (SP) method was developed by Barrows in 1968 for teaching purposes to assess the competence of medical doctors in a safe setting by means of a person trained to represent a disease [14,15]. It has been used in studies to assess the quality of care and decision-making in common clinical settings in several countries [16–29], and there are also useful guidelines for the reporting of research works in which this methodology is used [21].

The behaviour regarding the prescription of antimicrobials in MOAPs is not clear. The SP methodology can be used to evaluate prescriptions for the most common reasons for consultation leading to the prescription of antibiotics in ambulatory care, and it is also possible to measure adherence to clinical practice guidelines (CPGs).

The objective of this study was to record the prescriptions (type of antimicrobial, dose, route of administration and duration of treatment) in MOAPs in Mexico and to compare them with the CPGs for three clinical scenarios in adults: AP, AD and UAUTIs in adult women, represented by SP.

2. Results

A total of 280 clinical consultations with SP were given by different physicians. The distribution of medical consultations was: 101 (36.1%) for AP, 127 (45.4%) for AD and 52 (18.6%) for UAUTI. Most of the interactions took place at MOABCPs (238/280) and the rest in MOAIPs.

One hundred fifty-eight (56.4%) of the physicians were women and 122 (43.6%) were men. We found no differences in the pattern of antibiotic prescription between the sexes. The average seniority in the exercise of the profession of the consultant MD (calculated based on the year of issuance of their professional license) was 13.6 years. In terms of years of practice, 70 (25%) MDs had more than 20, 30 (10.7%) had between 10 and 19 and 166 (59.3%) had less than 10. The professional licenses of 14 MDs (5%) could not be found in the National Registry of Professions.

The median duration of the clinical interactions was 11 min (min: 7, max: 60). Diagnoses were given to all SPs along with their prescriptions, and all diagnoses were consistent with the condition simulated by the SPs. The median number of drugs in each prescription was 2 (minimum (min): 1; maximum (max): 5). Regarding the cost of the services rendered, 3 MOABCPs offered 'free medical guidance' at no cost; for the rest, the mean cost of the consultation was 2.0 USD (min: 1.5, max: 3).

A complete medical history and physical examination were performed in 174 (62.1%) of the clinical interactions, and in 106 of them (37.9%), the consultation focused on the current condition, and a minimal physical examination was performed. For the 101 AP scenarios, in 90 cases (89.1%), one or more antibiotics or antivirals were prescribed. The antibiotic group with the highest prescription pattern were aminopenicillins and benzylpenicillins (ampicillin, amoxicillin, amoxicillin/clavulanate, procaine and benzathine penicillin) with 30/90 prescriptions; followed by macrolides (erythromycin, azithromycin and clarithromycin) in 17/90 prescriptions and cephalosporins (cefalexin, cefuroxime and ceftriaxone) in 12/90 prescriptions. The group of antibiotics least prescribed for this clinical entity was the quinolones (norfloxacin, ciprofloxacin and levofloxacin). In 6/25 prescriptions for amantadine, an antibiotic was also prescribed (aminopenicillin) (Table 1). In 4/90 antibiotic prescriptions, a combination of an aminopenicillin plus a macrolide was indicated. In three SPs, although the diagnosis was bacterial pharyngitis, they did not receive antibiotics. For the rest of the SPs, the diagnoses were acute rhinopharyngitis (n = 35 (34.6%)), viral pharyngitis (n = 32 (31.6%)) or acute pharyngitis (n = 31 (30.6%)). In one SP, one MD used a delayed prescribing strategy (with a waiting period of 48 h), but the antibiotic to be used in case the symptoms persisted or worsened as ciprofloxacin.

Table 1. Antimicrobial prescriptions in 101 acute pharyngitis (AP) interactions.

Antimicrobial	n	%
Aminopenicillin/Benzylpenicillin	30	29.7
Macrolide	17	16.8
Cephalosporins	12	11.8
Quinolones	9	8.9
Clindamycin	1	0.9
Fosfomycin	1	0.9
Total with at least one antibiotic	70	69.3
Amantadine	25	24.7
No antibiotic	11	10.8

For the 127 AD scenarios, in 104 (81.9%), an antibiotic and/or antiparasitic drug was prescribed (Table 2). Four (3.9%) SPs received one antibiotic plus an antiparasitic drug or one of those antibiotics referred to as 'intestinal antiseptic' (nifuroxazide and neomycin) simultaneously; 23 (22.1%) did not receive an antibiotic, but for 13 of them, the diagnosis was different to AD: colitis (n = 6), inflammatory bowel disease (n = 4) or peptic acid disease (n = 3). Antiparasitic drugs included: albendazole, mebendazole, metronidazole, quinfamide, nitazoxanide and diiodohydroquinone.

Table 2. Antimicrobial prescription in 127 acute diarrhoea (AD) interactions.

Antimicrobial	n	%
TMP/SMZ	35	27.6
Quinolones	26	20.5
Aminopenicillin	4	3.1
Cephalosporins	3	2.4
Aminoglycoside	3	2.4
Tetracycline	2	1.6
Chloramphenicol	1	0.8
Macrolide	1	0.8
Total with at least one antibiotic	75	59
At least one antiparasitic drug	28	22
'Intestinal antiseptics'	14	11
No antibiotic	23	18.1

TMP/SMZ = trimethoprim–sulfamethoxazole.

For the 52 SPs simulating UAUTIs, in all but one, an antibiotic was prescribed (Table 3); in the case of the SP who did not receive antibiotics, the doctor requested urinalysis with a microbiological culture before prescribing an antibiotic. Quinolones were the most prescribed antibiotic, followed by nitrofurantoin and TMP/SMZ. In six SPs, two antibiotics were indicated: nalidixic acid plus norfloxacin; nalidixic acid plus cephalexin; TMP/SMZ plus nitrofurantoin; nalidixic acid plus gentamicin; nalidixic acid plus amikacin and ciprofloxacin plus nitrofurantoin.

Table 3. Antimicrobial prescription in 52 uncomplicated acute urinary tract infections (UAUTI) interactions.

Antimicrobial	n	%
Quinolones	38	73
Nitrofurantoin	8	15.4
TMP/SMZ	5	9.6
Cephalosporins	2	3.8
Aminopenicillin	1	1.9
Aminoglycoside	2	3.8
Macrolide	1	1.9
Total with at least one antibiotic	51	98
No antibiotic	1	1.9

Costs

The median total costs per prescription were similar for the three scenarios. The highest cost was for AP (median: 11.6 USD), followed by AD (median: 9.5 USD) and UAUTI (median: 9.4 USD (Figure 1).

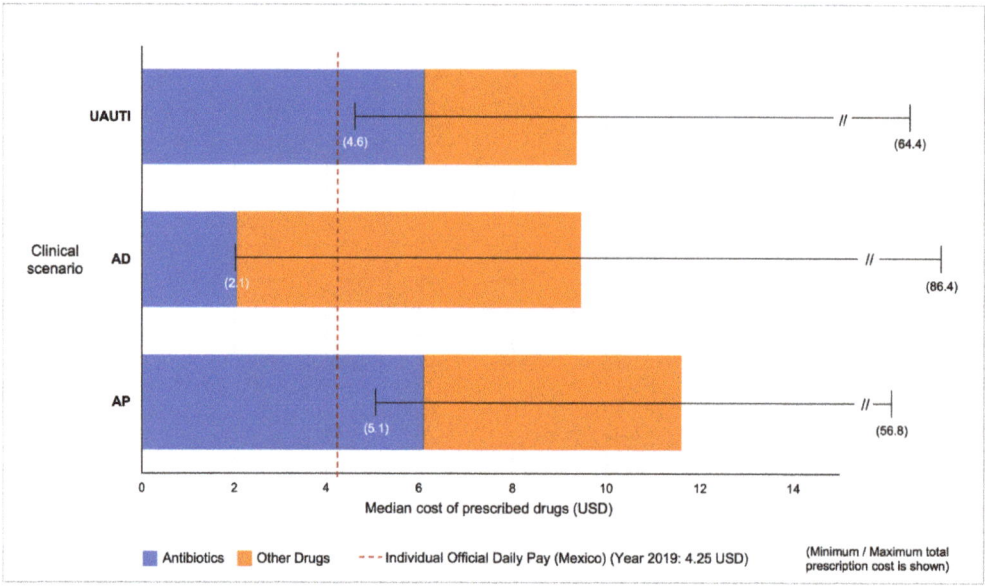

Figure 1. Cost of antimicrobials (antibiotics, antivirals, antiparasitic) and other drugs prescribed in the clinical scenarios: uncomplicated acute urinary tract infections (UAUTI), acute diarrhoea (AD) and acute pharyngitis (AP).

A great and diverse variety of other drugs not included or recommended in the CPGs were prescribed, such as mucolytics, expectorants, cough suppressants, steroids, bronchodilators, vitamins, centrally acting analgesics, anti-inflammatories, proton-pump inhibitors, lactobacilli, dopamine antagonists, antidiarrhoeal drugs (kaolin–pectin) and urine acidifiers. All these drugs contributed substantially to the final amount of each prescription, particularly for the AD scenario (Figure 1). Drugs prescribed in each interaction had a median of three (minimum 1-maximum 6). In the AP scenario, polypharmacy (5 or more drugs) was common and very diverse (16/101); examples of the combinations were as follows: loratadine/betamethasone plus nimesulide plus dextromethorphan plus vitamin C plus the antibiotic; ibuprofen/paracetamol plus amantadine plus dextromethorphan plus vitamin C plus the antibiotic; naproxen/paracetamol plus loratadine/betamethasone plus ambroxol plus the antibiotic.

3. Discussion

Despite clear recommendations in international and national guidelines for upper respiratory infections (URIs) (acute rhinopharyngitis (AR) or the common cold (CC)) and gastrointestinal diseases (acute diarrhoea (AD)), antibiotics are frequently prescribed for these conditions in outpatient settings [22–25]. Fleming-Dutra et al. [26] estimated the annual appropriate antibiotic prescription rate in the US for URIs. In all, acute respiratory conditions per 1000 population led to 221 antibiotic prescriptions (95% CI, 198–245) annually, but only 111 antibiotic prescriptions were estimated to be appropriate. In India, Kotwani et al. determined that during 2007 and 2008, patients with acute diarrhoea were prescribed at least one antibiotic in both public (171 of 398 (43%)) and private facilities (76 of 110 (69%)) [27], whereas the rate of antibiotic overuse in Thailand in adults with acute diarrhoea was 48.9% (86 of 176 patients) [28]. Appropriateness of antibiotic prescription is difficult to assess with certainty because important clinical data and risk factors are frequently lacking in the medical charts. The SP method makes it possible to gather relevant and real information on the quality of care. Satyanarayana S et al. summarised the experience of 3086 SP interactions in four countries representing cases of pulmonary tuberculosis, where providers prescribed medications that were unnecessary or harmful in 83% of the interactions; medications of interest were broad-spectrum antibiotics, fluoroquinolones and steroids [19]. In this study, volunteers were successful in representing the clinical scenario. Most of them received a diagnosis consistent with the signs and symptoms, so the training was adequate, and they appeared to be genuine patients. This strategy makes it possible to reproduce a situation in the daily life of an individual who goes to consultation and objectively obtains a result identical to that obtained with a real patient.

In Mexico, in May 2010, it was established by law that the sale and dispensing of antibiotics in private pharmacies may only be carried out with the presentation of a prescription [29]. Before this law was enacted, it was calculated that 40 to 60% of pharmacy customers self-medicated or asked for a recommendation from the pharmacy employee. After the law came into effect, the pharmacies, especially chain pharmacies, set up adjacent offices to offer very low-cost and free consultations, thus providing customers with full service. These offices satisfy a demand from the population, and the service they offer is considered satisfactory by users due to promptness and accessibility, while the pharmacy can continue to sell antibiotics. A study conducted in 1996 evaluated the prescriptive behaviour of pharmacy attendants, with simulated clients representing a gonorrhoea scenario. The attendants with no medical training prescribed adequate treatment in only 25% of the cases [30]. Researchers analysed the consumption of medicines in clients of private pharmacies and found that both by self-medication and by prescription, a wide variety of medicines were purchased: analgesics, antitussives, antibiotics, vitamins, herbal remedies, antidiarrhoeals, antiparasitic drugs and antihistamines, several of which in combinations that are not recommended [31]

Unfortunately, the use of antibiotics for the two most common causes of consultation (acute respiratory infection and acute diarrhoea) is like that reported in developing countries. In a systematic review by Li et al., the overall average of antibiotic prescriptions for upper respiratory tract infections was 83.7% (95%CI 80.6–86.4%) [32]. In our study, in the acute rhinopharyngitis scenario, all doctors made a correct diagnosis, but an antibiotic was prescribed in 9 out of 10 interactions. Most of the doctors who provided the consultations had less than 10 years of practice, so it is possible that this group was more familiar with the use of CPGs. Due to the design of the study, it was not feasible to explore this issue. In recent years, the management of CPGs has been a key point in the training programs and is included in every curriculum; current generations may be more familiar with its existence and use. However, some factors have been associated with antibiotic prescription, such as diagnosis of acute bronchitis, symptoms observed in the physical exam (fever, purulent sputum, tonsillar exudate) and the physician's perception of the patient's desire for antibiotics [33] In this study, all volunteers were healthy individuals and did not demand a prescription for an antibiotic. In addition to antibiotics, other prescribed drugs did not have clinical indications, such as antivirals, expectorants, mucolytics, bronchodilators and steroids.

In the acute diarrhoea scenario, our finding of an 82% antibiotic or antiparasitic prescription rate was higher than in other countries such as India [27]; a study conducted in New Delhi reported a prescription rate for antibiotics of 43% in the public sector and 69% in the private sector, in which the most commonly prescribed antibiotics were quinolones, followed by cephalosporins (cefuroxime and cefalexin) and in third place doxycycline. Increased prescribing in the private sector and lack of adherence to clinical practice guidelines are emphasised. In our study, the most prescribed drugs were TMP/SMZ and antiparasitic drugs, which are relatively inexpensive, but the final cost increases with all the medications added to the prescriptions.

Finally, the most common antibiotics prescribed for UAUTI in women were quinolones. The Mexican CPGs [24] note that these drugs should not be used as first-line treatment; however, it is stated that if there is no response to the drug initially indicated (nitrofurantoin or TMP/MSZ), the alternative is ciprofloxacin. Since it is accepted that it is unnecessary to take a urine culture before the antibiotic prescription, the aetiology would not be available to indicate a specific treatment in case of failure. Our volunteers have not prescribed the short-course treatment recommended in the guideline, which can significantly decrease the number of days of antimicrobial treatment.

If antibiotics are prescribed unnecessarily or used inappropriately, they can cause toxicity and other adverse effects, such as allergic reactions, gastrointestinal problems, headaches, and neurologic symptoms [34]. The patients or the institution that covers their care incurs additional expenses. Moreover, the inappropriate use of antibiotics by unlicensed individuals can contribute to the development of antimicrobial resistance. We found a non-negligible number (n = 14 (5%)) of physicians in the MOAPs practicing with a license that could not be verified as valid in the official databases. In these cases, the national regulatory authority (COFEPRIS) should suspend the activities of these medical offices, and those responsible must be held accountable.

Our study has several limitations. The number of interactions may seem small, but according to the sample size estimate, increasing the number of consultations probably would not lead to a different result. The assumptions used considered an even lower percentage of antimicrobial prescriptions. Factors that may have influenced the prescription of antibiotics by the physicians are not considered, among others, the load of the number of consultations and the hour of the day. It seems to be that an important factor is the economic interest of service providers that coercively influence their medical employees to increase the number of drugs listed in a prescription. The other is the limited consultation time available, which can lead the doctor to prescribe an antibiotic instead of educating the patient and explaining why it is not required.

In conclusion, the SP method allows prescription practices to be evaluated with objectivity and the identification of areas of opportunity to improve adherence to the CPGs and update their content. There is low adherence to CPGs in the primary care settings evaluated. Antimicrobial overuse is a considerable problem in common acute conditions (AP and AD), and apparently, the most frequent self-limited viral aetiology, which does not require antibiotics, is not considered. In UAUTIs, current antimicrobial resistance in uropathogens is also not considered, and several microbiological failures can be expected with the extensive use of quinolones.

4. Materials and Methods

This was a descriptive cross-sectional survey in which healthy medical and chemistry students were invited to participate. After review and approval by the institutional review board, volunteers who gave their consent were trained to represent one of the three clinical scenarios: AP, AD or UAUTI, according to the clinical description of the corresponding national CPG (Table 4) [22–24].

Table 4. Standardised patient clinical case scenarios and accepted recommendations according to national CPGs (References [22–24]).

Clinical Scenario	Symptoms	Management
Acute pharyngitis (AP)	-Sore throat -Dry cough -Runny nose -Conjunctival irritation (no secretion) -No fever Onset of symptoms: two days	Symptomatic treatment: paracetamol 500 mg orally every 8 h for 3–5 days or ;non-steroidal anti-inflammatory orally every 12 h for 3–5 days
Acute diarrhoea (AD)	-Abdominal pain -Loose stools (4–5 per day without mucus or blood) -Occasional nausea -No fever Onset of symptoms: 1 day	Oral rehydration solutions Astringent diet Watch for alarm signs of dehydration

Table 4. *Cont.*

Clinical Scenario	Symptoms	Management
Uncomplicated acute urinary tract infection in adult women (UAUTI)	-Dysuria -Urinary frequency and urgency -Abdominal discomfort -No fever -Onset of symptoms: 2 days	1st line treatment: (a) trimethoprim/sulfamethoxazole 160 mg/800 mg, twice daily for three days or nitrofurantoin 100 mg twice daily for 7 days. If after 3 day symptoms persist, request urine culture and initiate ciprofloxacin 250 mg twice daily for 3 days.

4.1. Procedure

Twenty-four research assistants were trained to act as SPs according to a script for each clinical scenario (AP, AD, UAUTI) in which signs and symptoms were described according to clinical practice guidelines [22–24], All participants were in good general health and had no prior experience as SPs or with the method; 18 were men (median age 29 years; interquartile range (IQR): 23–29) and 6 women (median age 23 years; IQR: 21–27). UAUTI was addressed only by the 6 women. In this method, the SP is a person acting a role. The training to represent the clinical cases was carried out in three sessions of 30 min each, supervised by a physician with clinical experience who was part of the research team. After the sessions, each participant simulated consultation with the instructor physician to ensure that the representation was consistent with the clinical scenarios. The advantage of the method is that a simulation can be reproduced for multiple participants, and the same simulation can be replicated with different actors [14].

Between May 2018 and January 2019, the SPs were randomly assigned to different MOABCPs and MOAIPs. After each visit, the participants recorded information related to the care received: duration of the medical consultation, characteristics of the medical interview and physical examination, indications and prescriptions. Drug prices were obtained through a specialised online search engine that includes the prices of medicines for at least 12 different pharmacies. For each drug, the average cost was obtained, as well as the minimum and maximum. Costs are shown in US dollars (USD); all costs were obtained in Mexican pesos (MXN) and the average exchange rate of 2019 was used (1 USD = 20 MXN).

4.2. Sample Size

A calculation was made with the estimated number of MOAPs in Mexico City's Metropolitan Area (n = 3360) [6] and the expected frequency of adequate antibiotic prescriptions for each scenario [23] as follows:

AP: 13% (95% CI, 7–22; confidence limit: 7%), a total of 86 visits.

AD: 9% (95% CI, 4–16; confidence limit: 5%), a total of 121 visits.

UAUTI: 75% (95% CI, 61–86; confidence limit: 10%), a total of 36 visits.

All the information from the registration forms of the medical consultations and prescriptions was captured in a database by the research group; the analysis of the information was performed through descriptive statistics with simple frequencies, percentages, median, interquartile range (IQR) and minimum and maximum values.

Author Contributions: Conceptualization, methodology, formal analysis, writing-original draft preparation, funding acquisition, review and editing, M.G.M.-N. Methodology, data curation, validation, formal analysis, funding acquisition, K.F.-M. Conceptualization, methodology, writing-original draft preparation, writing-review and editing, M.R.-Á. Conceptualization, methodology, writing-original draft preparation, funding acquisition, review and editing, Y.L.-V. Conceptualization, methodology, validation, formal analysis, writing-review and editing, J.L.S.-H. Conceptualization, methodology, validation, writing-review and editing, F.S.S. Conceptualization, methodology, formal analysis, funding acquisition, writing-review and editing, S.P.-d.-L.-R. All authors have read and agreed to the published version of the manuscript.

Funding: This project was funded with research resources from the Programa Universitario de Investigación en Salud (PUIS) and project number IN218220 from the Programa de Apoyo a Proyectos de Investigación e Innovación Tecnológica (PAPIIT), Universidad Nacional Autónoma de México (UNAM).

Institutional Review Board Statement: This study was conducted in accordance with the Declaration of Helsinki, and approved by the Institutional Review Board of the School of Medicine at the National Autonumus University of Mexico with the number FM/DI/108/2018 on 3 April 2018.

Informed Consent Statement: Informed consent was waived as the study involves no risks to participants, no procedures were performed as part of the research, and identifiable data was codified not included.

Data Availability Statement: The data presented in this study are available on request from the corresponding author.

Acknowledgments: The authors wish to thank Patricia Orduña Estrada and René Arredondo-Hernández for their feedback during the initial stage of the project and Mario Antonio Coello Santillanes and Christian Gibrán Ruiz Ramírez for their help in starting the simulated patient method for this study.

Conflicts of Interest: The authors declare that there are no conflict of interest regarding this study.

References

1. Gómez Dantés, O.; Sesma, S.; Becerril, V.M.; Knaul, F.M.; Arreola, H.; Frenk, J. Sistema de salud de México. *Salud Pública Méx.* **2011**, *53*, S220–S232.
2. Valdespino, J.L.; Olaiz, G.; López-Barajas, M.P.; Mendoza, L.; Palma, O.; Velázquez, O.; Tapia, R.; Sepúlveda, J. Encuesta Nacional de Salud 2000. Tomo I. Vivienda, Población y Utilización de Servicios de Salud. Instituto Nacional de Salud Pública. 2003. Available online: https://ensanut.insp.mx/informes/ENSA_tomo1.pdf (accessed on 3 January 2022).
3. Olaiz-Fernández, G.; Rivera-Dommarco, J.; Shamah-Levy, T.; Rojas, R.; Villalpando-Hernández, S.; Hernández-Avila, M.; Sepúlveda-Amor, J. Encuesta Nacional de Salud y Nutrición 2006. Instituto Nacional de Salud Pública. 2006. Available online: https://ensanut.insp.mx/informes/ensanut2006.pdf (accessed on 3 January 2022).
4. Gutiérrez, J.P.; Rivera-Dommarco, J.; Shamah-Levy, T.; Villalpando-Hernández, S.; Franco, A.; Cuevas-Nasu, L.; Romero-Martínez, M.; Hernández-Ávila, M. Encuesta Nacional de Salud y Nutrición 2012. Resultados Nacionales. Instituto Nacional de Salud Pública. 2012. Available online: https://ensanut.insp.mx/informes/ENSANUT2012ResultadosNacionales.pdf (accessed on 3 January 2022).
5. Chu, M.; Garcia-Cuellar, R. Farmacias Similares: Private and Public Health Care for the Base of the Pyramid in Mexico. Harvard Business School Case 307-092, January 2007. (Revised April 2011). Harvard Business School. Available online: https://hbsp.harvard.edu/product/307092-PDF-ENG (accessed on 3 January 2022).
6. Comisión Federal Para la Protección Contra Riesgos Sanitarios (COFEPRIS); Secretaría de Salud. Avanza la Estrategia Para Regular Consultorios en Farmacias (Comunicado de Prensa, 29/Ene/2014). Available online: https://www.gob.mx/cofepris/prensa/avanza-la-estrategia-para-regular-consultorios-en-farmacias-62847 (accessed on 3 January 2022).
7. Secretaría de Salud. Acuerdo por el que determinan los lineamientos a los que estará sujeta a la venta y dispensación de antibióticos. *Diario Oficial de la Federación*, 27 May 2010.
8. Fundación Mexicana Para la Salud (FUNSALUD). Estudio Sobre la Práctica de la Atención Médica en Consultorios Médicos Adyacentes a Farmacias Privadas. FUNSALUD. 2014. Available online: http://funsalud.org.mx/portal/wp-content/uploads/2015/07/Informe-final-CAF-v300615-e-book.pdf (accessed on 3 January 2022).
9. Lezama-Fernández, M.A. Consultorios adyacentes a farmacias privadas: Calidad de los servicios de salud y calidad de vida laboral (CAF). *Rev. Conamed* **2016**, *21*, 3–4. Available online: https://www.medigraphic.com/cgi-bin/new/resumen.cgi?IDARTICULO=79468 (accessed on 3 January 2022).
10. Díaz-Portillo, S.P.; Idrovo, A.J.; Dreser, A.; Bonilla, F.R.; Matías-Juan, B.; Wirtz, V.J. Consultorios adyacentes a farmacias privadas en México: Infraestructura y características del personal médico y su remuneración. *Salud Pública Méx.* **2015**, *57*, 320–328.
11. Perez-Cuevas, R.; Doubova, S.V.; Wirtz, V.J.; Servan-Mori, E.; Dreser, A.; Hernández-Ávila, M. Effects of the expansion of doctors' offices adjacent to private pharmacies in Mexico: Secondary data analysis of a national survey. *BMJ Open* **2014**, *4*, e004669. [CrossRef]
12. World Health Organization (WHO). The World Health Report 2006: Working Together for Health. WHO. Available online: https://apps.who.int/iris/handle/10665/43432 (accessed on 3 January 2022).
13. Comisión Federal Para la Protección Contra Riesgos Sanitarios (COFEPRIS); Secretaría de Salud. Informe de Rendición de Cuentas de Conclusión de la Administración 2012–2018. Available online: http://sipot.cofepris.gob.mx/Archivos/juridico/COFE/Informe_Consolidado.pdf (accessed on 3 January 2022).
14. Churchouse, C.; McCafferty, C. Standardized Patients Versus Simulated Patients: Is There a Difference? *Clin. Simul. Nurs.* **2012**, *8*, e363–e365. [CrossRef]

15. Austin, Z.; Gregory, P.; Tabak, D. Simulated patients vs. standardized patients in objective structured clinical examinations. *Am. J. Pharm. Educ.* **2006**, *70*, 119. [CrossRef]
16. Sylvia, S.; Shi, Y.; Xue, H.; Tian, X.; Wang, H.; Liu, Q.; Medina, A.; Rozelle, S. Survey using incognito standardized patients shows poor quality care in China's rural clinics. *Health Policy Plan* **2015**, *30*, 322–333. [CrossRef] [PubMed]
17. Ozuah, P.O.; Reznik, M. Using unannounced standardized patients to assess residents' competency in asthma severity classification. *Ambul. Pediatr.* **2008**, *8*, 139–142. [CrossRef]
18. Das, J.; Holla, A.; Das, V.; Mohanan, M.; Tabak, D.; Chan, B. In urban and rural India, a standardized patient study showed low levels of provider training and huge quality gaps. *Health Aff. (Millwood)* **2012**, *31*, 2774–2784. [CrossRef]
19. Satyanarayana, S.; Kwan, A.; Daniels, B.; Subbaraman, R.; McDowell, A.; Bergkvist, S.; Das, R.K.; Das, V.; Das, J.; Pai, M. Use of standardised patients to assess antibiotic dispensing for tuberculosis by pharmacies in urban India: A cross-sectional study. *Lancet Infect. Dis.* **2016**, *16*, 1261–1268. [CrossRef]
20. Miller, R.; Goodman, C. Do chain pharmacies perform better than independent pharmacies? Evidence from a standardised patient study of the management of childhood diarrhoea and suspected tuberculosis in urban India. *BMJ Glob. Health* **2017**, *2*, e000457. [CrossRef] [PubMed]
21. Howley, L.; Szauter, K.; Perkowski, L.; Clifton, M.; McNaughton, N.; on behalf of the Association of Standardized Patient Educators (ASPE). Quality of standardised patient research reports in the medical education literature: Review and recommendations. *Med. Educ.* **2008**, *42*, 350–358. [CrossRef] [PubMed]
22. Centro Nacional de Excelencia Tecnológica en Salud (CENETEC); Secretaría de Salud. Atención, Diagnóstico y Tratamiento de Diarrea Aguda en Adultos en el Primer Nivel de Atención (Guía de Referencia Rápida) (05 de octubre de 2015). Available online: https://www.gob.mx/salud/documentos/atencion-diagnostico-y-tratamiento-de-diarrea-aguda-en-adultos-en-el-primer-nivel-de-atencion-guia-de-referencia-rapida (accessed on 3 January 2022).
23. Centro Nacional de Excelencia Tecnológica en Salud (CENETEC); Secretaría de Salud. Guía de Práctica Clínica. Diagnóstico y tratamiento de Faringoamigdalitis Aguda. Evidencias y Recomendaciones (2009). Available online: http://www.cenetec-difusion.com/CMGPC/IMSS-073-08/ER.pdf (accessed on 3 January 2022).
24. Centro Nacional de Excelencia Tecnológica en Salud (CENETEC); Secretaría de Salud. Guía de Práctica Clínica. Diagnóstico y Tratamiento de la Infección Aguda, no Complicada del Tracto Urinario en la Mujer. Evidencias y Recomendaciones (2009). Available online: http://www.cenetec-difusion.com/CMGPC/IMSS-077-08/ER.pdf (accessed on 3 January 2022).
25. Smith, D.R.M.; Dolk, F.C.K.; Pouwels, K.B.; Christie, M.; Robotham, J.; Smieszek, T. Defining the appropriateness and inappropriateness of antibiotic prescribing in primary care. *J. Antimicrob. Chemother.* **2018**, *73* (Suppl. S2), ii11–ii18. [CrossRef]
26. Fleming-Dutra, K.E.; Hersh, A.L.; Shapiro, D.J.; Bartoces, M.; Enns, E.A.; File, T.M., Jr.; Finkelstein, J.A.; Gerber, J.S.; Hyun, D.Y.; Linder, J.A.; et al. Prevalence of Inappropriate Antibiotic Prescriptions Among US Ambulatory Care Visits, 2010–2011. *J. Am. Med. Assoc.* **2016**, *315*, 1864–1873. [CrossRef]
27. Kotwani, A.; Chaudhury, R.R.; Holloway, K. Antibiotic-prescribing practices of primary care prescribers for acute diarrhea in New Delhi, India. *Value Health* **2012**, *15* (Suppl. S1), S116–S119. [CrossRef]
28. Supcharassaeng, S.; Suankratay, C. Antibiotic prescription for adults with acute diarrhea at King Chulalongkorn Memorial Hospital, Thailand. *J. Med. Assoc. Thail.* **2011**, *94*, 545–550.
29. Pérez-Vega, A.I. Cumplimento Normativo en el Control de la Venta y la Dispensación de Antibióticos en Farmacias y Perspectivas en México en Combate a la Resistencia Antimicrobiana (RAM). *Boletin. Conamed.* **2018**, *4*, 17–20. Available online: http://www.conamed.gob.mx/gobmx/boletin/pdf/boletin22/Cumplimento.pdf (accessed on 3 January 2022).
30. Leyva-Flores, R.; Bronfman, M.; Erviti-Erice, J. Simulated clients in drugstores: Prescriptive behaviour of drugstore attendants. *J. Soc. Adm. Pharm.* **2000**, *17*, 151–158.
31. Leyva, R.; Erviti, J.; Bronfman, M.; Gassman, N. Consumo de medicamentos en farmacias privadas: Los medicamentos inseguros. In *Coords. Salud, Cambio Social y Política. Perspectivas Desde América Latina*; Bronfman, M., Castro, R., Eds.; Edamex: Mexico City, Mexico, 1999; pp. 493–508.
32. Li, J.; Song, X.; Yang, T.; Chen, Y.; Gong, Y.; Yin, X.; Lu, Z. A Systematic Review of Antibiotic Prescription Associated with Upper Respiratory Tract Infections in China. *Medicine* **2016**, *95*, e3587. [CrossRef]
33. McKay, R.; Mah, A.; Law, M.R.; McGrail, K.; Patrick, D.M. Systematic Review of Factors Associated with Antibiotic Prescribing for Respiratory Tract Infections. *Antimicrob. Agents Chemother.* **2016**, *60*, 4106–4118. [CrossRef]
34. Mohsen, S.; Dickinson, J.A.; Somayaji, R. Update on the adverse effects of antimicrobial therapies in community practice. *Can. Fam. Physician* **2020**, *66*, 651–659. [PubMed]

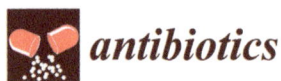

Article

Distinguishing Clinical *Enterococcus faecium* Strains and Resistance to Vancomycin Using a Simple In-House Screening Test

Natkamon Saenhom [1], Parichart Boueroy [1], Peechanika Chopjitt [1], Rujirat Hatrongjit [2] and Anusak Kerdsin [1,*]

[1] Faculty of Public Health, Kasetsart University Chalermphrakiat Sakon Nakhon Province Campus, Sakon Nakhon 47000, Thailand; natkamon030916@gmail.com (N.S.); parichart.bou@ku.th (P.B.); peechanika.c@ku.th (P.C.)

[2] Faculty of Science and Engineering, Kasetsart University Chalermphrakiat Sakon Nakhon Province Campus, Sakon Nakhon 47000, Thailand; Rujirat.ha@ku.th

* Correspondence: Anusak.ke@ku.th; Tel.: +66-42-725-023

Citation: Saenhom, N.; Boueroy, P.; Chopjitt, P.; Hatrongjit, R.; Kerdsin, A. Distinguishing Clinical *Enterococcus faecium* Strains and Resistance to Vancomycin Using a Simple In-House Screening Test. *Antibiotics* **2022**, *11*, 286. https://doi.org/10.3390/antibiotics11030286

Academic Editor: Carlos M. Franco

Received: 10 January 2022
Accepted: 18 February 2022
Published: 22 February 2022

Publisher's Note: MDPI stays neutral with regard to jurisdictional claims in published maps and institutional affiliations.

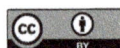
Abstract: Vancomycin-resistant enterococci (VRE) are a major concern as microorganisms with antimicrobial resistance and as a public health threat contributing significantly to morbidity, mortality, and socio-economic costs. Among VREs, vancomycin-resistant *Enterococcus faecium* (VREfm) is frequently isolated and is resistant to many antibiotics used to treat patients with hospital-acquired infection. Accurate and rapid detection of VREfm results in effective antimicrobial therapy, immediate patient isolation, dissemination control, and appropriate disinfection measures. An in-house VREfm screening broth was developed and compared to the broth microdilution method and multiplex polymerase chain reaction for the detection of 105 enterococci, including 81 VRE isolates (61 *E. faecium*, 5 *E. faecalis*, 10 *E. gallinarum*, and 5 *E. casseliflavus*). Verification of this screening broth on 61 VREfm, 20 other VRE, and 24 non-VRE revealed greater validity for VREfm detection. The accuracy of this broth was 100% in distinguishing *E. faecium* from other enterococcal species. Our test revealed 93.3% accuracy, 97.5% sensitivity, and 79.2% specificity compared with broth microdilution and PCR detecting *van* genes. The kappa statistic to test interrater reliability was 0.8, revealing substantial agreement for this screening test to the broth microdilution method. In addition, the in-house VREfm screening broth produced rapid positivity after at least 8 h of incubation. Application of this assay to screen VREfm should be useful in clinical laboratories and hospital infection control units.

Keywords: Enterococci; *Enterococcus faecium*; screening test; vancomycin

1. Introduction

Enterococci are known as opportunistic pathogens and a leading cause of hospital-acquired infections, especially vancomycin-resistant enterococci (VRE) that are a major concern regarding their antimicrobial resistance as a public health issue. The two major species that are well-known worldwide to cause human diseases and resistance to vancomycin are *Enterococcus faecium* and *E. faecalis* [1]. Of these two species, vancomycin-resistant *E. faecium* (VREfm) is more frequently isolated from patients with hospital-acquired infection than vancomycin-resistant *E. faecalis* and other species [1].

The World Health Organization (WHO) published their list of priority bacterial pathogens for which new antibiotics are urgently needed, and VREfm is listed in the high-priority category of antibiotic-resistant bacteria [2]. VREfm is widely distributed in hospitals around the world, with the prevalence varying according to geographical location. In the U.S., VREfm accounts for 82% of reported cases because vancomycin is rarely restricted and thus has widespread antibiotic use in hospitals [3–5]. In European countries, VREfm has shown increasing prevalence, from 10% in 2015 to 17.3% in 2018 [3]. In Asia, the prevalence of VREfm accounts for 22.4% of reported cases and is higher than for European countries but lower than for the U.S. [6]. Treatment options for invasive VREfm infections are very limited, resulting in high mortality [7]. Vancomycin resistance determinants due to the *vanA* and *vanB* genes are globally frequently reported in VRE, including in *E. faecium* clinical isolates [3,8].

A previous report discussed potential determinants influencing the future dissemination and control of antibiotic resistance and nominated the rapidity and accuracy of laboratory techniques that allowed for rapid identification of the infecting pathogen and antibiotic susceptibility testing [9]. Therefore, accurate and rapid detection of VRE, especially VREfm, support effective antimicrobial therapy, immediate patient isolation, and appropriate disinfection measures in hospitals. Many methods have been implemented to identify either VRE or VREfm, including conventional culture, real-time PCR, conventional PCR, and automated microbiology instruments, such as BD Phoenix (Becton, Dickinson and Company) or Vitek-2 (bioMerieux) [10,11]. Although some of these methods are rapid, easy to perform, and are accurate in identification or detection, many of these methods are expensive and have a high level of sophistication that requires operator experience and skill and special instrumentation. These constraints make such methods inappropriate in a laboratory with limited resources. Therefore, we developed an alternative assay to detect VREfm isolates at a low cost. The aim of this study was to compare an in-house VREfm screening broth with the broth microdilution method and multiplex PCR for the detection of VREfm. Our screening broth provides an alternative assay to detect VREfm isolates. This may be useful in laboratories where a large number of isolates must be screened at low cost and as such could reduce the costs associated with laboratory and infection control in hospitals with a high prevalence of VRE, especially VREfm.

2. Results

In this study, we compared the in-house VREfm screening broth using the broth microdilution method and multiplex PCR for the detection of VREfm. All tested enterococci were confirmed to the species level, *van* genes detected, and the MIC values determined of vancomycin. The screening broth was evaluated using the broth microdilution method and PCR assay in terms of specificity, sensitivity, accuracy, and Cohen's kappa coefficient.

2.1. Identification and Testing Vvancomycin-Resistant Strains

As shown in Table 1, among 105 enterococci confirmed using conventional biochemical tests and multiplex PCR (Figure 1), 71 were *E. faecium* isolates and 14 were *E. faecalis* isolates. The 20 *Enterococcus* spp. identified using conventional biochemical tests were *E. gallinarum* (*n* = 10), *E. casseliflavus* (*n* = 5), *E. mundtii* (*n* = 4), and *E. raffinosus* (*n* = 1). The multiplex PCR assay also detected *vanA* in 51 out of the 105 enterococci, consisting of 48 *E. faecium* and 3 *E. faecalis* isolates, respectively, whereas *vanB* were detected in 15 isolates, consisting of 13 *E. faecium* and 2 *E. faecalis* isolates. We detected *vanC1* in all *E. gallinarum* and *vanC2/C3* in all *E. casseliflavus*, whereas *vanA*, *vanB*, *vanC1*, or *vanC2/C3* genes were not detected in any of the *E. mundtii* and *E. raffinosus* samples.

The vancomycin MIC values indicated that 85.9% (61/71) of the *E. faecium* isolates were resistant to vancomycin (range 32–128 μg/mL) that were confirmed to be VRE according to their MIC values and the presence of either *vanA* or *vanB*, whereas the remaining 10 isolates were susceptible to vancomycin. Of the 14 *E. faecalis* isolates, only five were resistant to vancomycin (VREfs) by broth microdilution, with 3 isolates having an MIC value of 64 or 128 μg/mL, and they all carried *vanA*, while the remaining two *E. faecalis* isolates carrying *vanB* revealed an MIC value of 32 μg/mL. In contrast with the 20 *Enterococcus* spp., only 10 *E. gallinarum* and 5 *E. casseliflavus* isolates showed either intermediate or full resistance to vancomycin with MIC values in the range 8–64 μg/mL, whereas the rest were susceptible (vancomycin-susceptible enterococci, VSE). The results are summarized in Table 1.

Table 1. Results of minimal inhibitory concentration by broth microdilution and in-house VREfm screening broth to susceptibility of vancomycin on 105 enterococci in this study.

Enterococci	Total	*van* Gene	MIC Value (µg/mL)	N	MIC Interpretation	In-House VREfm Screening Broth						Sensitivity	Specificity
						Tube A (No Vancomycin)			Tube B (Containing Vancomycin)				
						Turbidity	Color	N	Turbidity	Color	N		
E. faecium (n = 71)	48	vanA	128	41	Resistance	+	Red	41	+	Red	41	100%	80%
			64	7		+	Red	7	+	Red	7		
	13	vanB	64	9		+	Red	9	+	Red	9		
			32	4		+	Red	4	+	Red	4		
	10	none	4	5	Susceptible	+	Red	5	+	Red	2		
			2	3		+	Red	3	-				
			1	2		+	Red	2	-				
E. faecalis (n = 14)	3	vanA	128	1	Resistance	+	Colorless	1	+	Colorless	1	100%	66.6%
	2	vanB	64	2		+	Colorless	2	+	Colorless	2		
			32	2		+	Colorless	2	+	Colorless	2		
	9	none	4	4	Susceptible	+	Colorless	4	+	Colorless	3		
			2	2		+	Colorless	2	-				
			1	1		+	Colorless	1	-				
			0.5	2		+	Colorless	2	-				
E. gallinarum (n = 10)	10	vanC1	64	1	Resistance	+	Colorless	1	+	Colorless	1	90%	ND*
			32	3	Resistance	+	Colorless	3	+	Colorless	3		
			16	2	Intermediate	+	Colorless	2	+	Colorless	2		
			8	4	Intermediate	+	Colorless	4	+	Colorless	3		
E. casseliflavus (n = 5)	5	vanC2/C3	32	1	Resistance	+	Colorless	1	+	Colorless	1	80%	ND*
			16	1	Intermediate	+	Colorless	1	+	Colorless	1		
			8	3	Intermediate	+	Colorless	3	+	Colorless	2		
E. muntidii (n = 4)	4	none	0.5	3	Susceptible	+	Colorless	3	-			ND*	100%
			0	1		+	Colorless	1	-				
E. raffinosus (n = 1)	1	none	0.25	1	Susceptible	+	Colorless	1	-			ND*	100%
Total	**105**			**105**				**105**			**84**		

* ND = No data because denominator is zero.

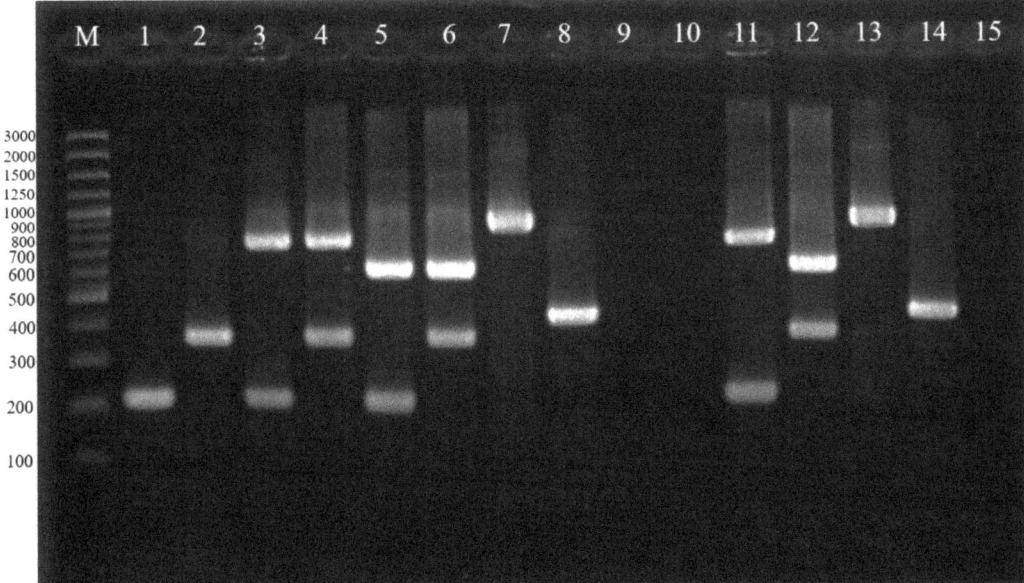

Figure 1. Agarose gel electrophoresis of PCR-amplified products from local enterococci (lane 1–10) and reference enterococci (lane 11–14). *E. faecium* (lane 1), *E. faecalis* (lane 2), *E. faecium* carrying *vanA* (lane 3), *E. faecalis* carrying *vanA* (lane 4), *E. faecium* carrying *vanB* (lane 5), *E. faecalis* carrying *vanB* (lane 6), *E. gallinarum* carrying *vanC1* (lane 7), *E. casseliflavus* carrying *vanC2/C3* (lane 8), *E. muntdii* (lane 9), *E. raffinosus* (lane 10), *E. faecium* ATCC BAA-2316 carrying *vanA* (lane 11), *E. faecalis* ATCC51299 carrying *vanB* (lane 12), *E. gallinarum* ATCC49608 carrying *vanC1* (lane 13), *E. casseliflavus* ATCC700668 carrying *vanC2/C3* (lane 14), and blank control (lane 15). A 100-bp DNA ladder is shown in lane M.

2.2. Evaluation of In-House VREfm Screening Broth

The in-house VREfm screening broth determined resistance to vancomycin based on turbidity and distinguished *E. faecium* from other enterococci based on color changes. The broth was used in two tubes (A and B). Tube A did not contain vancomycin, whereas tube B did (6 μg/mL vancomycin). Basically, all enterococci, including those that were vancomycin not-susceptible or susceptible, could grow in tube A, while growth in tube B depended on their resistance to the antibiotic. *E. faecium* could produce β-galactosidase, the enzyme degraded to Salmon-Gal that produced a red product, whereas the other *Enterococcus* spp. did not (Figure 2).

We verified this screening broth using broth microdilution as a reference method on 105 enterococci. These included 61 VREfm, 5 VREfs, 4 vancomycin-resistant *E. gallinarum* (VREg), and one vancomycin-resistant *E. casseliflavus* (VREc), while the other 34 isolates consisted of vancomycin-intermediate isolates (6 *E. gallinarum*, VIEg; and 4 *E. casseliflavus*, VIEc) and vancomycin-susceptible *E. faecalis* (VSEfs; $n = 9$), *E. faecium* (VSEfm; $n = 10$), *E. mundtii* (VSEm; $n = 4$), and *E. raffinosus* (VSEr; $n = 1$). As shown in Table 1, all VREfm showed turbidity and the presence of red color in both tubes. The other VREs (VREfs, VREg, VREc) showed turbidity but with no color in either tube.

We found 5 VSEs (2 were VSEfm and 3 were VSEfs) that produced a positive result in tube B (containing vancomycin), indicating that they were vancomycin-resistant based on the screening broth. Indeed, they were susceptible to vancomycin based on broth microdilution with an MIC value of 4 μg/mL for all isolates (Table 1). In contrast, one isolate each of VIEg and VIEc showed neither turbidity nor color in tube B, although they showed intermediate resistance to vancomycin with an MIC value of 8 μg/mL (Table 1).

This suggested that our test had variation with the borderline MIC cut-off for some intermediate isolates, especially for VIEg or VIEc that carried *vanC*. However, there was good correlation of our screening broth and broth microdilution to indicate vancomycin resistance at MIC ≥16 µg/mL.

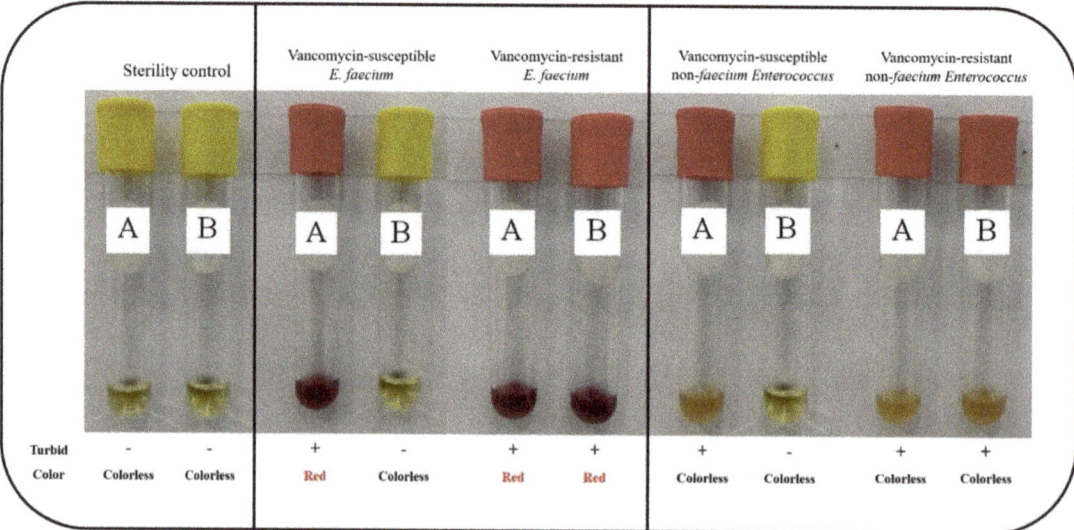

Figure 2. Interpretation of in-house VREfm screening broth for vancomycin-resistant enterococci (VRE) and vancomycin-susceptible enterococci (VSE).

The screening broth could identify *E. faecium* by producing the red color in all 71 isolates, while all the other species of *Enterococcus* (*n* = 34) were colorless. This demonstrated that the accuracy of this broth-based method was 100% for identification of *E. faecium* according to multiplex PCR assay. However, determination of vancomycin resistance and presence of *van* genes revealed 93.3% accuracy, 97.5% sensitivity, and 79.2% specificity (Tables 2 and 3). The kappa statistic to test interrater reliability showed 0.8 for this screening test. Based on the kappa criterion, our in-house VREfm screening broth had substantial agreement (values in the range 0.61–0.80) to the broth microdilution and PCR detecting *van* genes as the reference method. In addition, our in-house VREfm screening broth showed rapid positivity after at least 8 h of incubation, and the cost per test (2 tubes) was USD 0.9 or EUR 0.8.

Table 2. Validity of in-house VREfm screening broth to determine vancomycin resistance compared with broth microdilution.

In-House Screening Broth	Broth Microdilution		Validity
	Positive (Vancomycin Not-Susceptible) *	Negative (Vancomycin Susceptible)	
Positive (vancomycin resistance)	79	5	Accuracy = 93.3%
Negative (vancomycin susceptible)	2	19	
Validity	Sensitivity = 97.5%	Specificity = 79.2%	

* Vancomycin not-susceptible = intermediate or fully resistant to vancomycin.

Table 3. Validity of in-house VREfm screening broth to determine vancomycin resistance compared with PCR detecting *van* genes.

In-House Screening Broth	PCR		Validity
	vanA, vanB, vanC1/C2/C3	None	
Positive (vancomycin resistance)	79	5	Accuracy = 93.3%
Negative (vancomycin susceptible)	2	19	
Validity	Sensitivity = 97.5%	Specificity = 79.2%	

3. Discussion

VREfm has a global impact as a threat to public health according to the WHO, and it contributes significantly to morbidity, mortality, and the socio-economic costs of healthcare-acquired infection [2,12]. For example, the daily costs of contact isolation (considering only gloves and gowns) for each VREfm patient in a ward and an intensive care unit (ICU) were USD 10.8 and USD 17.3, respectively [13]. With the mean duration of isolation of 25 and 41.5 days for the ward and the ICU, respectively, a total cost was estimated to be USD 270 and USD 718, respectively [13]. Another study revealed that the overall hospital costs of blood-stream infection were significantly higher in VREfm cases (EUR 80,465) compared to VSEfm (EUR 51,365) and VSEfs (EUR 31,122) cases [14]. Screening is recommended for patients at high risk of VRE colonization to prevent and control the transmission of VRE. Our study successfully developed an in-house VREfm screening test to distinguish VREfm from other VRE and VSE isolates.

Validity testing based on the kappa coefficient demonstrated that our screening broth had strong agreement in the determination of VRE (especially VREfm) but false-positive or false-negative results may occur in either VIEg/VIEc or VSE isolates with low MIC values of about 8 or 4 µg/mL, respectively. For the false-positives in 5 VSE with MIC at 4 µg/mL, the actual MIC may be 6 or 7 µg/mL because the broth microdilution technique applied two-fold dilution of vancomycin that started from 0.25 µg/mL and produced 0.5, 1, 2, 4, 8, 16, 32, 64, and 128 µg/mL. The gap between 4 and 8 µg/mL may have contained the exact MIC for these 5 false-positive VSE isolates according to our screening broth, which contained 6 µg/mL of vancomycin, and so allowed these 5 isolates to grow. However, the false-negatives involving VIEg and VIEc had MIC values of 8 µg/mL (Table 2) and were PCR-positive for *vanC* (Table 3) but did not grow in tube B of the screening broth, even though we repeated both the broth microdilution and screening tests. The explanation for this has not been elucidated but it may depend on the strain characteristics or the low concentration of inoculum used that retarded bacterial growth under marginal conditions.

Another study evaluated chromogenic agar to screen VRE based on the different colors of colonies for either VREfm or VREfs [15]. A false-positive was detected in the medium with non-enterococci, such as *Staphylococcus sciuri*, *Streptococcus mutans*, or other enterococci (*E. casseliflavus* and *E. raffinosus*) [15]. Cross-reactivity of our screening broth may have occurred with *S. sciuri*, as mentioned in another study [15]. Performing catalase and Gram-stain testing of presumptive VRE isolates should increase the specificity. Notably, our screening broth identified *E. faecium* based on degradation of 6-chloro-3-indoxyl-β-D-galactopyranoside by its β-galactosidase. This enzyme is also present in some species of enteroccoci, such as *E. malodoratus*, *E. saccharolyticus*, *E. villorum*, and *E. dispar*; however, these species have very low prevalence in hospitals, and their resistance to vancomycin is very rare [16,17]. To increase the efficiency and rapidity of VREfm screening among patients, the screening broth should be further studied and validated on clinical specimens directly. In addition, our screening broth has some limitations, including that it does not diagnose other pathogenic enterococci, such as *E. faecalis*, and does not specify the MIC. Furthermore, the broth could not be detected where there were strains resistant to teicoplanin only. Therefore, further development of this screening broth should be carried out to identify *E. faecalis*, *E. gallinarum*, or *E. casseliflavus*, to specify the MIC values, and to determine whether it is possible to detect teicoplanin-resistant strains.

Resistance to vancomycin in *enterococci* is mediated by the *van* genes, with *vanA*, *vanB*, *vanC*, *vanD*, *vanE*, *vanG*, *vanL*, *vanM*, and *vanN* having been identified to date; in particular, *vanA* and *vanB* are predominant worldwide [18]. In the current study, all clinical VREfm and VREfs carried either *vanA* or *vanB*, which conferred high resistance to vancomycin with an MIC range of 32–128 µg/mL. Most of them carried *vanA* (77.3%). Accordingly, the specific character of *vanA*-carrying enterococci showed high resistance to vancomycin (MIC $\geq$ 64 µg/mL) and teicoplanin (MIC $\geq$8 µg/mL) [19]. The high prevalence of *vanA*-harboring *E. faecium* or *E. faecalis* observed in the current study was similar to reports for China, Japan, Iran, the Netherlands, Germany, Italy, Australia, Tunisia, Brazil, and Canada [18,20–28].

The annual estimated laboratory costs were projected to be USD 19,074 for 6372 patients screened in a pediatric hospital between 2010 and 2014 in Turkey [13]. Therefore, screening priorities should be based on the prevalence of infection and the financial resources of the institution. The previous study revealed laboratory cost per specimen for rectal swab culture and PCR was USD 2.7 and USD 40.5, respectively [13]. The cost per test (2 tubes) for our assay was USD 0.9 or EUR 0.8, whereas the cost of the gold standard is about USD 2.7–3.0 or EUR 2.4–2.6. Application of this assay for VRE screening from pure culture should be useful for clinical laboratories and hospital infection control units where there is high prevalence of VRE to provide prompt information to facilitate the rapid control of VRE dissemination in hospitals and more rapid implementation of isolation precautions regarding VRE carriage or infection to other patients, as well as reducing the cost.

4. Materials and Methods

4.1. Bacterial Strains

In total, 105 enterococci, consisting of 71 *E. faecium*, 14 *E. faecalis*, and 20 other *Enterococcus* spp., were used in this study. These enterococci were isolated and sent by hospitals for further confirmation by the Public Health Microbiological Laboratory Service of the Faculty of Public Health, Kasetsart University Chalermphrakiat Sakon Nakhon province campus under the Emerging Antimicrobial Resistant Bacteria Surveillance Program (EARB). *E. faecium* ATCC BAA-2316 (*vanA*), *E. faecalis* ATCC51299 (*vanB*), *E. gallinarum* ATCC49608 (*vanC1*), and *E. casseliflavus* ATCC700668 (*vanC2/C3*) were used as controls in the multiplex PCR assay. *E. faecalis* ATCC29212 and *E. faecium* ATCC BAA-2316 were used as the control for the broth microdilution. In addition, *E. faecium* ATCC BAA-2316, *E. faecium* ATCC19434 and *E. faecalis* ATCC29212 were used for controls for the in-house VREfm screening broth.

4.2. Microbiological Analysis

Each isolate was cultured on sheep blood agar at 37 °C for 18 h and identified using a conventional biochemical test, including arabinose utilization, resistance to 6.5% NaCl, bile esculin degradation, and PYR (pyrrolidonyl β-naphthylamide) degradation [16], and multiplex PCR assay to simultaneously identify *E. faecium* and *E. faecalis*, as well as the vancomycin-resistant genes; *vanA*, *vanB*, *vanC1*, and *vanC2/C3*, that were developed in our laboratory [29,30]. Genomic DNA from all isolates was extracted using a NucleoSpin® Tissue Kit (Macherey-Nagel, Germany) according to the manufacturer's instructions. The PCR reaction mixtures contained 1X JumpStart™ REDTaq® ReadyMix™ Reaction Mix (Sigma-Aldrich, MO, USA) and 0.4 µM of each primer pair (IDT, Singapore; Table 4). The following PCR thermocycling parameters were used: initial activation of DNA polymerase at 95 °C for 3 min; 30 cycles of denaturation at 95 °C for 30 s, primer annealing at 55 °C for 30 s, and extension at 72 °C for 1.15 min; with a final extension at 72 °C for 5 min. The PCR products were resolved using gel electrophesis for 30 min on 2% agarose gels (Vivantis, Selangor, Malaysia) in 0.5× TBE buffer (Vivantis, Malaysia). The gels were stained with ethidium bromide (Sigma-Aldrich, MO, USA) and visualized under ultraviolet light using a

GeneGenius Bioimaging System (SynGene, Maryland, USA). The sizes of the PCR products were determined by comparison with a molecular size standard (GeneRuler™ 100 bp Plus DNA ladder, Thermo Fisher Scientific, Waltham, MA, USA) as shown in Figure 1.

Table 4. Primers used in multiplex PCR in current study.

Primer Name	Sequence (5′-3′)	Target	PCR Product Size (bp)	Reference
E. faecium-FL1	GAAAAAACAATAGAAGAATTAT	*sodA*	215	[29]
E. faecium-FL2	TGCTTTTTTGAATTCTTCTTTA			
E. faecalis-FM1	ACTTATGTGACTAACTTAACC	*sodA*	360	
E. faecalis-FM2	TAATGGTGAATCTTGGTTTGG			
vanA-A1	GGGAAAACGACAATTGC	*vanA*	732	[30]
vanA-A2	GTACAATGCGGCCGTTA			
vanB-B1	ATGGGAAGCCGATAGTC	*vanB*	635	
vanB-B2	GATTTCGTTCCTCGACC			
vanC1-C1	GGTATCAAGGAAACCTC	*vanC1*	822	
vanC1-C2	CTTCCGCCATCATAGCT			
vanC2/3-D1	CTCCTACGATTCTCTTG	*vanC2/C3*	438	
vanC2/3-D2	CGAGCAAGACCTTTAAG			

Susceptibility to vancomycin was performed to determine minimal inhibitory concentration (MIC) using broth microdilution according to the current CLSI guidelines [31]. A 0.5 McFarland standard suspension of the isolate was made from culture grown on Muller Hinton agar plates (BD BBL, Bergen County, NJ, USA). The interpretation of MIC followed the criteria in the CLSI 2021 guidelines, namely $\leq$4 mg/mL is susceptible, 8–16 mg/mL is intermediate, and $\geq$32 mg/mL indicates resistance [31]. Standard enterococci strains of *E. faecalis* ATCC 29212 (*van* absence) and *E. faecium* ATCC BAA-2316 (*vanA* presence) were used for quality control for the broth microdilution.

4.3. In-House VREfm Screening Broth

This screening broth was prepared using 2 tubes (A and B). Tube A (1 mL) contained 1.85% Brain Heart Infusion broth (Merck, Kenilworth, NJ, USA) and 0.2% 6-chloro-3-indoxyl-β-D-galactopyranoside (Salmon-Gal; GoldBio, St. Louis, MO, USA). This concentration of Salmon-Gal was selected experimentally based on our optimization (data not shown). Tube B (1 mL) consisted of the same ingredients as tube A and also contained vancomycin (Sigma-Aldrich, St. Louis, MO, USA) at 6 µg/mL according to the 2021 CLSI guideline recommendation for VRE screening. Interpretation is shown in Figure 2. A 0.1-mL amount of inoculum at a concentration of 0.5 McFarland was inoculated into the broth.

4.4. Statistical Analysis

Diagnostic measures were calculated, such as sensitivity, specificity, and accuracy of each test. The kappa statistic was calculated to evaluate the associations and levels of agreement of the data [32].

5. Conclusions

We successfully developed an in-house VREfm screening broth to distinguish *E. faecium* from other *Enterococcus* spp., and to determine resistance to vancomycin in a single assay. This alternative screening procedure for VREfm could be useful for hospital infection control.

Author Contributions: Conceptualization, A.K.; methodology, N.S., P.B., R.H.; validation, A.K., P.C., and N.S.; formal analysis, N.S.; investigation, N.S.; resources, A.K.; data curation, A.K., N.S.; writing—original draft preparation, A.K., P.C., N.S., R.H.; writing—review and editing, A.K., P.B.; supervision, A.K.; funding acquisition, A.K., N.S. All authors have read and agreed to the published version of the manuscript.

Funding: This research was funded by a research grant from Research and Researchers for Industries (RRI), National Research Council of Thailand (NRCT) and U & V Holding (Thailand) Co., Ltd. with grant number: NRCT5-RRI63002.

Institutional Review Board Statement: Not applicable.

Informed Consent Statement: Not applicable.

Data Availability Statement: No new data were created or analyzed in this study. Data sharing is not applicable to this article.

Conflicts of Interest: The authors declare no conflict of interest.

References

1. O'Driscoll, T.; Crank, C.W. Vancomycin-resistant enterococcal infections: Epidemiology, clinical manifestations, and optimal management. *Infect. Drug Resist.* **2015**, *8*, 217–230. [PubMed]
2. Tacconelli, E.; Carrara, E.; Savoldi, A.; Harbarth, S.; Mendelson, M.; Monnet, D.L.; Pulcini, C.; Kahlmeter, G.; Kluytmans, J.; Carmeli, Y.; et al. WHO Pathogens Priority List Working Group. Discovery, research, and development of new antibiotics: The WHO priority list of antibiotic-resistant bacteria and tuberculosis. *Lancet Infect. Dis.* **2018**, *18*, 318–327. [CrossRef]
3. Rios, R.; Reyes, J.; Carvajal, L.P.; Rincon, S.; Panesso, D.; Echeverri, A.M.; Dinh, A.; Kolokotronis, S.O.; Narechania, A.; Tran, T.T.; et al. Genomic epidemiology of vancomycin-resistant Enterococcus faecium (VREfm) in Latin America: Revisiting the global VRE population structure. *Sci. Rep.* **2020**, *10*, 5636. [CrossRef]
4. Paladino, J.A.; Sunderlin, J.L.; Adelman, M.H.; Singer, M.E.; Schentag, J.J. Observations on vancomycin use in U.S. hospitals. *Am. J. Health Syst. Pharm.* **2007**, *64*, 1633–1641. [CrossRef]
5. Kühn, I.; Iversen, A.; Finn, M.; Greko, C.; Burman, L.G.; Blanch, A.R.; Vilanova, X.; Manero, A.; Taylor, H.; Caplin, J.; et al. Occurrence and relatedness of vancomycin-resistant enterococci in animals, humans, and the environment in different European regions. *Appl. Environ. Microbiol.* **2005**, *71*, 5383–5890. [CrossRef]
6. Shrestha, S.; Kharel, S.; Homagain, S.; Aryal, R.; Mishra, S.K. Prevalence of vancomycin-resistant enterococci in Asia-A systematic review and meta-analysis. *J. Clin. Pharm.* **2021**, *46*, 1226–1237. [CrossRef] [PubMed]
7. Linden, P.K. Treatment options for vancomycin-resistant enterococcal infections. *Drugs* **2002**, *62*, 425–441. [CrossRef] [PubMed]
8. Raza, T.; Ullah, S.R.; Mehmood, K.; Andleeb, S. Vancomycin resistant Enterococci: A brief review. *J. Pak. Med. Assoc.* **2018**, *68*, 768–772.
9. Bassetti, M.; Poulakou, G.; Ruppe, E.; Bouza, E.; Van Hal, S.J.; Brink, A. Antimicrobial resistance in the next 30 years, humankind, bugs and drugs: A visionary approach. *Intensive Care Med.* **2017**, *43*, 1464–1475. [CrossRef]
10. Metan, G.; Zarakolu, P.; Unal, S. Rapid detection of antibacterial resistance in emerging Gram-positive cocci. *J. Hosp. Infect.* **2005**, *61*, 93–99. [CrossRef]
11. Endtz, H.P.; Van Den Braak, N.; Van Belkum, A.; Goessens, W.H.; Kref, D.; Stroebel, A.B.; Verbrugh, H.A. Comparison of eight methods to detect vancomycin resistance in enterococci. *J. Clin. Microbiol.* **1998**, *36*, 592–594. [CrossRef] [PubMed]
12. Gorrie, C.; Higgs, C.; Carter, G.; Stinear, T.P.; Howden, B. Genomics of vancomycin-resistant Enterococcus faecium. *Microb. Genom.* **2019**, *5*, e000283. [CrossRef] [PubMed]
13. Ulu-Kilic, A.; Özhan, E.; Altun, D.; Perçin, D.; Güneş, T.; Alp, E. Is it worth screening for vancomycin-resistant Enterococcus faecium colonization? Financial burden of screening in a developing country. *Am. J. Infect. Control.* **2016**, *44*, e45–e49. [CrossRef] [PubMed]
14. Kramer, T.S.; Remschmidt, C.; Werner, S.; Behnke, M.; Schwab, F.; Werner, G.; Gastmeier, P.; Leistner, R. The importance of adjusting for enterococcus species when assessing the burden of vancomycin resistance: A cohort study including over 1000 cases of enterococcal bloodstream infections. *Antimicrob. Resist. Infect. Control* **2018**, *7*, 133. [CrossRef]
15. Kallstrom, G.; Doern, C.D.; Dunne, W.M., Jr. Evaluation of a chromogenic agar under development to screen for VRE colonization. *J. Clin. Microbiol.* **2010**, *48*, 999–1001. [CrossRef]
16. Teixeira, L.M.; Carvalho, M.G.S.; Shewmaker, P.L.; Facklam, R.R. Enterococcus. In *Manual of Clinical Microbiology*, 10th ed.; Versalovic, J., Carroll, K.C., Funke, G., Jorgensen, J.H., Landry, M.L., Warnock, D.W., Eds.; ASM Press: Washington, DC, USA, 2011; pp. 350–364.
17. Adhikari, L. High-level aminoglycoside resistance and reduced susceptibility to vancomycin in nosocomial enterococci. *J. Glob. Infect. Dis.* **2010**, *2*, 231–235. [CrossRef]

18. Zhou, W.; Zhou, H.; Sun, Y.; Gao, S.; Zhang, Y.; Cao, X.; Zhang, Z.; Shen, H.; Zhang, C. Characterization of clinical enterococci isolates, focusing on the vancomycin-resistant enterococci in a tertiary hospital in China: Based on the data from 2013 to 2018. *BMC Infect. Dis.* **2020**, *20*, 356. [CrossRef]
19. Gold, H.S. Vancomycin-resistant enterococci: Mechanisms and clinical observations. *Clin. Infect. Dis.* **2001**, *33*, 210–219. [CrossRef]
20. Arredondo-Alonso, S.; Top, J.; Corander, J.; Willems, R.J.L.; Schürch, A.C. Mode and dynamics of vanA-type vancomycin resistance dissemination in Dutch hospitals. *Genome Med.* **2021**, *13*, 9. [CrossRef]
21. Hughes, A.; Ballard, S.; Sullivan, S.; Marshall, C. An outbreak of vanA vancomycin-resistant Enterococcus faecium in a hospital with endemic vanB VRE. *Infect. Dis. Health* **2019**, *24*, 82–91. [CrossRef]
22. Correa-Martinez, C.L.; Tönnies, H.; Froböse, N.J.; Mellmann, A.; Kampmeier, S. Transmission of vancomycin-resistant enterococci in the hospital setting: Uncovering the patient-environment interplay. *Microorganisms* **2020**, *8*, 203. [CrossRef] [PubMed]
23. Armin, S.; Zahedani, S.S.; Rahbar, M.; Azimi, L. Prevalence and resistance profiles of vancomycin-resistant enterococcal isolates in Iran; An Eight-month Report from Nine Major Cities. *Infect. Disord. Drug Targets* **2020**, *20*, 828–833. [CrossRef] [PubMed]
24. Dziri, R.; El Kara, F.; Barguellil, F.; Ouzari, H.I.; El Asli, M.S.; Klibi, N. Vancomycin-resistant Enterococcus faecium in Tunisia: Emergence of novel clones. *Microb. Drug Resist.* **2019**, *25*, 469–474. [CrossRef] [PubMed]
25. Fioriti, S.; Simoni, S.; Caucci, S.; Morroni, G.; Ponzio, E.; Coccitto, S.N.; Brescini, L.; Cirioni, O.; Menzo, S.; Biavasco, F.; et al. Trend of clinical vancomycin-resistant enterococci isolated in a regional Italian hospital from 2001 to 2018. *Braz. J. Microbiol.* **2020**, *51*, 1607–1613. [CrossRef]
26. Fujiya, Y.; Harada, T.; Sugawara, Y.; Akeda, Y.; Yasuda, M.; Masumi, A.; Hayashi, J.; Tanimura, N.; Tsujimoto, Y.; Shibata, W.; et al. Transmission dynamics of a linear vanA-plasmid during a nosocomial multiclonal outbreak of vancomycin-resistant enterococci in a non-endemic area, Japan. *Sci. Rep.* **2021**, *11*, 14780. [CrossRef]
27. Resende, M.; Caierão, J.; Prates, J.G.; Narvaez, G.A.; Dias, C.A.; d'Azevedo, P.A. Emergence of vanA vancomycin-resistant Enterococcus faecium in a hospital in Porto Alegre, South Brazil. *J. Infect. Dev. Ctries* **2014**, *8*, 160–167. [CrossRef]
28. Simner, P.J.; Adam, H.; Baxter, M.; McCracken, M.; Golding, G.; Karlowsky, J.A.; Nichol, K.; Lagacé-Wiens, P.; Gilmour, M.W.; Canadian Antimicrobial Resistance Alliance (CARA); et al. Epidemiology of vancomycin-resistant enterococci in Canadian hospitals (CANWARD study, 2007 to 2013). *Antimicrob. Agents Chemother.* **2015**, *59*, 4315–4317. [CrossRef]
29. Jackson, C.R.; Fedorka-Cray, P.J.; Barrett, J.B. Use of a genus- and species-specific multiplex PCR for identification of enterococci. *J. Clin. Microbiol.* **2004**, *42*, 3558–3565. [CrossRef]
30. Pérez-Hernández, X.; Méndez-Alvarez, S.; Claverie-Martín, F. A PCR assay for rapid detection of vancomycin-resistant enterococci. *Diagn. Microbiol. Infect. Dis.* **2002**, *42*, 273–277. [CrossRef]
31. Clinical and Laboratory Standards Institute. *Performance Standards for Antimicrobial Susceptibility Testing*, 31st ed.; CLSI Document M100; Clinical and Laboratory Standards Institute: Wayne, PA, USA, 2021.
32. McHugh, M.L. Interrater reliability: The kappa statistic. *Biochem. Med.* **2012**, *22*, 276–282. [CrossRef]

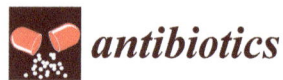

antibiotics

Article

Multiplex PCR Detection of Common Carbapenemase Genes and Identification of Clinically Relevant *Escherichia coli* and *Klebsiella pneumoniae* Complex

Rujirat Hatrongjit [1,*], Peechanika Chopjitt [2], Parichart Boueroy [2] and Anusak Kerdsin [2]

[1] Faculty of Science and Engineering, Kasetsart University Chalermphrakiat Sakon Nakhon Province Campus, Sakon Nakhon 47000, Thailand
[2] Faculty of Public Health, Kasetsart University Chalermphrakiat Sakon Nakhon Province Campus, Sakon Nakhon 47000, Thailand
* Correspondence: rujirat.ha@ku.th

Abstract: Carbapenem-resistant *Enterobacterales* (CRE) species are top priority pathogens according to the World Health Organization. Rapid detection is necessary and useful for their surveillance and control globally. This study developed a multiplex polymerase chain reaction (mPCR) detection of the common carbapenemase genes NDM, KPC, and OXA-48-like, together with identification of *Escherichia coli*, and distinguished a *Klebsiella pneumoniae* complex to be *K. pneumoniae*, *K. quasipneumoniae*, and *K. variicola*. Of 840 target *Enterobacterales* species, 190 *E. coli*, 598 *K. pneumoniae*, 28 *K. quasipneumoniae*, and 23 *K. variicola*. with and without NDM, KPC, or OXA-48-like were correctly detected for their species and carbapenemase genes. In contrast, for the *Enterobacterales* species other than *E. coli* or *K. pneumoniae* complex with carbapenemase genes, the mPCR assay could detect only NDM, KPC, or OXA-48-like. This PCR method should be useful in clinical microbiology laboratories requiring rapid detection of CRE for epidemiological investigation and for tracking the trends of carbapenemase gene dynamics.

Keywords: PCR; carbapenemase; NDM; KPC; OXA-48-like; *Escherichia coli*; *Klebsiella pneumoniae* complex

Citation: Hatrongjit, R.; Chopjitt, P.; Boueroy, P.; Kerdsin, A. Multiplex PCR Detection of Common Carbapenemase Genes and Identification of Clinically Relevant *Escherichia coli* and *Klebsiella pneumoniae* Complex. *Antibiotics* **2023**, *12*, 76. https://doi.org/10.3390/antibiotics12010076

Academic Editor: Nicholas Dixon

Received: 29 November 2022
Revised: 15 December 2022
Accepted: 30 December 2022
Published: 31 December 2022

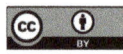
1. Introduction

The current emergence of carbapenem-resistant *Enterobacterales* (CRE) is an especially concerning antimicrobial resistant (AMR) threat that can result in an important clinical problem associated with resistance to many last-resort antibiotics, making it difficult to treat and leading to high mortality rates and expensive hospital stays [1]. The World Health Organization (WHO) considers the growing AMR issue one of the three major public health challenges of the 21st century, responsible for healthcare costs, long hospitalizations, treatment failures, and death [2]. In addition, the WHO has listed CRE as critical priority pathogens, necessitating the development of new antibiotics against such organisms [3]. The *Enterobacterales*, especially *Escherichia coli*, *Klebsiella pneumoniae*, and *Enterobacter cloacae*, are major causes of hospital-acquired infections that have spread around the globe [1,4].

CRE develops antibiotic resistance through several mechanisms, including through the main mechanism of production of carbapenemases which are enzymes that degrade carbapenem antibiotics [4,5]. They can be divided into CRE with and CRE without carbapenemase production [1,4,5]. Carbapenemase-producing CRE (CP-CRE) are more associated with higher levels of antimicrobial resistance, worse outcomes, and rapid spread via plasmid transmission among bacterial strains, while non-carbapenemase-producing CRE (non-CP-CRE) have been associated with asymptomatic carriage and perhaps less person-to-person transmission [1,6]. Among the carbapenemase types, NDM, OXA-48-like, IMP, VIM, and KPC have been commonly found in different parts of the world [2,4,5]. KPC is the most common carbapenemase in the United States, China, Italy, Greece, and the

UK, whereas NDM has now spread worldwide [4,5,7]. VIM and IMP are most prevalent in Southern Europe and Asia, while OXA-48-like is most prevalent in the Mediterranean region, Europe, and Asia, including India, China, Vietnam, and Thailand [4–7]. Of these carbapenemase types, NDM, KPC, and OXA-48-like have been very frequently detected worldwide [4,5,7]. Furthermore, the major *Enterobacterales* carriers of these carbapenemases are *E. coli* and *K. pneumoniae* [4–6].

Surveillance is a crucial element of national prevention and control strategies to control dissemination of CP-CRE. Several countries have systems to monitor acquired carbapenem resistance [8]. For example, diagnostic laboratories in England have a duty to report carbapenemase-producing Gram-negative bacteria isolated from human samples to Public Health England [8]. Therefore, rapid detection and reporting of CP-CRE is one of the top priorities of clinical microbiology laboratories. Recently, there have been increasing numbers of tests available for carbapenemase detection, including colorimetric tests, immunochromatographic assays, matrix-assisted laser desorption ionization-time of flight MS-based tests, phenotypic and molecular methods [9,10]. However, the Clinical and Laboratory Standards Institute (CLSI) recommends the modified carbapenem inactivation method (mCIM), Carba NP, and molecular assay, such as PCR, to determine CP-CRE [11].

PCR is a technique with high accuracy and a rapid turnaround time that is currently inexpensive. Several studies have developed a multiplex PCR (mPCR) to detect the relevant carbapenemase genes [12–16]. However, there is no current PCR approach that detects both carbapenemase genes and *Enterobacterales* species in the same reaction. Herein, we developed an mPCR assay to detect the most prevalent carbapenemase genes, including KPC, NDM, and OXA-48-like, and identify *E. coli*, *K. pneumoniae*, *K. quasipneumoniae*, and *K. variicola* in the same reaction. This mPCR technique could be applied usefully in clinical diagnostic laboratories to determine both common CRE species and the relevant carbapenemase genes at the same time, as well as reducing the turnaround time and saving on costs.

2. Results and Discussion

In the current study, an mPCR assay was designed to detect common carbapenemase genes and, frequently, the *Enterobacterales* species carrying those genes. *E. coli* and *K. pneumoniae* complex (*K. pneumoniae*, *K. quasipneumoniae*, *K. variicola*), NDM, OXA-48-like, and KPC, which are common carbapenemase genes disseminated globally, were the target for this mPCR assay. According to several studies, *K. pneumoniae*- and *E. coli*-carrying NDM, KPC, and OXA-48-like, were prevalent in the Netherlands, Spain, the USA, Thailand, China, Korea, Tunisia, Iran, Nepal, and India [6,17–27]. This assay could be applied in these countries, especially in Asia, where there are high prevalence levels of these bacteria carrying the aforementioned carbapenemase genes.

We demonstrated the potential utility of the mPCR assay to detect either *E. coli* or *K. pneumoniae* complex with and without carbapenemase genes. The mPCR assay identified the *E. coli* and *K. pneumoniae* complex together with detected NDM, OXA-48-like, and KPC in the same reaction (Figure 1 and Table 1). Our mPCR assay could distinguish the *K. pneumoniae* complex into *K. pneumoniae*, *K. quasipneumoniae*, and *K. variicola* (Figure 1). In the case of *E. coli*, *K. pneumoniae*, *K. quasipneumoniae*, and *K. variicola* without carbapenemase genes, the mPCR assay could identify the species correctly with no carbapenemase genes NDM, OXA-48-like, or KPC (Table 1). In addition, the mPCR assay detected NDM, KPC, or OXA-48-like in *C. fruendii*, *C. werkmanii*, *E. cloacae*, and *E. asburiae*, without bands of *E. coli* or the *K. pneumoniae* complex (Table 1). A limitation of this mPCR assay is that it could not identify *C. freundii*, *E. cloacae*, *E. asburiae*, and *Enterobacterales* species other than the 4 mPCR target organisms. The expansion of this mPCR to detect other *Enterobacterales* species should be the subject of future investigations. In addition, no cross reactivity was observed in other bacteria except the target bacteria and carbapenemase genes.

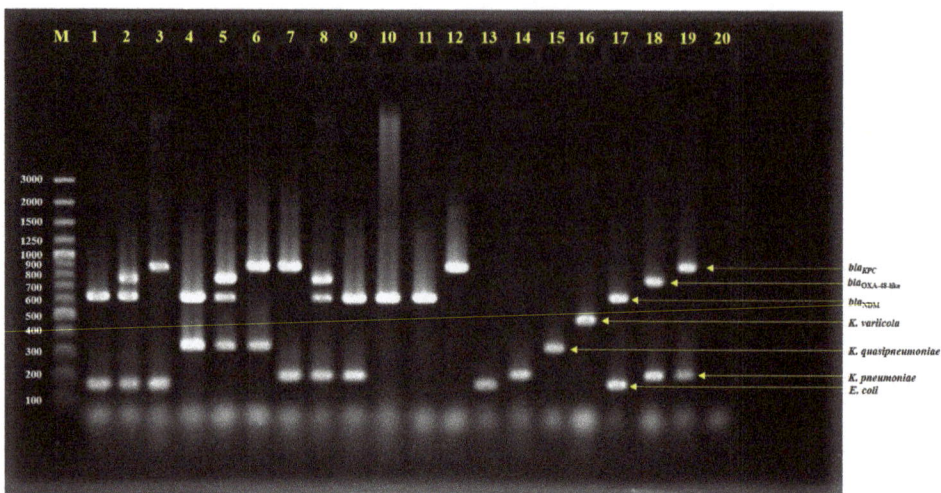

Figure 1. Agarose gel electrophoresis of multiplex PCR-amplified products; lane 1 = Isolate No. C76 (*E. coli* with NDM), lane 2 = Isolate No. C163 (*E. coli* with NDM and OXA-48-like), lane 3 = Isolate No. C1992 (*E. coli* with KPC), lane 4 = Isolate No. C34 (*K. quasipneumoniae* with NDM), lane 5 = Isolate No. C110 (*K. quasipneumoniae* with NDM and OXA-48-like), lane 6 = Isolate No. AMR353 (*K. quasipneumoniae* with KPC), lane 7 = Isolate No. C1985 (*K. pneumoniae* with KPC), lane 8 = Isolate No. C73 (*K. pneumoniae* with NDM and OXA-48-like), lane 9 = Isolate No. C75 (*K. pneumoniae* with NDM), lane 10 = Isolate No. C19 (*E. cloacae* with NDM), lane 11 = Isolate No. C487 (*C. freundii* with NDM), lane 12 = Isolate No. C2135 (*E. asburiae* with KPC), lane 13 = *E. coli* ATCC25922, lane 14 = *K. pneumoniae* ATCC27335, lane 15 = *K. quasipneumoniae* ATCC700603, lane 16 = *K. variicola* ATCC-BAA830, lane 17 = *E. coli* ATCC-BAA2469 (contain NDM), lane 18 = *K. pneumoniae* ATCC-BAA2524 (contain OXA-48), lane 19 = *K. pneumoniae* ATCC-BAA1705 (contain KPC), lane 20 = negative control, and lane M = 100 bp DNA ladder.

Table 1. *Enterobacterales* species used in this study and mPCR results.

Bacteria	Carbapenemase Gene	N	mPCR Detection						
			E. coli	*K. pneumoniae*	*K. quasipneumoniae*	*K. variicola*	NDM	OXA-48-like	KPC
E. coli (*n* = 191)	NDM-1	43	+				+		
	NDM-3	1	+				+		
	NDM-4	4	+				+		
	NDM-5	109	+				+		
	NDM-7	1	+				+		
	OXA-48	1	+					+	
	OXA-181	10	+					+	
	KPC-2	1	+						+
	IMP-6	1	+						
	NDM-1 + OXA-181	1	+				+	+	
	none	20	+						

Table 1. *Cont.*

Bacteria	Carbapenemase Gene	N	mPCR Detection						
			E. coli	*K. pneumoniae*	*K. quasip-neumoniae*	*K. variicola*	NDM	OXA-48-like	KPC
K. pneumoniae (*n* = 598)	NDM-1	201		+			+		
	NDM-4	1		+			+		
	NDM-5	5		+			+		
	NDM-9	1		+			+		
	OXA-48	13		+				+	
	OXA-181	147		+				+	
	OXA-232	77		+				+	
	KPC-2	1		+					+
	IMP-14	5		+					
	GES-5	1		+					
	NDM-1 + OXA-181	11		+			+	+	
	NDM-1 + OXA-232	114		+			+	+	
	NDM-1 + GES-5	1		+			+		
	none	20		+					
K. quasip-neumoniae (*n* = 28)	NDM-1	12			+		+		
	IMP-14	2			+				
	NDM-1 + OXA-181	2			+		+	+	
	none	12			+				
K. variicola (*n* = 23)	none	23				+			
K. oxytoca (*n* = 10)	none	10							
K. aerogenes (*n* = 20)	none	20							
E. cloacae (*n* = 20)	NDM-1	5					+		
	OXA-181	1						+	
	none	14							
E. asburiae (*n* = 1)	KPC-2	1							+
C. freundii (*n* = 13)	NDM-1	3					+		
	none	10							
C. werkmanii (*n* = 5)	NDM-1	5					+		
S. enterica (*n* = 20)	none	20							
S. marcescens (*n* = 10)	none	10							

+ = mPCR positive; blank = mPCR negative.

In addition, we also tried to use the mPCR to directly detect the *E. coli* and *K. pneumoniae* complex together with detected NDM, OXA-48-like, and KPC from pure colonies. As shown in Figure 2, the colony PCR has successfully detected representative strains. This is an alternative method for laboratories because it is not necessary to purify DNA from bacteria growths, and shortens the time and renders unnecessary the equipment required for DNA purification.

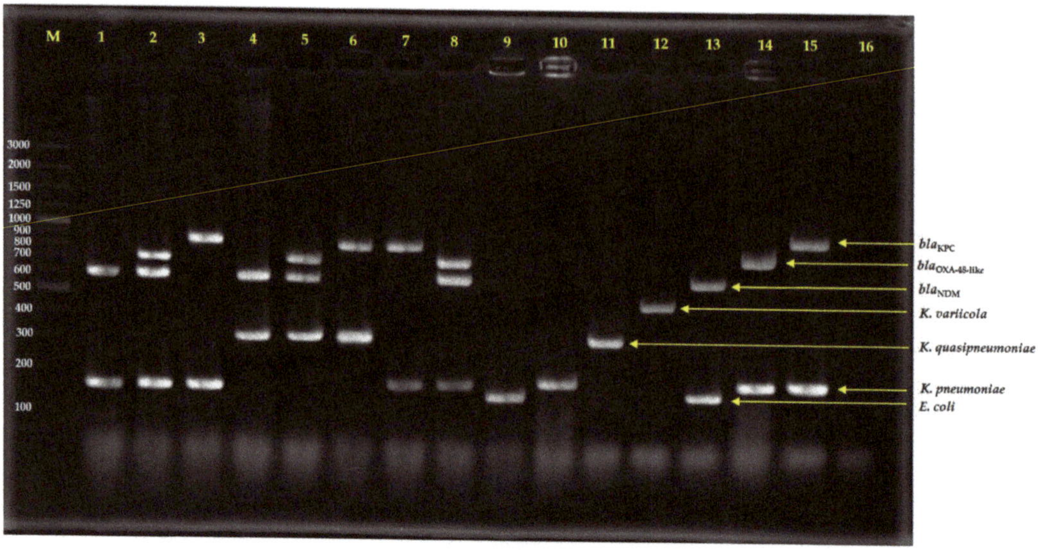

Figure 2. Agarose gel electrophoresis of multiplex PCR-amplified products from direct colonies; lane 1 = Isolate No. C76 (*E. coli* with NDM), lane 2 = Isolate No. C163 (*E. coli* with NDM and OXA-48-like), lane 3 = Isolate No. C1992 (*E. coli* with KPC), lane 4 = Isolate No. C34 (*K. quasipneumoniae* with NDM), lane 5 = Isolate No. C110 (*K. quasipneumoniae* with NDM and OXA-48-like), lane 6 = Isolate No. AMR353 (*K. quasipneumoniae* with KPC), lane 7 = Isolate No. C1985 (*K. pneumoniae* with KPC), lane 8 = Isolate No. C73 (*K. pneumoniae* with NDM and OXA-48-like), lane 9 = *E. coli* ATCC25922, lane 10 = *K. pneumoniae* ATCC27335, lane 11 = *K. quasipneumoniae* ATCC700603, lane 12 = *K. variicola* ATCC-BAA830, lane 13 = *E. coli* ATCC-BAA2469 (contain NDM), lane 14 = *K. pneumoniae* ATCC-BAA2524 (contain OXA-48), lane 15 = *K. pneumoniae* ATCC-BAA1705 (contain KPC), lane 16 = negative control, and lane M = 100 bp DNA ladder.

The spread of CP-CRE is a global threat to public health. Among CP-CREs, the carbapenemase genes, NDM, OXA-48-like, and KPC, are widely spread globally, as mentioned above. Several phenotypic and genotypic techniques have been applied to detect CRE and CP-CRE [28]. It is vital to diagnose CP-CRE early to undertake the appropriate measures to prevent transmission and to help in implementing effective countermeasures at an appropriate time to initiate early treatment interventions. In addition, the plasmids harboring carbapenemase genes can be transmitted easily among patients. Therefore, a method which can search for genetically diverse CP-CRE isolates would be useful in terms of epidemiological investigation and in tracking the trends of carbapenemase gene dynamics.

PCR is an ideal tool that saves on costs, is rapid, and can identify the type of carbapenemase genes to trace epidemiological dynamics, be proactive in the control and prevention of spread, and provide prompt treatment [12–16]. However, the currently available PCR-detectable carbapenemase genes have not identified the bacterial species [12–16]. Our mPCR assay allows for the rapid testing of common carbapenemase genes (NDM, KPC, OXA-48-like) together with identification of clinical *E. coli* and *K. pneumoniae* complex isolates that frequently harbor these genes; furthermore, the assay does not require prior phenotypical characterization, thus constituting a rapid and valuable tool in the management of infections in hospitals. However, this mPCR has limitations due to the fact that it does not detect IMP genes. The IMP gene is more prevalent in Asia and the South Pacific region than other continents [29]. Therefore, future research directions should include developing this mPCR to detect IMP genes.

3. Materials and Methods

3.1. Bacterial Strains

As shown in Table 1, this study included 780 *Enterobacterales* strains with known species and carbapenemase genes based on whole-genome sequencing from another study [26,30]: 578 *K. pneumoniae*, 16 *K. quasipneumoniae*, 171 *E. coli*, 6 *Enterobacter cloacae*, 1 *Enterobacter asburiae*, 5 *Citrobacter werkmanii*, and 3 *Citrobacter freundii*.

An additional 159 *Enterobacterales* species without carbapenemase genes including 20 *E. coli*, 20 *K. pneumoniae*, 10 *K. oxytoca*, 23 *K. variicola*, 12 *K. quasipneumoniae*, 20 *K. aerogenes*, 14 *E. cloacae*, 10 *Serratia marcescens*, 20 *Salmonella enterica*, and 10 *C. freundii*, were identified at the species level using conventional biochemical tests; PCR-detected carbapenemase genes described elsewhere were included in the current study [31–33]. These bacterial isolates were resistant to either carbapenems or cephalosporins.

We also included reference strains of other bacterial species to evaluate possible non-specific reactions. These strains consisted of: *Achromobacter xylosoxidans* ATCC27061, *Pseudomonas aeruginosa* ATCC9027, *Acinetobacter baumannii* ATCC19606, *Burkholderia cepacia* LMG0122, *Haemophilus influenzae* ATCC10211, *Elizabethkingia meningoseptica* ATCC13253, *Micrococcus luteus* ATCC10240, *Bacillus subtilis* ATCC6633, *Staphylococcus aureus* ATCC700698, *Enterococcus faecalis* ATCC29212, *Streptococcus pneumoniae* ATCC33400, *Leuconostoc lactis* ATCC19256, and *Listeria monocytogenes* ATCC7644. In addition, *E. coli* ATCC-BAA2469 (NDM-1), *K. pneumoniae* ATCC-BAA2524 (OXA-48), *K. pneumoniae* ATCC-BAA1705 (KPC), *K. quasipneumoniae* ATCC700603, and *K. variicola* ATCC-BAA830 were used for PCR reaction control.

The bacterial stains from stock at −80 °C were cultured overnight on sheep blood agar and incubated at 37 °C before performing the DNA extraction.

3.2. Primer Design

As shown in Table 2, only primers for NDM and *E. coli* were designed in the current study. The NDM and *E. coli uidA* were retrieved from GenBank under accession numbers NC_023908 and S69414, respectively. These sequences were used as the templates for design of primers by using Primer-BLAST program (http://www.ncbi.nlm.nih.gov/tools/primer-blast/; accessed on 9 December 2022).

Table 2. Primers used for detection of antibiotic resistance genes.

Primer Name	Sequences (5′—3′)	Final Conc. of Primers (μM)	Species/Gene	PCR Product Size (bp)	Reference
KpnWaaQ-F	CGG ATC CTG GTC ATT AAG CTG	0.5	*K. pneumoniae*	217	[34]
KpnWaaQ-R	ATT GCA TCT TCA GCT GAT ACC TTT	0.5			
KpnCpxLEN-F	CAC GCT GCG YAA ACT ACT GAC YGC GCA GCA	0.5	*K. variicola*	489	[35]
KpnCpxOKP-F	GGC CGG YGA GCG GGG CTC A	0.5	*K. quasipneumoniae*	348	
KpnCpxDeO-R *	AGA AGC ATC CTG CTG TGC G	1.0	*K. quasipneumoniae* and *K. variicola*	-	

Table 2. *Cont.*

Primer Name	Sequences (5′—3′)	Final Conc. of Primers (µM)	Species/Gene	PCR Product Size (bp)	Reference
ECuidA-F	GGG AAT GGT GAT TAC CGA CGA AAA CGG C	0.1	*E. coli*	175	This study
ECuidA-R	ACA GAC GCG TGG TTA CAG TCT TGC G	0.1			
NDM-F	AAC GGT TTG GCG ATC TGG TTT TC	0.7	*bla*NDM	627	This study
NDM-R	GGC GGA ATG GCT CAT CAC GAT C	0.7			
Oxa-48F	TTG GTG GCA TCG ATT ATC GG	0.7	*bla*OXA-48-like	733	[36]
Oxa-48R	GAG CAC TTC TTT TGT GAT GGC	0.7			
KPC-F	ATG TCA CTG TAT CGC CGT CT	0.5	*bla*KPC	893	[37]
KPC-R	TTT TCA GAG CCT TAC TGC CC	0.5			

* This primer is a reverse primer for KpnCpxOKP-F and KpnCpxLEN-F.

3.3. Multiplex PCR

Bacterial genomic DNA samples were extracted using ZymoBIOMICS DNA Kits (Zymo Research, CA, USA), following the manufacturer's instruction. The PCR reaction mixture (25 µL) contained a 1× JumpStart REDTaq ReadyMix (Sigma) and each primer (Table 2). The list of primers used in the mPCR are also presented in Table 2 [34–37]. The PCR reaction was performed as follows: initial activation of DNA polymerase at 95 °C for 3 min, plus 35 cycles of denaturation at 95 °C for 30 sec, primer annealing and extension at 62.5 °C for 1.30 min, and a final extension at 72 °C for 5 min. A negative control was included in each run, consisting of the same reaction mixture but with water instead of template DNA.

The PCR products (5 µL) were analyzed using gel electrophoresis on 1.5% (w/v) agarose gel in 0.5 × TBE buffer at a constant voltage of 100 V for 30 min (Mupid exU system; Takara; Tokyo, Japan). The gels were stained with ethidium bromide and visualized under ultraviolet light (GeneGenius Bioimaging System; SynGene; Cambridge, UK). The sizes of the PCR products were determined by comparison with molecular-sized standards (GeneRuler™ 100 bp Plus DNA ladder; Thermo Fisher Scientific; Vilnius, Lithuania).

3.4. Colony PCR

Bacteria were cultured on Tryptic Soy Agar for 18 h at 37 °C. A small amount of pure colony was picked up using a toothpick and then suspended in the PCR reaction mixture of each tube. The PCR reaction and gel electrophoresis were done as described above.

4. Conclusions

The mPCR assay developed in the current study could detect NDM, KPC, and OXA-48-like together with distinguishing *E. coli*, *K. pneumoniae*, *K. quasipneumoniae*, and *K. variicola* in a single reaction. It should be useful for clinical microbiology laboratories requiring the rapid detection of CRE as one of the critical priority pathogens according to the WHO.

In addition, the developed assay should be useful for epidemiological investigation and tracking the trends of carbapenemase gene dynamics.

Author Contributions: Conceptualization, R.H. and A.K.; methodology, R.H.; validation, A.K.; formal analysis, R.H. and P.C.; resources, R.H. and A.K.; writing—original draft preparation, R.H., P.C. and P.B.; writing—review and editing, R.H. and A.K.; supervision, A.K.; funding acquisition, R.H. and A.K. All authors have read and agreed to the published version of the manuscript.

Funding: This research was funded by Kasetsart University, Bangkok, Thailand under the research program of Establishment of Knowledge and Innovation Products for Detection of Antimicrobial Resistant Bacteria.

Institutional Review Board Statement: Not applicable because this study did not involve humans or animals.

Informed Consent Statement: Not applicable.

Data Availability Statement: Not applicable.

Acknowledgments: The Kasetsart University Research and Development Institute (KURDI) provided English editing and the article processing charge (APC).

Conflicts of Interest: The authors declare no conflict of interest.

References

1. Suay-García, B.; Pérez-Gracia, M.T. Present and Future of Carbapenem-resistant *Enterobacteriaceae* (CRE) Infections. *Antibiotics* **2019**, *8*, 122. [CrossRef] [PubMed]
2. Neidhöfer, C.; Buechler, C.; Neidhöfer, G.; Bierbaum, G.; Hannet, I.; Hoerauf, A.; Parčina, M. Global Distribution Patterns of Carbapenemase-Encoding Bacteria in a New Light: Clues on a Role for Ethnicity. *Front. Cell Infect. Microbiol.* **2021**, *11*, 659753. [CrossRef]
3. World Health Organization WHO Priority Pathogens List for R&D of New Antibiotics. 2017. Available online: http://www.who.int/bulletin/volumes/94/9/16-020916.pdf (accessed on 20 November 2022).
4. Logan, L.K.; Weinstein, R.A. The Epidemiology of Carbapenem-Resistant Enterobacteriaceae: The Impact and Evolution of a Global Menace. *J. Infect. Dis.* **2017**, *215*, S28–S36. [CrossRef] [PubMed]
5. Hansen, G.T. Continuous Evolution: Perspective on the Epidemiology of Carbapenemase Resistance among Enterobacterales and Other Gram-Negative Bacteria. *Infect. Dis. Ther.* **2021**, *10*, 75–92. [CrossRef]
6. Paveenkittiporn, W.; Lyman, M.; Biedron, C.; Chea, N.; Bunthi, C.; Kolwaite, A.; Janejai, N. Molecular epidemiology of carbapenem-resistant *Enterobacterales* in Thailand, 2016–2018. *Antimicrob. Resist. Infect. Control* **2021**, *10*, 88. [CrossRef] [PubMed]
7. van Duin, D.; Doi, Y. The global epidemiology of carbapenemase-producing Enterobacteriaceae. *Virulence* **2017**, *8*, 460–469. [CrossRef]
8. Patel, B.; Hopkins, K.L.; Freeman, R.; People, D.; Brown, C.S.; Robotham, J.V. Carbapenemase-producing Enterobacterales: A challenge for healthcare now and for the next decade. *Infect. Prev. Pract.* **2020**, *2*, 100089. [CrossRef]
9. Baeza, L.L.; Pfennigwerth, N.; Greissl, C.; Göttig, S.; Saleh, A.; Stelzer, Y.; Gatermann, S.G.; Hamprecht, A. Comparison of five methods for detection of carbapenemases in Enterobacterales with proposal of a new algorithm. *Clin. Microbiol. Infect.* **2019**, *25*, 1286-e9. [CrossRef]
10. Tamma, P.D.; Opene, B.N.; Gluck, A.; Chambers, K.K.; Carroll, K.C.; Simner, P.J. Comparison of 11 Phenotypic Assays for Accurate Detection of Carbapenemase-Producing *Enterobacteriaceae*. *J. Clin. Microbiol.* **2017**, *55*, 1046–1055. [CrossRef]
11. Clinical Laboratory Standard Institute. Performance standards for antimicrobial susceptibility testing. In *CLSI Supplement M100*, 32nd ed.; Clinical Laboratory Standard Institute: Wayne, PA, USA, 2022. ISBN 978-1-68440-066-9.
12. Poirel, L.; Walsh, T.R.; Cuvillier, V.; Nordmann, P. Multiplex PCR for detection of acquired carbapenemase genes. *Diagn. Microbiol. Infect. Dis.* **2011**, *70*, 119–123. [CrossRef]
13. Smiljanic, M.; Kaase, M.; Ahmad-Nejad, P.; Ghebremedhin, B. Comparison of in-house and commercial real time-PCR based carbapenemase gene detection methods in *Enterobacteriaceae* and non-fermenting gram-negative bacterial isolates. *Ann. Clin. Microbiol. Antimicrob.* **2017**, *16*, 48. [CrossRef]
14. Watahiki, M.; Kawahara, R.; Suzuki, M.; Aoki, M.; Uchida, K.; Matsumoto, Y.; Kumagai, Y.; Noda, M.; Masuda, K.; Fukuda, C.; et al. Single-Tube Multiplex Polymerase Chain Reaction for the Detection of Genes Encoding Enterobacteriaceae Carbapenemase. *Jpn. J. Infect. Dis.* **2020**, *73*, 166–172. [CrossRef]
15. Cerezales, M.; Biniossek, L.; Gerson, S.; Xanthopoulou, K.; Wille, J.; Wohlfarth, E.; Kaase, M.; Seifert, H.; Higgins, P.G. Novel multiplex PCRs for detection of the most prevalent carbapenemase genes in Gram-negative bacteria within Germany. *J. Med. Microbiol.* **2021**, *70*, 001310. [CrossRef]
16. Yoshioka, N.; Hagiya, H.; Deguchi, M.; Hamaguchi, S.; Kagita, M.; Nishi, I.; Akeda, Y.; Tomono, K. Multiplex Real-Time PCR Assay for Six Major Carbapenemase Genes. *Pathogens* **2021**, *10*, 276. [CrossRef]

17. Vlek, A.L.; Frentz, D.; Haenen, A.; Bootsma, H.J.; Notermans, D.W.; Frakking, F.N.; de Greeff, S.C.; Leenstra, T. ISIS-AR study group. Detection and epidemiology of carbapenemase producing *Enterobacteriaceae* in the Netherlands in 2013–2014. *Eur. J. Clin. Microbiol. Infect. Dis.* **2016**, *35*, 1089–1096. [CrossRef]

18. Hernández-García, M.; Pérez-Viso, B.; Carmen Turrientes, M.; Díaz-Agero, C.; López-Fresneña, N.; Bonten, M.; Malhotra-Kumar, S.; Ruiz-Garbajosa, P.; Cantón, R. Characterization of carbapenemase-producing Enterobacteriaceae from colonized patients in a university hospital in Madrid, Spain, during the R-GNOSIS project depicts increased clonal diversity over time with maintenance of high-risk clones. *J. Antimicrob. Chemother.* **2018**, *73*, 3039–3043. [CrossRef]

19. Sekar, R.; Srivani, S.; Kalyanaraman, N.; Thenmozhi, P.; Amudhan, M.; Lallitha, S.; Mythreyee, M. New Delhi Metallo-β-lactamase and other mechanisms of carbapenemases among Enterobacteriaceae in rural South India. *J. Glob. Antimicrob. Resist.* **2019**, *18*, 207–214. [CrossRef]

20. Dziri, O.; Dziri, R.; Ali, E.L.; Salabi, A.; Chouchani, C. Carbapenemase Producing Gram-Negative Bacteria in Tunisia: History of Thirteen Years of Challenge. *Infect. Drug Resist.* **2020**, *13*, 4177–4191. [CrossRef]

21. Gurung, S.; Kafle, S.; Dhungel, B.; Adhikari, N.; Thapa Shrestha, U.; Adhikari, B.; Banjara, M.R.; Rijal, K.R.; Ghimire, P. Detection of OXA-48 Gene in Carbapenem-Resistant *Escherichia coli* and *Klebsiella pneumoniae* from Urine Samples. *Infect. Drug Resist.* **2020**, *13*, 2311–2321. [CrossRef]

22. Han, R.; Shi, Q.; Wu, S.; Yin, D.; Peng, M.; Dong, D.; Zheng, Y.; Guo, Y.; Zhang, R.; Hu, F. China Antimicrobial Surveillance Network (CHINET) Study Group. Dissemination of Carbapenemases (KPC, NDM, OXA-48, IMP, and VIM) among Carbapenem-Resistant *Enterobacteriaceae* Isolated From Adult and Children Patients in China. *Front. Cell Infect. Microbiol.* **2020**, *10*, 314. [CrossRef]

23. Kim, S.H.; Kim, G.R.; Jeong, J.; Kim, S.; Shin, J.H. Prevalence and Characteristics of Carbapenemase-Producing *Enterobacteriaceae* in Three Tertiary-Care Korean University Hospitals between 2017 and 2018. *Jpn. J. Infect. Dis.* **2020**, *73*, 431–436. [CrossRef] [PubMed]

24. Solgi, H.; Nematzadeh, S.; Giske, C.G.; Badmasti, F.; Westerlund, F.; Lin, Y.L.; Goyal, G.; Nikbin, V.S.; Nemati, A.H.; Shahcheraghi, F. Molecular Epidemiology of OXA-48 and NDM-1 Producing *Enterobacterales* Species at a University Hospital in Tehran, Iran, between 2015 and 2016. *Front. Microbiol.* **2020**, *11*, 936. [CrossRef] [PubMed]

25. Castanheira, M.; Deshpande, L.M.; Mendes, R.E.; Doyle, T.B.; Sader, H.S. Prevalence of carbapenemase genes among carbapenem-nonsusceptible *Enterobacterales* collected in US hospitals in a five-year period and activity of ceftazidime/avibactam and comparator agents. *JAC. Antimicrob. Resist.* **2022**, *4*, dlac098. [CrossRef] [PubMed]

26. Takeuchi, D.; Kerdsin, A.; Akeda, Y.; Sugawara, Y.; Sakamoto, N.; Matsumoto, Y.; Motooka, D.; Ishihara, T.; Nishi, I.; Laolerd, W.; et al. Nationwide surveillance in Thailand revealed genotype-dependent dissemination of carbapenem-resistant *Enterobacterales*. *Microb. Genom.* **2022**, *8*, 000797. [CrossRef] [PubMed]

27. Thapa, A.; Upreti, M.K.; Bimali, N.K.; Shrestha, B.; Sah, A.K.; Nepal, K.; Dhungel, B.; Adhikari, S.; Adhikari, N.; Lekhak, B.; et al. Detection of NDM Variants (bla_{NDM-1}, bla_{NDM-2}, bla_{NDM-3}) from Carbapenem-Resistant *Escherichia coli* and *Klebsiella pneumoniae*: First Report from Nepal. *Infect. Drug Resist.* **2022**, *15*, 4419–4434. [CrossRef] [PubMed]

28. Osei Sekyere, J.; Govinden, U.; Essack, S.Y. Review of established and innovative detection methods for carbapenemase-producing Gram-negative bacteria. *J. Appl. Microbiol.* **2015**, *119*, 1219–1233. [CrossRef]

29. Matsumura, Y.; Peirano, G.; Motyl, M.R.; Adams, M.D.; Chen, L.; Kreiswirth, B.; DeVinney, R.; Pitout, J.D. Global Molecular Epidemiology of IMP-Producing Enterobacteriaceae. *Antimicrob. Agents Chemother.* **2017**, *61*, e02729-16. [CrossRef]

30. Kerdsin, A.; Deekae, S.; Chayangsu, S.; Hatrongjit, R.; Chopjitt, P.; Takeuchi, D.; Akeda, Y.; Tomono, K.; Hamada, S. Genomic characterization of an emerging bla_{KPC-2} carrying Enterobacteriaceae clinical isolates in Thailand. *Sci. Rep.* **2019**, *9*, 18521. [CrossRef]

31. Abbott, S. *Klebsiella, Enterobacter, Citrobacter, Serratia, Plesiomonas*, and other Enterobacteriaceae. In *Manual of Clinical Microbiology*, 10th ed.; Versalovic, J., Carroll, K., Funke, G., Jorgensen, J., Landry, M.L., Warnock, D., Eds.; ASM Press: Washington, DC, USA, 2011; Volume 2, pp. 639–657.

32. Hatrongjit, R.; Kerdsin, A.; Akeda, Y.; Hamada, S. Detection of plasmid-mediated colistin-resistant and carbapenem-resistant genes by multiplex PCR. *MethodsX* **2018**, *5*, 532–536. [CrossRef]

33. Phetburom, N.; Boueroy, P.; Chopjitt, P.; Hatrongjit, R.; Akeda, Y.; Hamada, S.; Nuanualsuwan, S.; Kerdsin, A. *Klebsiella pneumoniae* Complex Harboring *mcr-1*, *mcr-7*, and *mcr-8* Isolates from Slaughtered Pigs in Thailand. *Microorganisms* **2021**, *9*, 2436. [CrossRef]

34. Pechorsky, A.; Nitzan, Y.; Lazarovitch, T. Identification of pathogenic bacteria in blood cultures: Comparison between conventional and PCR methods. *J. Microbiol. Methods* **2009**, *78*, 325–330. [CrossRef]

35. Fonseca, E.L.; Ramos, N.D.; Andrade, B.G.; Morais, L.L.; Marin, M.F.; Vicente, A.C. A one-step multiplex PCR to identify *Klebsiella pneumoniae*, *Klebsiella variicola*, and *Klebsiella quasipneumoniae* in the clinical routine. *Diagn. Microbiol. Infect. Dis.* **2017**, *87*, 315–317. [CrossRef]

36. Poirel, L.; Heritier, C.; Tol'un, V.; Nordmann, P. Emergence of oxacillinase-mediated resistance to imipenem in *Klebsiella pneumoniae*. *Antimicrob. Agents. Chemother.* **2004**, *48*, 15–22. [CrossRef]
37. Bradford, P.A.; Bratu, S.; Urban, C.; Visalli, M.; Mariano, N.; Landman, D.; Rahal, J.J.; Brooks, S.; Cebular, S.; Quale, J. Emergence of carbapenem-resistant *Klebsiella* species possessing the class A carbapenem-hydrolyzing KPC-2 and inhibitor-resistant TEM-30 beta-lactamases in New York City. *Clin. Infect. Dis.* **2004**, *39*, 55–60. [CrossRef]

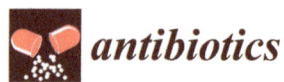

Article

Genotypic Diversity, Antibiotic Resistance, and Virulence Phenotypes of *Stenotrophomonas maltophilia* Clinical Isolates from a Thai University Hospital Setting

Orathai Yinsai, Manu Deeudom and Kwanjit Duangsonk *

Department of Microbiology, Faculty of Medicine, Chiang Mai University, Chiang Mai 50200, Thailand
* Correspondence: kwanjit.d@cmu.ac.th; Tel.: +66-81-4734854

Abstract: *Stenotrophomonas maltophilia* is a multidrug-resistant organism that is emerging as an important opportunistic pathogen. Despite this, information on the epidemiology and characteristics of this bacterium, especially in Thailand, is rarely found. This study aimed to determine the demographic, genotypic, and phenotypic characteristics of *S. maltophilia* isolates from Maharaj Nakorn Chiang Mai Hospital, Thailand. A total of 200 *S. maltophilia* isolates were collected from four types of clinical specimens from 2015 to 2016 and most of the isolates were from sputum. In terms of clinical characteristics, male and aged patients were more susceptible to an *S. maltophilia* infection. The majority of included patients had underlying diseases and were hospitalized with associated invasive procedures. The antimicrobial resistance profiles of *S. maltophilia* isolates showed the highest frequency of resistance to ceftazidime and the lower frequency of resistance to chloramphenicol, levofloxacin, trimethoprim/sulfamethoxazole (TMP/SMX), and no resistance to minocycline. The predominant antibiotic resistance genes among the 200 isolates were the *smeF* gene (91.5%), followed by bla_{L1} and bla_{L2} genes (43% and 10%), respectively. Other antibiotic resistance genes detected were *floR* (8.5%), *intI1* (7%), *sul1* (6%), *mfsA* (4%) and *sul2* (2%). Most *S. maltophilia* isolates could produce biofilm and could swim in a semisolid medium, however, none of the isolates could swarm. All isolates were positive for hemolysin production, whereas 91.5% and 22.5% of isolates could release protease and lipase enzymes, respectively. In MLST analysis, a high degree of genetic diversity was observed among the 200 *S. maltophilia* isolates. One hundred and forty-one sequence types (STs), including 130 novel STs, were identified and categorized into six different clonal complex groups. The differences in drug resistance patterns and genetic profiles exhibited various phenotypes of biofilm formation, motility, toxin, and enzymes production which support this bacterium in its virulence and pathogenicity. This study reviewed the characteristics of genotypes and phenotypes of *S. maltophilia* from Thailand which is necessary for the control and prevention of *S. maltophilia* local spreading.

Keywords: *Stenotrophomonas maltophilia*; mutilocus sequence typing; antibiotic resistance; multidrug resistance; biofilm; motility; toxin; enzyme

Citation: Yinsai, O.; Deeudom, M.; Duangsonk, K. Genotypic Diversity, Antibiotic Resistance, and Virulence Phenotypes of *Stenotrophomonas maltophilia* Clinical Isolates from a Thai University Hospital Setting. *Antibiotics* **2023**, *12*, 410. https://doi.org/10.3390/antibiotics12020410

Academic Editors: Anusak Kerdsin, Jinquan Li, Jonathan Frye and Alastair Hay

Received: 8 December 2022
Revised: 16 February 2023
Accepted: 16 February 2023
Published: 18 February 2023

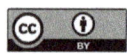
1. Introduction

Stenotrophomonas maltophilia is a Gram-negative obligate aerobic bacillus that is often recovered from various environments such as soil, plant, water, and drinking water [1–3]. It is widely recognized as an opportunistic pathogen that can cause severe infections in hospitalized patients, especially those with severely impaired immune systems, including those with HIV infection and malignancy, chemotherapy-treated patients, and patients who used immune suppressive drugs [4–6]. *S. maltophilia* infections have been increasingly reported worldwide [1,6,7]. In several countries, most cases are nosocomial infections, that are caused by the contamination of medical equipment and water systems in hospitals [8–10].

S. maltophilia produces many virulence factors that contribute to infection [11]. It usually forms biofilm as a means of attaching to the surface of medical equipment, like respirators and catheters, which promotes their survivability and pathogenicity [1,11]. Another factor is flagella, which are used for motility, and can stimulate the host's immune response [12]. This bacterium has extracellular enzymes that are released to promote pathogenesis, such as proteases, lipases, esterase, DNase, Rnase, and fibrolysin [6,13]. Due to the exceptional innate antimicrobial resistance of the species and acquired resistance to numerous antimicrobial drugs, treating *S. maltophilia*, infections can be challenging [14]. The multidrug resistance mechanisms of *S. maltophilia* are the production of drug-degrading enzymes and efflux pumps, as well as the transport proteins involved in the extrusion of drugs [15]. TMP/SMX is the first-line treatment for *S. maltophilia* infections, however, substantial rates of TMP/SMX resistance have been increasingly reported [7]. Levofloxacin and minocycline are additional antibiotics against *S. maltophilia* [16].

Recent investigations have revealed the high genetic diversity among *S. maltophilia* strains isolated in different parts of the world [17]. Molecular methods are used to provide evidence of epidemiological relationships between isolates. These methods are also an important tool in the investigation of the spread of *S. maltophilia* infections all over the world. There are a number of studies about *S. maltophilia* genotypes in many countries, which help in the understanding of the epidemiology and clonality of bacteria. Nowadays, many methods have been developed to clarify bacterial genetic background. The gold standard technique is multilocus sequence typing (MLST). MLST is a procedure for the characterization of bacterial species, using seven housekeeping genes' internal fragment sequences. MLST is used to provide a portable, accurate, and highly discriminating typing system that can be used for most bacteria and some other organisms [18]. The unique allele sequences of the seven housekeeping genes were defined as allelic profiles or STs [19]. Phenotypic characterization of *S. maltophilia* includes growth rate, biofilm formation, motility, mutation frequencies, antibiotic resistance, virulence, and pathogenicity. These phenotypic factors are required to give more understanding of the relationship between genotypic patterns and phenotypes within the bacterial population.

S. maltophilia from different countries or regions may have different genotypic properties with the divergence of virulence genes, drug resistance genes, and mobile genetic elements [20–23]. These genotypic differences may contribute to the differences in phenotypic properties, e.g., morphology, bacterial pathogenesis and virulence, drug resistance property, gene exchange or gene transfer, enzyme production, and biofilm formation. During the last decade, *S. maltophilia* has been recovered with increasing frequency at Maharaj Nakorn Chiang Mai Hospital, a 1400-bed university-affiliated hospital in Chiang Mai, Thailand [24]. Moreover, published data is rarely available on the epidemiology and characteristics of *S. maltophilia* in Thailand [25].

Therefore, this study aims to characterize clinical information, genotypes, and phenotypes of *S. maltophilia* isolated from Maharaj Nakorn Chiang Mai Hospital. The investigation includes molecular classification based on housekeeping gene allelic patterns using MLST, and the identification of antibiotic resistance genes such as β-lactamase encoding genes, efflux pump encoding genes, and the integrase gene. In addition, the phenotypic properties of *S. maltophilia*, including antibiotic resistance patterns, biofilm formation, motility, and enzyme production were investigated.

2. Results

2.1. Bacterial Collection and Clinical Characteristics

A total of 200 *S. maltophilia* nonrepetitive isolates were randomly collected from Maharaj Nakorn Chiang Mai Hospital, Chiang Mai, Thailand for six months. In our collection, 199 isolates were collected from patients and one isolate, from a hospital environment (fluid from the dialysis unit). All clinical isolates were obtained from four different sources and most of the isolates were from sputum ($n = 152$; 76%), while others were from body fluids ($n = 21$; 10.5%), pus ($n = 20$; 10.0%), and urine ($n = 6$; 3.0%).

Among *S. maltophilia*-infected patients, 192 patient information could be accessed (Table 1). In total, 117 male patients (60.94%) and 75 female patients (39.06%) were included. The age of the youngest patient was one month, and the oldest patient was 99 years. The average of the ages was 54.61 ± 28.14 years, and the aged people (≥65 years) were the most affected group (*n* = 79; 41.15%).

Table 1. Demographic and clinical characteristics, and risk factors of respiratory tract infections due to *S. maltophilia*.

Characteristics	No. of Patients (%) (*n* = 192)	No. of Respiratory Infection (*n* = 148)	No. of Non-Respiratory Inection (*n* = 44)	*p* Value
Age				
Range	1 M–99 Y	1 M–99 Y	6 M–89 Y	
Pediatrics (<15)	32 (16.67)	30	2	0.308
Aged (≥65)	79 (41.15)	62	17	**0.031**
Mean ± SD	54.61Y ± 28.14	52.94 ± 29.78	55.82 ± 22.14	
Gender: Male	117 (60.94)	91	26	0.398
Underlying Diseases and Comorbidities				
Malignancy	56 (29.17)	40	16	**0.041**
CNS and cerebrovascular diseases	36 (18.75)	31	5	**0.040**
Urinary tract infection	34 (17.71)	28	6	**0.044**
Hypertension	33 (17.19)	22	11	0.129
Cardiovascular diseases	28 (14.58)	24	4	**0.043**
Diabetes	25 (13.02)	20	5	0.281
Chronic kidney disease	20 (10.42)	20	3	0.391
Chronic pulmonary diseases	18 (9.38)	12	6	0.401
Chronic viral infections	11 (5.73)	8	3	0.677
Predisposing factors				
Invasive procedures	190 (98.96)	147	43	0.183
Intravenous catheter	116 (60.42)	79	37	**0.040**
Urinary catheter	46 (23.96)	41	5	0.129
Suction catheter	98 (51.04)	80	18	0.258
Endotracheal intubation	57 (29.69)	39	18	0.148
Gastrostomy (feeding) intubation	38 (19.79)	32	6	0.529
Surgery	56 (29.17)	40	16	**0.046**
Chemotherapy, Radiotherapy	19 (9.90)	12	7	**0.031**
Amputation	5 (2.60)	2	3	
Organ transplant	3 (1.56)	2	1	
Dialysis	5 (2.60)	5	0	
Hospitalization	190 (98.96)	147	43	
Medical wards				
General medicine	53 (27.60)	44	9	
Pediatric	33 (17.19)	31	2	
General surgery	24 (12.5)	14	10	
Emergency surgery	17 (8.85)	11	6	
Orthopedics	9 (4.69)	7	2	
Neurosurgery	3 (1.56)	3	0	
Others	51 (26.56)	37	14	
Patient in ICU of each ward	78 (40.63)	71	7	**0.001**

p value < 0.05 was considered to be significant; *p* value in bold letter = significant; M = Month; Y = Year; ICU = intensive care unit.

All patients had at least one underlying illness and were exposed to predisposing factors such as invasive procedures, surgery, chemotherapy, and radiotherapy. The most common underlying diseases and comorbidities were malignancy (*n* = 56; 29.17%), CNS and cerebrovascular diseases (*n* = 36; 18.75%), and urinary tract infections (*n* = 28; 17.71%). One hundred and ninety patients were hospitalized (98.96%) in different wards, including general medicine (*n* = 53; 27.60%), pediatric (*n* = 33; 17.19%), general surgery (*n* = 24; 12.5%), emergency surgery (n = 17; 8.85%), orthopedics (n = 9; 4.69%), neurosurgery (n = 3; 1.56%), and other wards (n = 51; 26.56%).

Since the majority of the isolates were obtained from respiratory specimens, risk factors associated with respiratory tract infection were evaluated. The patients who were significantly more likely to develop respiratory tract infections included aged patients, patients with malignancy, CNS and cerebrovascular diseases, and cardiovascular diseases (Table 1). Furthermore, the respiratory group had a significantly higher number of patients who were exposed to intravenous catheters, surgery, chemotherapy, and radiotherapy, and were admitted to the intensive care unit.

2.2. Antibiotic Susceptibility and Antibiotic Resistances

The MIC results show that *S. maltophilia* was highly resistant to CAZ (n = 155; 77.5%). All the isolates that showed a lower resistance frequency were observed to C (n = 36; 18%), LEV (n = 18; 9%), TMP/SMX (n = 15; 7.5%), and no resistance to minocycline. The MIC range, MIC_{50}, and MIC_{90} values are shown in Table 2. From all of the isolates, 37 isolates were susceptible to all antibiotics tested. On the contrary, 20 isolates were resistant to three or more antibiotics, hence exhibiting a multidrug-resistant (MDR) phenotype.

Table 2. Antibiotic susceptibility of *S. maltophilia* isolates.

Antibiotic	MIC (µg/mL)			Susceptibility (%)		
	MIC Range	MIC_{50}	MIC_{90}	S	I	R
Trimethoprim/ Sulfamethoxazole * (TMP/SMX)	0.047/0.893 → 32/608	0.19/3.61	0.5/9.5	185 (92.5)	0	15 (7.5)
Levofloxacin ** (LEV)	0.5 → 32	2	4	163 (81.5)	19 (9.5)	18 (9.0)
Ceftazidime ** (CAZ)	2 → 128	128	>128	21 (10.5)	24 (12.0)	150 (77.5)
Chloramphenicol ** (C)	4 → 128	16	32	67 (33.5)	97 (48.5)	36 (18)
Minocycline ** (MH)	0.5 → 4	0.5	2	200 (100)	0	0

MIC, A minimal inhibitory concentration value used breakpoint establishing by CLSI for *S. maltophilia*, document M100 ED29 [26]; MIC range, A minimal inhibitory concentration from the lowest value to highest value; MIC_{50}, A minimum concentration value at which 50% of the isolates were inhibited; MIC_{90}, A minimum concentration value at which 90% of the isolates were inhibited; * MIC determination was defined by MIC test strip; ** MIC determination was defined by agar dilution; S, Susceptible, I, Intermediate, R, Resistant; TMP/SMX, trimethoprim/sulfamethoxazole; LEV, levofloxacin; CAZ, ceftazidime; C, chloramphenicol; MH, minocycline.

Antibiotic susceptibility results revealed six antibiotypes: TMP/SMX resistance, LEV resistance, CAZ resistance, C resistance, nonresistance, and MDR. Most isolates in the TMP/SMX and LEV resistances also exhibited MDR phenotypes at a high rate (86.67% and 72.22% of isolates tested, respectively). MDR phenotypes were found in a lower percentage of C resistance (64.52%). On the contrary, the majority of CAZ-resistant isolates exhibited a non-MDR phenotype at a higher rate than MDR (Table S1). However, non-MDR negatively correlated with all of the antibiotic-resistant groups, whereas the MDR phenotype showed a positively correlated with three antibiotic-resistant groups, except CAZ resistance.

Antibiotic resistance phenotypes in *S. maltophilia* varied between specimens. The majority of sputum isolates (88.08%) were resistant to CAZ and have a lower proportion of the isolates that are resistant to C (21.85%), TMP/SMX (6.63%), and LEV (7.28%). Sixteen out of twenty isolates from pus were resistant to CAZ (80.0%), two isolates were resistant to C (20.0%), and none were resistant to TMP/SMX and LEV. All isolates from body fluid were resistant to CAZ and four isolates were resistant to C and TMP/SMX. However, resistance to LEV, was not found. All of the isolates from urine were resistant to CAZ and four out of six isolates were resistant to C, TMP/SMX, and LEV. Minocycline was the most active compound tested against our isolates with no resistance among all isolates or specimens

(MIC$_{50}$ of 0.5 µg/mL and MIC$_{90}$ of 2.0 µg/mL). Interestingly, only one isolate from the hospital environment did not show resistance properties to any of the drugs tested.

2.3. Detection of Antibiotic Resistance Genes

The detection of antibiotic resistance genes is shown in Table 3. The *smeF* gene was found in the majority of the isolates (91.5%), while *sul2*, *floR*, and *mfsA* were only found in a few (2%, 4%, and 4.5%, respectively). The *bla*$_{L1}$ and *sul1* genes were found in greater proportion (43% and 6%) among resistant groups than the *bla*$_{L2}$ and *sul2* genes (10% and 2%). The *intI1* gene, on the other hand, was found in all resistant groups. The majority of the *sul1-2* and *intI1* positive isolates were also TMP/SMX resistant.

Table 3. Antibiotic resistance genes among *S. maltophilia* isolates are stratified into six resistance groups.

Antibiotic Resistance	Total of Isolates *	Antibiotic Resistance Genes							
		smeF	*bla*$_{L1}$	*bla*$_{L2}$	*sul1*	*sul2*	*intI1*	*floR*	*mfsA*
		No. of Isolate (%)							
All isolates	200 (100)	183 (91.5)	86 (43)	20 (10)	12 (6)	4 (2)	14 (7)	8 (4)	9 (4.5)
TMP/SMX resistance	15 (7.5)	15 (100)	12 (80.0)	1 (6.67)	12 (80.0)	4 (26.67)	14 (93.33)	5 (33.33)	1 (6.67)
LEV resistance	18 (9)	16 (88.89)	7 (38.89)	1 (5.56)	4 (22.22)	2 (11.11)	5 (27.78)	2 (11.11)	2 (11.11)
CAZ resistance	157 (78.5)	123 (78.34)	80 (50.96)	19 (12.1)	12 (7.64)	4 (5.09)	13 (8.28)	12 (7.64)	7 (4.46)
C resistance	31 (15.5)	30 (96.77)	11 (35.48)	2 (6.45)	10 (32.26)	3 (9.68)	11 (35.48)	4 (12.90)	2 (6.45)
Non-resistance	37 (18.5)	37 (100)	6 (16.22)	1 (2.70)	0	0	0	5 (13.51)	0
MDR	20 (10)	20 (100)	11 (55)	1 (5)	10 (50)	3 (15)	12 (60)	4 (20)	2 (10)

Eight antibiotic resistance genes were detected among total *S. maltophilia* isolates and six resistant groups; * Number and percentage of the isolates of total and each antibiotic resistances; TMP/SMX, trimethoprim/sulfamethoxazole; LEV, levofloxacin; CAZ, ceftazidime; C, chloramphenicol; MDR, multidrug resistance.

2.4. Biofilm Formation

The results from the biofilm formation assay showed that most of the isolates are strong biofilm producers (*n* = 146; 73%), whereas one strain (0.5%) did not form biofilm. Moderate biofilm was formed by 31 isolates (15.5%), while 22 strains were weak biofilm producers (11.0%) (Table 4). The comparison of biofilm formation efficiency among the six drug-resistant groups revealed that isolates in the nonresistant group produced significantly more biofilm than isolates in the TMP/SMX, C, and MDR groups (Figure 1A). In all drug resistance patterns, the majority of isolates produced strong biofilm levels, followed by moderate and weak levels, respectively. The biofilm formation capability of isolates, compared among four types of specimens, was not significantly different (Figure 1B).

2.5. Motility

Swimming motility was observed in most of the isolates. Twenty-one (10.5%) isolates were nonmotile, while 73 (36.5%) exhibited weak motility, and 86 (43.0%) moderate motility (Table 4). Swimming motility was compared in the six drug resistance patterns. Swimming efficiency was significantly higher in nonresistant and CAZ-resistant isolates than in TMP/SMX, C, and MDR isolates (Figure 2A). In all antibiotic resistance patterns, the majority of isolates could swim moderately or weakly, followed by no swimming and strongly swim, respectively. When the isolates from different types of specimens were compared, it was discovered that the swimming ability of the isolates from pus (high viscosity environment) was significantly higher than the isolates from other specimens (Figure 2B). However, swarming motility was not detected in any of the isolates.

Antibiotics **2023**, *12*, 410

Table 4. Virulence phenotypes of *S. maltophilia* isolates stratified on the different resistance groups.

Antibiotic Resistance	Biofilm Formation				Swimming Motility				Toxin and Enzymes			
	Non	Weak	Moderate	Strong	Non	Weak	Moderate	Strong	α-Hemolys in	β-Hemolys in	Protease	Lipase
						Number of Isolate (%)						
All isolates	1 (0.5)	22 (11)	31 (15.5)	146 (73)	21 (10.5)	73 (36.5)	81 (40.5)	25 (12.5)	106 (53)	94(47)	183 (91.5)	45 (22.5)
TMP/SMX resistance	0	2 (13.33)	6 (40)	7 (46.67)	6 (40)	8 (53.33)	0	1 (6.67)	11 (73.33)	4 (26.67)	11 (73.33)	2 (13.33)
LEV resistance	0	1 (5.56)	4 (22.22)	13 (72.22)	6 (33.33)	5 (27.78)	6 (33.33)	1 (5.55)	9 (50)	9 (50)	14 (77.78)	3 (16.67)
CAZ resistance	1 (0.64)	20 (12.74)	28 (17.83)	108 (68.79)	18 (11.46)	63 (40.13)	55 (35.03)	21 (13.38)	89 (56.69)	68 (43.31)	144 (91.72)	35 (22.29)
C resistance	0	5 (16.13)	7 (22.58)	19 (61.29)	8 (25.8)	12 (38.71)	9 (29.03)	2 (6.45)	15 (48.39)	16 (51.61)	25 (80.65)	8 (5.10)
Non-resistance	0	2 (5.4)	3 (8.10)	32 (86.49)	2 (5.4)	10 (27.02)	22 (59.46)	3 (8.11)	21 (56.76)	16 (43.24)	34 (91.89)	5 (13.51)
MDR	0	2 (10)	7 (35)	11 (55)	7 (35)	8 (40)	4 (20)	1 (5)	11 (55)	9 (45)	19 (95)	4 (20)

Three virulent phenotypes were detected among total *S. maltophilia* isolates and six resistant groups: TMP/SMX, trimethoprim/sulfamethoxazole; LEV, levofloxacin; CAZ, ceftazidime; C, chloramphenicol; and MDR, multidrug resistance.

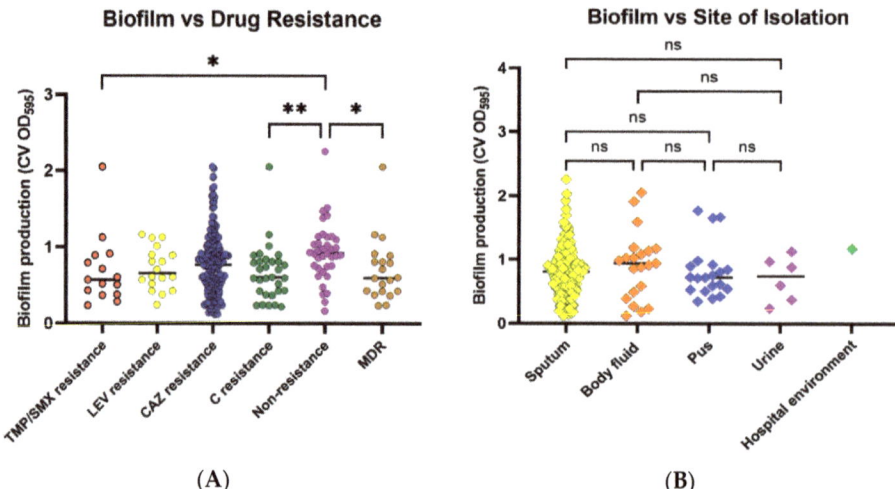

Figure 1. Biofilm formation by *S. maltophilia* isolates. Biofilm formation was evaluated using a crystal violet assay by measuring crystal violet absorbance (CV OD) at 595 nm. Biofilm formation capabilities were investigated among various antibiotic-resistant groups (**A**) and sites of isolation (**B**). Antibiotic-resistant groups included trimethoprim/sulfamethoxazole (TMP/SMX) resistance, levofloxacin (LEV) resistance, ceftazidime (CAZ) resistance, chloramphenicol (C) resistance, nonresistance, and multidrug resistance (MDR). Each symbol showed the mean OD_{595} value with the median line of each distribution. Statistical significance at Fisher's exact test: * $p < 0.05$, ** $p < 0.01$. ns = non-significant.

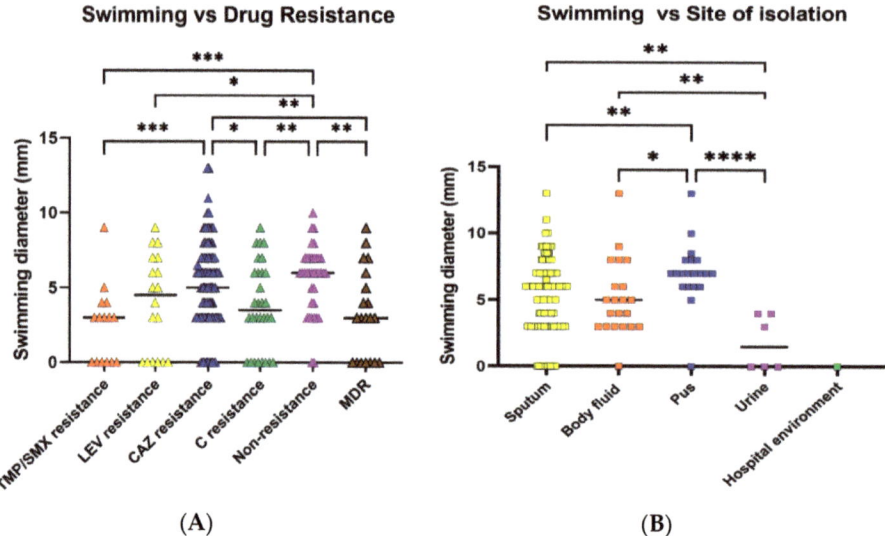

Figure 2. Swimming motility of *S. maltophilia* isolates. Swimming motility was evaluated by measuring the swimming zone diameter in a semi-solid medium (0.3% agar). Swimming efficacies were investigated in various antibiotic-resistant groups (**A**) and sites of isolation (**B**). Each symbol showed the mean swimming diameter with the median line of each distribution. A percentage of isolates belonged to each group. Statistical significance at Fisher's exact test: * $p < 0.05$, ** $p < 0.01$, *** $p < 0.001$, **** $p < 0.0001$.

2.6. Toxin and Enzyme Production

Screening of toxin and enzyme production revealed that all isolates could produce hemolysin after an incubation time of 48 h on a 5% sheep's blood agar plate. In 53% of the isolates (n = 106), a greenish zone appeared around the bacterial colony, indicating that those isolates could produce α-hemolysin, while 94 isolates (47%) could produce β-hemolysin. Protease enzyme was found in 183 of 200 isolates (91.5%), whereas lipase production was observed in 22.5% of isolates (n = 45) after 48 h. Among the various drug resistance patterns, isolates in the majority of groups produced more α-hemolysis than β-hemolysis. Protease-positive isolates were common in all antibiotic resistance groups, while a few isolates produced lipase enzymes (Table 4). There were 21 isolates capable of producing all three enzymes. These isolates were obtained from sputum (17 isolates), fluid (3 isolates), and pus (1 isolate), in that order.

2.7. Correlation of Antibiotic Resistance

The relationship between antibiotic resistance genotypes and phenotypes showed that the presence of *sul1*, *sul2*, *intI1*, and *floR* genes (Figure 3) were positively correlated with each other as shown in high Spearman *r* values. Among antibiotic-resistant groups, C resistance was correlated with TMP/SMX resistance (Spearman *r* = 0.50, *p* < 0.0001) and LEV resistance (Spearman *r* = 0.46, *p* < 0.0001), but not with CAZ resistance (Spearman *r* = 0.01, *p* = 0.0001). Furthermore, a positive correlation was discovered between the presence of drug-resistance genes and antibiotic-resistance properties. TMP/SMX resistance was linked to the presence of *sul1*, *sul2*, *intI1*, and *floR*. Chloramphenicol resistance was also found to be associated with the *sul1* and *intI1* genes.

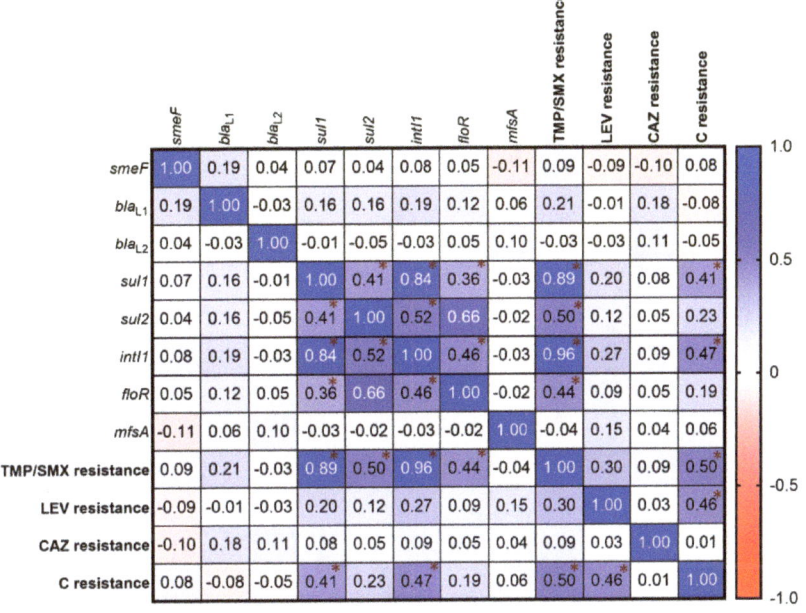

Figure 3. Correlation matrix of *S. maltophilia* antibiotic resistances. The relationships were determined by Spearman correlation coefficients. A heat map shows the Spearman *r* value indicating a correlation between the presence of drug-resistance genes and drug-resistant phenotypes. The gradient of positive and negative values shows a positive correlation (Blue) and a negative correlation (Red). Asterisk (*) shows the *r* value exhibiting the significant correlation. A statistical significance of the correlation was set at *p* < 0.05.

2.8. MLST Analysis and Clonal Complexes

S. maltophilia allelic profiles revealed 141 STs across 200 isolates. The profiles were created using different patterns of allelic numbers at seven different loci. There were 11 STs among 16 isolates; ST3, ST4, ST24, ST27, ST28, ST77, ST91, ST208, ST210, ST212 and ST511 have been reported on database previously. However, 130 STs among 184 isolates were reported for the first time in this study (ST365, ST376, ST605, ST609, ST611, ST613, ST615, ST618-619, ST621, ST626-628, ST631-632, ST634, ST639, ST643-648, ST651, ST656-660, ST663-669, ST671-675, ST678-681, ST684-688, ST692, ST697-698, ST700, ST703-705, ST709, ST713-714, ST718, ST720-721, ST731, ST736-738, ST745, ST748-750, ST752-754, ST756-764, ST766-770, ST773, ST775, ST777, ST780-785, ST788-808, and ST810-818). These 130 new STs and allelic profiles from Thailand have been submitted to PubMLST (https://pubmlst.org/organisms/stenotrophomonas-maltophilia accessed on 7 December 2022). The most common ST was ST619, which was found in six isolates, followed by ST672 and ST749 in five isolates, respectively. Additionally, the ST type of the isolates from the hospital environment (ST793) was similar to the isolate from human fluid in this collection.

Clonal complexes were studied using goeBURST analysis. *S. maltophilia* isolates from this study were classified into six clonal groups, based on the variation of allelic profiles (Figure 4) The six clonal groups exhibited different genotypes and phenotypes. Characteristics of the majority of isolates in each group are shown in Table 5. The population distribution of *S. maltophilia* worldwide was also analyzed as a minimum-spanning tree, using all *S. maltophilia* in the MLST database. *S. maltophilia* from Thailand was distributed in many branches of the tree as shown in Figure 5. *S. maltophilia* isolates from Thailand (e.g., ST646, ST709, ST818) were found to be closely related to *S. maltophilia* from Asian countries such as China, Korea, and Japan (classified in the same branch). Similarly, some of the isolates (e.g., ST365, ST635, ST700, and ST734) are related to those from Europe and America such as isolates from the UK, France, Mexico, and the USA.

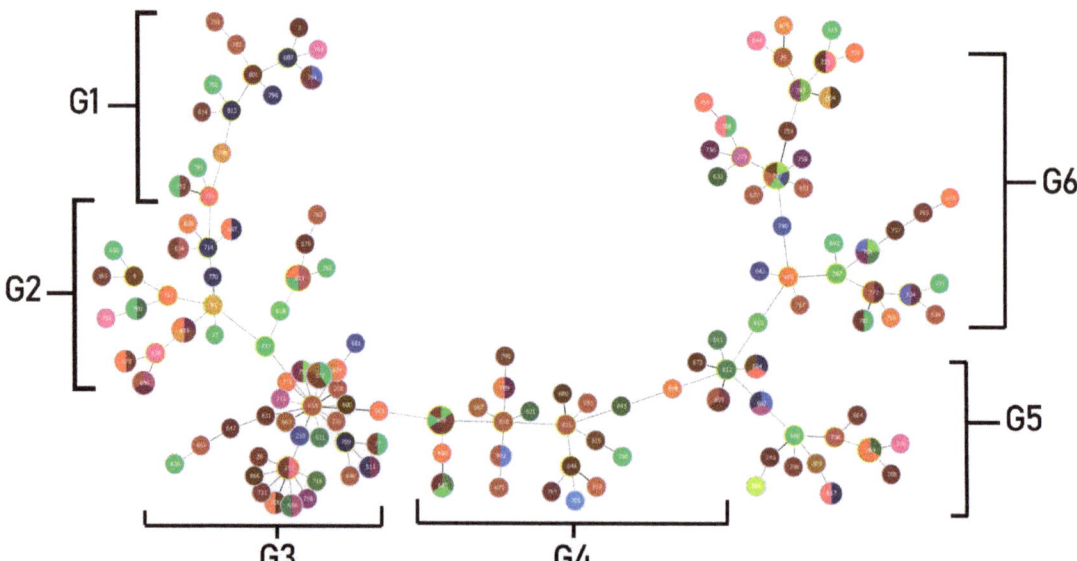

Figure 4. Minimum spanning tree (MST) generated for 200 Thai *S. maltophilia* isolates. The tree was created using PHYLOViZ online software with the goeBURST algorithm. Isolates are represented by different colors and STs are shown in circles. The name of each ST is labeled as the number in the center of the circles. Six clonal complex groups were revealed as G1 (Group 1)–G6 (Group 6).

Table 5. Genotypic and phenotypic characteristics of *S. maltophilia* isolates in each clonal complex.

Clonal * Complex	Sequence Types **	Specimens (Sources of Isolates)	Genotypes and Phenotypes Exhibited by Most of the Isolates				
			Drug [a] Resistance	Drug Resistance [b] Gene	Biofilm Formation	Swimming Motility	Toxin and [c] Enzymes Production
Group 1	3, 761, 762, 748, 750, 752, 753, 785, 796, 801, 807, 813, 814	Sputum, Fluid	1–2 drugs	1–2 genes	Strong producer	Weak swimming	2 types
Group 2	4, 27, 91, 363, 365, 613, 618, 619, 628, 634, 656, 660, 678, 686, 687, 697, 714, 737, 760, 770, 784	Sputum, Fluid, Pus, Urine	2–4 drugs	2–4 genes	Moderate and strong producer	Weak to moderate swimming	2 types
Group 3	28, 208, 212, 624, 626, 631, 647, 657, 658, 663, 665, 666, 668, 681, 700, 718, 720, 731, 738, 775, 791	Sputum, Fluid, Pus, Urine	1–3 drugs	0–5 genes (most isolates contained 2 genes)	Strong producer	Weak swimming	2 types
Group 4	621, 645, 648, 659, 667, 671, 673, 680, 685, 688, 697, 698, 705, 764, 789, 795, 802, 803, 808, 811, 812, 816, 818	Sputum, Fluid, Pus, Urine	0–1 drug	1 gene	Strong producer (All isolates)	Moderate swimming	2 types
Group 5	367, 605, 609, 627, 632, 643, 651, 692, 749, 754, 756, 757, 758, 759, 763, 766, 767, 773, 777, 781, 788, 790, 799, 810	Sputum, Fluid, Pus	1 drug	2 genes	Strong producer	Moderate to strong swimming	3 types
Group 6	376, 664, 669, 736, 745, 768, 769, 798, 805, 806, 817	Sputum, Fluid, Pus	1 drug	1 gene	Strong producer (All isolates)	Weak, moderate and strong (found in similar rate)	2–3 types

* Six clonal complex groups of *S. maltophilia* Thai isolates were classified using PHYLOViZ software; ** *S. maltophilia* STs belong to six clonal complex groups; [a] Number of drug resistance property; [b] Number of drug resistance genes; [c] Number of toxin and enzymes which were produced by each group.

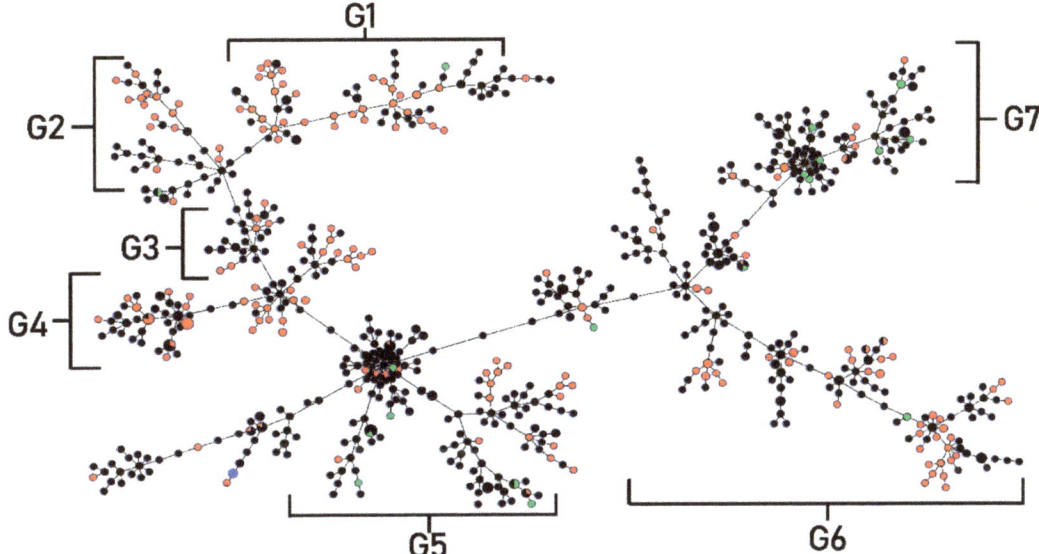

Figure 5. Phylogenetic tree of global *S. maltophilia* isolates based on MLST allelic profile variation. The minimal spanning tree was created using PHYLOViZ online software with the goeBURST algorithm and the analysis considered 995 isolates reported in the *S. maltophilia* MLST database. The population distribution of the isolates worldwide is shown. Countries are shown in different colors and STs in each circle. Isolates from Thailand are represented by pink circles and are distributed all around the branches of the tree.

3. Discussion

S. maltophilia infection has become an important, emerging opportunistic pathogen, which has been increasingly reported worldwide [13]. Thailand also has reported a large number of *S. maltophilia* infections, but the characterization of this pathogen of concern is rarely found [24].

In this study, 200 *S. maltophilia* isolates were collected from Maharaj Nakorn Chiang Mai Hospital, Thailand during six months of collection. Most of the isolates were collected from sputum. The collection of isolates in a short period of time indicates that the incidence of *S. maltophilia* respiratory tract infections in Thailand is high compared to other regions of the world [25,27–32].

The clinical information showed that male and elderly patients were more susceptible to *S. maltophilia* infection, frequently distributed in the general medicine ward. The majority of isolates were from hospitalized patients who suffered from underlying illnesses associated with invasive procedures. The patients with respiratory tract infections exhibited a higher proportion of risk factors than non-respiratory tract infection patients. The retrospective studies from China and the USA also reported demographic and clinical characteristics of *S. maltophilia* infection, similar to this study [33,34]. These findings should serve as a reminder to clinicians to focus more on *S. maltophilia* infection control in specific population groups [33]. However, the isolates from this study were collected at the high prevalence period, however, the obtained data were not up to date. The efficient strategy of infection control should be carried out together with the information from the recent isolates in further study.

Antibiotic susceptibility revealed that the high resistance incidence to CAZ of Thai *S. maltophilia* was distinguished, compared to the global trend [35]. Although TMP/SMX is the current drug of choice for *S. maltophilia* treatment with a high sensitivity (79–96%), the resistance has been raised worldwide (30–48%) [16,36–39]. The isolates of our study showed a similar rate of TMP/SMX resistance to those of global isolates [34]. Minocycline is the most active antibiotic against the isolates from our study and another geological region of Thailand and China [33,40].

It must be noted that our *S. maltophilia* isolates from urinary tract infections are highly resistant to antibiotics compared to isolates from other specimen sources, which is similar to a study by Hamdi et al. from Minnesota, USA [41]. According to antibiotic susceptibility patterns, there were six antibiotypes in which isolates with TMP/SMX and LEV resistance appeared to have MDR phenotypes in higher proportion than isolates with C and CAZ resistances. This result was consistent with the study of Zhao et al., which found that TMP/SMX resistance was a signal of multidrug resistance [42].

Numerous molecular processes contribute to *S. maltophilia*'s widespread antibiotic resistance. The *smeDEF* genes are an efflux pump encoding protein complex of *S. maltophilia*, that are involved in quinolones, chloramphenicol, and tetracyclines resistances [5]. In our findings, *smeF* was the most common gene (91.5%) among our collection of isolates, of which 89% of them were LEV and C resistance. The bla_{L1} gene, a Zn^{2+}-dependent metalloenzyme that can hydrolyze β-lactams [43], was found in 43% of isolates, and most of them (78.34%) were resistant to CAZ, suggesting that the role of the bla_{L1} gene is contributing to β-lactam resistance of this *S. maltophilia* collection. Meanwhile, bla_{L2} (a serine active-site cephalosporinase [43]) showed a less important role in CAZ resistance similar to other collections of southern Thailand and Iran [25,44]. Our findings showed that *sul1* and *intI1* were detected in six percent and seven percent of isolates, respectively. All of the *sul1* and *intI1* positive isolates were resistant to TMP/SMX, indicating that TMP/SMX resistance was mediated by *sul1* and class one integron integrase genes [45,46]. Bostanghadiri et al. similarly found a higher rate of *sul1*-positive strains among isolates from Iran [44]. In addition, the Florfenicol/chloramphenicol resistance gene, *floR*, and a major facilitator superfamily (MFS) of the efflux pump gene, *mfsA* could also be detected in eight and eight point five percent of *S. maltophilia* collection. The correlation analysis revealed that *sul1*, *sul2*,

IntI1, and *floR* genes are positively correlated to each other and involved with TMP/SMX resistant phenotypes, similar to a prior study from Nigeria [47].

Among *S. maltophilia* virulence factors, biofilm plays an important role in the survivability and virulence of many bacteria, as is found in *S. maltophilia*. In this study, all *S. maltophilia* isolates were able to produce biofilm and most of them were strong biofilm producers (73.0%). Interestingly, the nonresistance showed significantly higher level of biofilm formation compared to the other groups. There were similar findings in 2020, which found that non-MDR *S. maltophilia* exhibited higher biofilm formation capacity compared to MDR phenotypes [48]. This suggested that biofilm-forming *S. maltophilia* isolates depended less frequently on antibiotic resistance for survival as those isolates do not need the biologically costly expression of antibiotic resistance to survive in an environment, such as a hospital setting [48].

In the study of motility, most of the isolates exhibited weak or moderate levels of swimming phenotypes, however, none of the isolates were able to swarm, which is similar to some other studies [49,50]. Surprisingly, *S. maltophilia* isolates from urine exhibited significantly less swimming capability than isolates from other sources. This incidence may be affected by the different densities of biological environments, in which, the bacterium swims faster in a suspension with more viscosity (e.g., sputum, pus, and body fluid) [51]. Moreover, the transitions between motility and adherent state were found in UTI-causing bacteria which helped the improved colonization of bacteria to the upper urinary tract [52]. In our study, all *S. maltophilia* isolates could produce hemolysin, and α-hemolysin was frequently detected, while most of the isolates in our collection were able to produce protease (91.5%), whereas the number of lipase-producing isolates were found in a lower proportion of isolates (22.5%).

The study of the genetic relationship and MLST analysis in *S. maltophilia* isolates from Chiang Mai, Thailand showed high diversity in allelic profiles. The majority of isolates contained new allelic sequences that have never been reported before. We submitted to an international database and reported 130 novel STs. This study also found 11 STs that were previously reported in the studies from Japan, Korea, and Germany [5,19,53], especially ST77, which was distributed widely throughout the world. The MLST profiles of *S. maltophilia* from several countries even in the recent study from Iran were similar to this study in terms of the great diversity of STs in a single hospital [44,54,55].

Moreover, our study included one isolate from a hospital environment, and this isolate belongs to ST739, which is the same ST as the one isolate from a human patient. This incidence supported the study of Gideskog et al. which found the clonal relationship between isolates from patients and hospital settings, which help them achieve infection control by replacing contaminated devices [56]. The *S. maltophilia* outbreak most likely depended on the environmental spread and further study of the genetic relationship between isolates from specimens and hospital environments is required to promote an understanding of the *S. maltophilia* hospital outbreak and control the infection.

From genetic population analysis of global *S. maltophilia*, seven major clonal complexes exhibited that *S. maltophilia* from Thailand was closely related to *S. maltophilia* from other countries such as China, South Korea, Japan, and the USA. Interestingly, Thai isolates were dominant and found as founders in some branches of clonal complexes which were considered to be ancestors and a reservoir of *S. maltophilia*. However, this assumption needs to be confirmed with genetic population data of a larger number of *S. maltophilia* from Thailand. The clonal complex analysis of Thai isolates identified six major different groups based on different allelic sequences and multilocus variants. Each group carried different antibiotic resistance genes and exhibited different phenotypes. Therefore, there was no association between genetic lineages and *S. maltophilia* phenotypes. Similarly, the novel STs had been identified from a previous study and they also found differences in resistance and virulence genes in their collection [57]. The association of clonal complex and particular specimens of isolation were not observed, except the isolates from urine which were found in the same clonal complex and correlated with the MDR phenotype.

There are a number of limitations to this study. In order to understand the epidemiology of *S. maltophilia* isolates in hospitals and implement infection control strategies, additional studies that include more recent isolates and environmental sampling are required. Moreover, additional epidemiological multicenter studies in Thailand with extended surveillance are required to better characterize the prevalence and spread of nosocomial infections linked to *S. maltophilia*.

4. Materials and Methods

4.1. Bacterial Collection, Culture, and Clinical Information

S. maltophilia isolates were randomly collected from the Microbiology Unit, Diagnostic Laboratory, Maharaj Nakorn Chiang Mai Hospital, Chiang Mai, Thailand for six months, from October 2015 to March 2016. This collection included clinical isolates which were isolated from various patient specimens and environmental isolate which was collected from a hospital environment. Each isolate was collected per one patient or one environmental sample and must be the dominant bacteria with significant numbers, not a contaminant. All the isolates were identified by a microbiology unit, and diagnostic laboratory using mass spectrometry (MALDI Biotyper®, Bruker Corp., Billerica, MA, USA). Bacterial isolates were cultured on Luria Bertani (LB) agar and incubated overnight at 37 °C. Bacterial stocks are preserved at −80 °C in LB broth containing 20% skimmed milk. This study used *Escherichia coli* ATCC 25922, *Pseudomonas aeruginosa* ATCC 27853, and *Proteus mirabilis* FL118 as control strains. Additionally, demographic information and clinical characteristics including age, gender, underlying diseases, comorbidities, predisposing factors, hospitalization, and medical wards of 192 included patients from our collection were recorded.

4.2. Species Confirmation by 23S rRNA PCR

Total DNA was extracted from each isolate by using a Thermo Scientific™ GnenJET nucleic acid purification kit (Thermo Fisher Scientific Inc., Waltham, MA, USA) according to the instruction of the manufacturer. All *S. maltophilia* isolates in this study were confirmed by PCR using specific primers to the 23S rRNA encoding gene (Forward primer: 5′ GCTGGATTGGTTCTAGGAAAACGC 3′; Reverse primer: 5′ ACGCAGTCACTCCTTGCG 3′). Twenty microliters of PCR reaction total volume contains 10 μL of 2X master mix solution (iNtRON Biotechnology Inc., Burlington, MA, USA), 5 μM of each primer condition, and 100 ng of DNA template. Amplification was performed as previously described [58].

4.3. Antibiotic Susceptibility

Antimicrobial susceptibility testing of *S. maltophilia* was determined by minimal inhibitory concentration (MIC) using the agar dilution method and MIC test strip. Four antibiotics including levofloxacin (LEV), ceftazidime (CAZ), chloramphenicol (C), and minocycline (MN) were tested by agar dilution. *S. maltophilia* colony suspension was prepared and adjusted equivalent to McFarland no. 0.5 before diluting 1:10 and inoculating on antibiotic-contained MHA using a multipoint inoculator. MIC of TMP/SMX was determined by MIC test strip (TMP/SMX = 1/19, 0.002–32 μg/mL) (Liofilchem s.r.l., Abruzzo, Italy). The bacterial suspension was similarly prepared as agar dilution and was swabbed onto an MHA plate (no drug). *E. coli* ATCC 25922 and *P. aeruginosa* ATCC 27853 were used as quality control strains and the results were interpreted according to Clinical and Laboratory Standards Institute (CLSI) guidelines [26]. Isolates resistant to at least three antibiotics were considered MDR [59,60].

4.4. Detection of Drug Resistance Genes

PCR assays were used to detect eight antibiotic resistance genes, including bla_{L1}/bla_{L2} genes, *smeF*, *sul1/sul2*, *IntI1*, *floR*, and *mfsA*. All primers used are listed in Supplementary Table S2 [25,30,50,61–65]. The PCR reaction and conditions were carried out as previously described [25]. The amplicons were detected and visualized under ultraviolet light using a 1.5% agarose gel stained with Redsafe (iNtRON Biotechnology Inc., MA, USA).

4.5. Biofilm Formation Assay

Overnight culture of *S. maltophilia* in a tryptic soy broth (TSB) at 37 °C was diluted at 100-fold dilution and was transferred into a 96-well plate. After washing and removing bacterial planktonic cells by PBS, the plate was heat fixed at 60 °C for 15 min and stained with 0.1% crystal violet for 5 min. After that, the plate was rinsed three times with water and then 30% acetic acid was added to dissolve the dyed pellet. Biofilm formation capability was observed by measuring optical density (OD) at 595 nanometers. Their observed optical density was classified as follows: no biofilm producer (OD ≤ OD negative control (ODc); weak biofilm producer (ODc ≤ OD ≤ 2 × ODc); moderate biofilm producer (2 × ODc ≤ OD ≤ 4 × ODc); and as a strong biofilm producer (OD > 4 × ODc). The negative controls were wells that contained culture medium alone. *P. aeruginosa* ATCC 27853 was used as a positive control for biofilm production [66].

4.6. Motility Test

Ten microliters of bacterial overnight culture in TSB were dropped and stabbed into a swimming medium (containing 10 g/L tryptone, 5 g/L NaCl, 3 g/L agar) and dropped on a swarming medium (containing 8 g/L nutrient broth, 5 g/L). As for the interpretation of the swarming test, a positive result was observed by a transparent growth zone appearing around a bacterial colony. The swimming zones on media were measured in millimeters (mm) and classified by the following criteria: no swimming motility (<3 mm); weak swimming motility (3–5 mm); moderate swimming motility (6–8 mm); and strong swimming motility (≥9 mm) [67]. Positive control strains for these swimming and swarming tests were *E. coli* ATCC 25922 and *P. mirabilis* FL118.

4.7. Screening of Toxin and Enzymes Production

Production of toxins and enzymes by *S. maltophilia* was determined as previously described [50]. The isolates were streaked on agar media containing substrates for each enzyme. To test protease enzyme production, the bacterium was inoculated on Mueller Hinton (MH) agar containing 3% skimmed milk and incubated at 37 °C. At 24 h of incubation, the clear zone around the colonies was observed from isolates that could produce protease.

S. maltophilia isolates were inoculated on Tryptic Soy (TS) agar containing 1% tween 80, the lipase substrate, and incubated at 37 °C to detect lipase activity. At 48 h, the appearance of a turbid halo zone around colonies indicated a positive outcome. The isolate was streaked on 5% sheep blood agar and incubated at 37 °C for 48 h to detect hemolytic activity. Positive results were seen for β-hemolysin producers when a transparent zone appeared around colonies, and for α-hemolysin producers when a greenish zone appeared around colonies [68].

4.8. Multi-Locus Sequence Typing (MLST) Analysis

MLST analysis of *S. maltophilia* was performed as previously described by Kaiser et al. [19]. The alleles at each of the seven loci defined the allelic profile or ST. PCR was performed on *S. maltophilia* isolates using specific primers to seven housekeeping genes, namely, *atpD*, *gapA*, *guaA*, *mutM*, *nuoD*, *ppsA*, and *recA*. The primer sequences and PCR condition was set as described by Kaiser et al. PCR products were purified using a Thermo Scientific GeneJET PCR Purification Kit (Thermo Fisher Scientific Inc., MA, USA) and were sequenced. The nucleotide sequences of seven housekeeping genes were compared to the reference sequences on the PubMLST database (https://pubmlst.org/smaltophilia/: accessed on 16 October 2017) for identifying the allelic number of each locus and the classifying STs.

4.9. Statistical Analysis

Each microbiological assay was performed at least in duplicate and repeated three times. Mean ± SD was used for the continuous variables. The statistical significance of the difference between groups of the test was calculated by one-way ANOVA and Fisher's exact test. Continuous variables from demographic and clinical data were analyzed using a Student's *t* test or the Mann–Whitney *U* test. Correlation analyses were determined by the Spearman test. All statistical tests and graphs were evaluated by GraphPad Prism version 9.1.1. The statistical significance was considered when $p < 0.05$. For genetic population and clonal complex analysis, all given STs were classified into clonal groups by PHYLOViZ software version 2.0 (https://online.phyloviz.net/index: accessed on 23 April 2018), based on the goeBURST algorithm.

5. Conclusions

This study revealed demographic, genotypic, and phenotypic characteristics of *S. maltophilia* isolates from a Northern Thailand hospital during the period of the highest prevalence. Infection with *S. maltophilia* can occur in hospitalized patients with a variety of comorbidities and risk factors. We underline a high degree of genetic diversity among the isolates and this is the first report on numerous novel STs of *S. maltophilia* collection in Thailand. Most of the isolates carried many drug-resistance genes and showed a highly resistant rate to several antibiotics, especially, the isolates that were resistant to the drug of choice (TMP/SMX), exhibited MDR phenotype, and also produced various virulence factors. *S. maltophilia* isolates of Thailand were found to be genetically related to *S. maltophilia* from other countries, of which Thai isolates were dominant and found to be a founder. The data obtained from this study contribute to a better understanding of *S. maltophilia* characteristics in Thailand, which is necessary for *S. maltophilia* infection control and prevention.

Supplementary Materials: The following supporting information can be downloaded at: https://www.mdpi.com/article/10.3390/antibiotics12020410/s1, Table S1: MDR and non-MDR phenotypes of *S. maltophilia* isolates. Table S2: Primer pairs used in the detection of antibiotic resistance genes among *S. maltophilia* isolates. References [25,30,50,64–68] are cited in the supplementary materials.

Author Contributions: Conceptualization, O.Y. and K.D.; methodology, O.Y. and K.D.; software, O.Y.; validation, O.Y., K.D., and M.D.; formal analysis, K.D.; investigation, O.Y. and K.D.; resources, K.D.; data curation, O.Y. and K.D.; writing—original draft preparation, O.Y. and K.D.; writing—review and editing, O.Y.; visualization, O.Y., M.D., and K.D.; supervision, K.D.; project administration, K.D.; funding acquisition, K.D. All authors have read and agreed to the published version of the manuscript.

Funding: This research was funded by the National Research Council of Thailand and the Faculty of Medicine, Chiang Mai University grant no 153-2562 PD10/2559.

Institutional Review Board Statement: Not applicable.

Informed Consent Statement: Not applicable.

Data Availability Statement: The new allele types and new sequence types of *S. maltophilia* in the present study were deposited in PubMLST: https://pubmlst.org/organisms/stenotrophomonas-maltophilia accessed on 7 December 2022.

Acknowledgments: The authors would like to express our appreciation to Banyong Kantawa from the Diagnostic Laboratory of Maharaj Nakorn Chiang Mai Hospital who provided an *S. maltophilia* collection. We give special thanks to the curator of the MLST database for assigning our new sequence types.

Conflicts of Interest: The funders had no role in the design of the study; in the collection, analyses, or interpretation of data; in the writing of the manuscript; or in the decision to publish the results.

References

1. Adegoke, A.A.; Stenström, T.A.; Okoh, A.I. *Stenotrophomonas maltophilia* as an emerging ubiquitous pathogen: Looking beyond contemporary antibiotic therapy. *Front. Microbiol.* **2017**, *8*, 2276. [CrossRef] [PubMed]
2. Singhal, L.; Kaur, P.; Gautam, V. *Stenotrophomonas maltophilia*: From trivial to grievous. *Indian J. Med. Microbiol.* **2017**, *35*, 469–479. [CrossRef] [PubMed]
3. Looney, W.J.; Narita, M.; Mühlemann, K. *Stenotrophomonas maltophilia*: An emerging opportunist human pathogen. *Lancet Infect. Dis.* **2009**, *9*, 312–323. [CrossRef]

4. Caylan, R.; Kaklikkaya, N.; Aydin, K.; Aydin, F.; Yilmaz, G.; Ozgumus, B.; Koksal, I. An epidemiological analysis of *Stenotrophomonas maltophilia* strains in a university hospital. *Jpn. J. Infect. Dis.* **2004**, *57*, 37–40. [PubMed]
5. Chang, Y.T.; Lin, C.Y.; Chen, Y.H.; Hsueh, P.R. Update on infections caused by *Stenotrophomonas maltophilia* with particular attention to resistance mechanisms and therapeutic options. *Front. Microbiol.* **2015**, *6*, 893. [CrossRef]
6. Gajdács, M.; Urbán, E. Prevalence and Antibiotic Resistance of *Stenotrophomonas maltophilia* in Respiratory Tract Samples: A 10-Year Epidemiological Snapshot. *Health Serv. Res. Manag. Epidemiol.* **2019**, *6*, 2333392819870774. [CrossRef]
7. Mojica, M.F.; Humphries, R.; Lipuma, J.J.; Mathers, A.J.; Rao, G.G.; Shelburne, S.A.; Fouts, D.E.; Van Duin, D.; Bonomo, R.A. Clinical challenges treating *Stenotrophomonas maltophilia* infections: An update. *JAC Antimicrob. Resist.* **2022**, *4*, dlac040. [CrossRef]
8. Looney, W.J. Role of *Stenotrophomonas maltophilia* in hospital-acquired infection. *Br. J. Biomed. Sci.* **2005**, *62*, 145–154. [CrossRef]
9. Guyot, A.; Turton, J.F.; Garner, D. Outbreak of *Stenotrophomonas maltophilia* on an intensive care unit. *J. Hosp. Infect.* **2013**, *85*, 303–307. [CrossRef]
10. Cervia, S.J.; Ortolano, A.G.; Canonica, P.F. Hospital tap water as a source of *Stenotrophomonas maltophilia* infection. *Clin. Infect. Dis.* **2008**, *46*, 1485–1487. [CrossRef]
11. Trifonova, A.; Strateva, T. *Stenotrophomonas maltophilia*—A low-grade pathogen with numerous virulence factors. *Infect. Dis.* **2019**, *51*, 168–178. [CrossRef]
12. de Oliveira-Garcia, D.; Dall'Agnol, M.; Rosales, M.; Azzuz, A.C.; Alcántara, N.; Martinez, M.B.; Girón, J.A. Fimbriae and adherence of *Stenotrophomonas maltophilia* to epithelial cells and to abiotic surfaces. *Cell Microbiol.* **2003**, *5*, 625–636. [CrossRef]
13. Brooke, J.S. Advances in the Microbiology of *Stenotrophomonas maltophilia*. *Clin. Microbiol. Rev.* **2021**, *34*, e0003019. [CrossRef] [PubMed]
14. Igbinosa, E.O.; Oviasogie, F.E. Multiple antibiotics resistant among environmental isolates of *Stenotrophomonas maltophilia*. *J. Appl. Sci. Environ. Manag.* **2014**, *18*, 255–261. [CrossRef]
15. Kwa, A.L.; Low, J.G.; Lim, T.P.; Leow, P.C.; Kurup, A.; Tam, V.H. Independent predictors for mortality in patients with positive *Stenotrophomonas maltophilia* cultures. *Ann. Acad. Med. Singap.* **2008**, *37*, 826–830. [CrossRef]
16. Gibb, J.; Wong, D.W. Antimicrobial Treatment Strategies for *Stenotrophomonas maltophilia*: A Focus on Novel Therapies. *Antibiotics* **2021**, *10*, 1226. [CrossRef] [PubMed]
17. Gherardi, G.; Creti, R.; Pompilio, A.; Di Bonaventura, G. An overview of various typing methods for clinical epidemiology of the emerging pathogen *Stenothophomonas maltophilia*. *Diagn. Microbiol. Infect. Dis.* **2015**, *81*, 219–226. [CrossRef] [PubMed]
18. Maiden, M.C.; Bygraves, J.A.; Feil, E.; Morelli, G.; Russell, J.E.; Urwin, R.; Zhang, Q.; Zhou, J.; Zurth, K.; Caugant, D.A.; et al. Multilocus sequence typing: A portable approach to the identification of clones within populations of pathogenic microorganisms. *Proc. Natl. Acad. Sci. USA* **1998**, *95*, 3140–3145. [CrossRef]
19. Kaiser, S.; Biehler, K.; Jonas, D.A. A *Stenotrophomonas maltophilia* multilocus sequence typing scheme for inferring population structure. *J. Bacteriol.* **2009**, *191*, 2934–2943. [CrossRef]
20. Zając, O.M.; Tyski, S.; Laudy, A.E. Phenotypic and Molecular Characteristics of the MDR Efflux Pump Gene-Carrying *Stenotrophomonas maltophilia* Strains Isolated in Warsaw, Poland. *Biology* **2022**, *11*, 105. [CrossRef]
21. Crossman, L.C.; Gould, V.C.; Dow, J.M.; Vernikos, G.S.; Okazaki, A.; Sebaihia, M.; Saunders, D.; Arrowsmith, C.; Carver, T.; Peters, N.; et al. The complete genome, comparative and functional analysis of *Stenotrophomonas maltophilia* reveals an organism heavily shielded by drug resistance determinants. *Genome Biol.* **2008**, *9*, R74. [CrossRef] [PubMed]
22. Ryan, R.; Monchy, S.; Cardinale, M.; Taghavi, S.; Crossman, L.; Avison, B.M.; Berg, G.; van der Lelie, D.; Dow, J.M. The versatility and adaptation of bacteria from the genus *Stenotrophomonas*. *Nat. Rev. Microbiol.* **2009**, *7*, 514–525. [CrossRef] [PubMed]
23. Gil-Gil, T.; Martínez, J.L.; Blanco, P. Mechanisms of antimicrobial resistance in *Stenotrophomonas maltophilia*: A review of current knowledge. *Expert Rev. Anti. Infect. Ther.* **2020**, *18*, 335–347. [CrossRef]
24. Diagnostic Laboratory, Maharaj Nakorn Chiang Mai Hospital. Antibiotic Susceptibility Testing Summary Report of Important Organisms from Wards. 2016. Available online: https://www.med.cmu.ac.th/hospital/lab/2011/index.php?option=com_content&view=article&layout=edit&id=87 (accessed on 3 June 2017).
25. Paopradit, P.; Srinitiwarawong, K.; Ingviya, N.; Singkhamanan, K.; Vuddhakul, V. Distribution and characterization of *Stenotrophomonas maltophilia* isolates from environmental and clinical samples in Thailand. *J. Hosp. Infect.* **2017**, *97*, 185–191. [CrossRef] [PubMed]
26. CLSI. *Performance Standards for Antimicrobial Susceptibility Testing*, 29th ed.; CLSI Supplement M100; Clinical and Laboratory Standards Institute: Wayne, PA, USA, 2019.
27. Neela, V.; Rankouhi, S.Z.; van Belkum, A.; Goering, R.V.; Awang, R. *Stenotrophomonas maltophilia* in Malaysia: Molecular epidemiology and trimethoprim-sulfamethoxazole resistance. *Int. J. Infect. Dis.* **2012**, *16*, 603–607. [CrossRef]
28. Jia, W.; Wang, J.; Xu, H.; Li, G. Resistance of *Stenotrophomonas maltophilia* to fluoroquinolones: Prevalence in a university hospital and possible mechanisms. *Int. J. Environ. Res. Public Health* **2015**, *12*, 5177–5195. [CrossRef]
29. Gallo, S.W.; Figueiredo, T.P.; Bessa, M.C.; Pagnussatti, V.E.; Ferreira, C.A.; Oliveira, S.D. Isolation and characterization of *Stenotrophomonas maltophilia* isolates from a brazilian hospital. *Microb. Drug Resist.* **2016**, *22*, 688–695. [CrossRef]
30. Waters, V.; Atenafu, E.G.; Lu, A.; Yau, Y.; Tullis, E.; Ratjen, F. Chronic *Stenotrophomonas maltophilia* infection and mortality or lung transplantation in cystic fibrosis patients. *J. Cyst. Fibros.* **2013**, *12*, 482–486. [CrossRef]

31. Herrera-Heredia, S.A.; Pezina-Cantú, C.; Garza-González, E.; Bocanegra-Ibarias, P.; Mendoza-Olazarán, S.; Morfín-Otero, R.; Camacho-Ortiz, A.; Villarreal-Treviño, L.; Rodríguez-Noriega, E.; Paláu-Davila, L.; et al. Risk factors and molecular mechanisms associated with trimethoprim-sulfamethoxazole resistance in *Stenotrophomonas maltophilia* in Mexico. *J. Med. Microbiol.* **2017**, *66*, 1102–1109. [CrossRef]

32. Gülmez, D.; Hasçelik, G. *Stenotrophomonas maltophilia*: Antimicrobial resistance and molecular typing of an emerging pathogen in a Turkish university hospital. *Clin. Microbiol. Infect.* **2005**, *11*, 880–886. [CrossRef]

33. Duan, Z.; Qin, J.; Liu, Y.; Li, C.; Ying, C. Molecular epidemiology and risk factors of *Stenotrophomonas maltophilia* infections in a Chinese teaching hospital. *BMC Microbiol.* **2020**, *20*, 294. [CrossRef]

34. Samonis, G.; Karageorgopoulos, D.E.; Maraki, S.; Levis, P.; Dimopoulou, D.; Spernovasilis, N.A.; Kofteridis, D.P.; Falagas, M.E. *Stenotrophomonas maltophilia* infections in a general hospital: Patient characteristics, antimicrobial susceptibility, and treatment outcome. *PLoS ONE* **2012**, *7*, e37375. [CrossRef]

35. Farrell, D.J.; Sader, H.S.; Jones, R.N. Antimicrobial susceptibilities of a worldwide collection of *Stenotrophomonas maltophilia* isolates tested against tigecycline and agents commonly used for *S. maltophilia* infections. *Antimicrob. Agents Chemother.* **2010**, *54*, 2735–2737. [CrossRef]

36. Rhee, J.Y.; Choi, J.Y.; Choi, M.J.; Song, J.H.; Peck, K.R.; Ko, K.S. Distinct groups and antimicrobial resistance of clinical *Stenotrophomonas maltophilia* complex isolates from Korea. *J. Med. Microbiol.* **2013**, *62*, 748–753. [CrossRef]

37. Wu, H.; Wang, J.T.; Shiau, Y.R.; Wang, H.Y.; Lauderdale, T.L.; Chang, S.C.; TSAR Hospitals. A multicenter surveillance of antimicrobial resistance on *Stenotrophomonas maltophilia* in Taiwan. *J. Microbiol. Immunol. Infect.* **2012**, *45*, 120–126. [CrossRef] [PubMed]

38. Hu, L.F.; Gao, L.P.; Ye, Y.; Chen, X.; Zhou, X.T.; Yang, H.F.; Liiu, Y.Y.; Mei, Q.; Li, J.B. Susceptibility of *Stenotrophomonas maltophilia* clinical strains in China to antimicrobial combinations. *J. Chemother.* **2014**, *26*, 282–286. [CrossRef]

39. Çalışkan, A.; Çopur Çicek, A.; Aydogan Ejder, N.; Karagöz, A.; Kirişc, İ.Ö.; Kılıç, S. The Antibiotic sensitivity of *Stenotrophomonas maltophilia* in a 5-year period and investigation of clonal outbreak with PFGE. *J. Infect. Dev. Ctries.* **2019**, *13*, 634–639. [CrossRef] [PubMed]

40. Insuwanno, W.; Kiratisin, P.; Jitmuang, A. *Stenotrophomonas maltophilia* infections: Clinical characteristics and factors associated with mortality of hospitalized patients. *Infect. Drug Resist.* **2020**, *13*, 1559–1566. [CrossRef]

41. Hamdi, A.M.; Fida, M.; Abu Saleh, O.M.; Beam, E. *Stenotrophomonas* bacteremia antibiotic susceptibility and prognostic determinants: Mayo Clinic 10-year experience. *Open Forum Infect. Dis.* **2020**, *7*, ofaa008. [CrossRef] [PubMed]

42. Zhao, S.; Yang, L.; Liu, H.; Gao, F. *Stenotrophomonas maltophilia* in a university hospital of traditional Chinese medicine: Molecular epidemiology and antimicrobial resistance. *J. Hosp. Infect.* **2017**, *96*, 286–289. [CrossRef]

43. Avison, M.B.; Higgins, C.S.; von Heldreich, C.J.; Bennett, P.M.; Walsh, T.R. Plasmid location and molecular heterogeneity of the L1 and L2 β-lactamase genes of *Stenotrophomonas maltophilia*. *Antimicrob. Agents Chemother.* **2001**, *45*, 413–419. [CrossRef] [PubMed]

44. Bostanghadiri, N.; Ghalavand, Z.; Fallah, F.; Yadegar, A.; Ardebili, A.; Tarashi, S.; Pournajaf, A.; Mardaneh, J.; Shams, S.; Hashemi, A. Characterization of phenotypic and genotypic diversity of *Stenotrophomonas maltophilia* strains isolated from selected hospitals in Iran. *Front. Microbiol.* **2019**, *29*, 1191. [CrossRef] [PubMed]

45. Kaur, P.; Gautam, V.; Tewari, R. Distribution of class 1 integrons, *sul1* and *sul2* genes among clinical isolates of *Stenotrophomonas maltophilia* from a tertiary care hospital in North India. *Microb. Drug Resist.* **2015**, *21*, 380–385. [CrossRef] [PubMed]

46. Le, T.H.; Ng, C.; Chen, H.; Yi, X.Z.; Koh, T.H.; Barkham, T.M.; Zhou, Z.; Gin, K.Y. Occurrences and Characterization of Antibiotic-Resistant Bacteria and Genetic Determinants of Hospital Wastewater in a Tropical Country. *Antimicrob. Agents Chemother.* **2016**, *60*, 7449–7456. [CrossRef]

47. Adelowo, O.O.; Osuntade, A.I. Class 1 Integron, Sulfonamide and Florfenicol Resistance Genes in Bacteria from Three Unsanitary Landfills, Ibadan, Nigeria. *J. Microbiol. Infect. Dis.* **2019**, *9*, 34–42. [CrossRef]

48. Pompilio, A.; Ranalli, M.; Piccirilli, A.; Perilli, M.; Vukovic, D.; Savic, B.; Krutova, M.; Drevinek, P.; Jonas, D.; Fiscarelli, E.V.; et al. Biofilm formation among *Stenotrophomonas maltophilia* isolates has clinical relevance: The ANSELM prospective multicenter study. *Microorganisms* **2020**, *9*, 49. [CrossRef] [PubMed]

49. Pompilio, A.; Crocetta, V.; Ghosh, D.; Chakrabarti, M.; Gherardi, G.; Vitali, L.A.; Fiscarelli, E.; Di Bonaventura, G. *Stenotrophomonas maltophilia* phenotypic and genotypic diversity during a 10-year colonization in the lungs of a cystic fibrosis patient. *Front. Microbiol.* **2016**, *7*, 1551. [CrossRef] [PubMed]

50. Tanimoto, K. *Stenotrophomonas maltophilia* strains isolated from a university hospital in Japan: Genomic variability and antibiotic resistance. *J. Med. Microbiol.* **2013**, *62*, 565–570. [CrossRef]

51. Zöttl, A.; Yeomans, J.M. Enhanced bacterial swimming speeds in macromolecular polymer solutions. *Nat. Phys.* **2019**, *15*, 554–558. [CrossRef]

52. Luterbach, C.L.; Mobley, H. Cross talk between MarR-like transcription factors coordinates the regulation of motility in uropathogenic *Escherichia coli*. *Infect. Immun.* **2018**, *86*, e00338-18. [CrossRef]

53. Bender, J.; Flieger, A. Lipases as pathogenicity factors of bacterial pathogens of humans. In *Handbook of Hydrocarbon and Lipid Microbiology*; Timmis, K.N., Ed.; Springer: Berlin/Heidelberg, Germany, 2010; pp. 3241–3258.

54. Cho, H.H.; Sung, J.Y.; Kwon, K.C.; Koo, S.H. Expression of Sme efflux pumps and multilocus sequence typing in clinical isolates of *Stenotrophomonas maltophilia*. *Ann. Lab. Med.* **2012**, *32*, 38–43. [CrossRef]

55. Emami, S.; Nowroozi, J.; Abiri, R.; Mohajeri, P. Multilocus Sequence Typing for Molecular Epidemiology of *Stenotrophomonas maltophilia* Clinical and Environmental Isolates from a Tertiary Hospital in West of Iran. *Iran Biomed. J.* **2022**, *26*, 142–152.

56. Gideskog, M.; Welander, J.; Melhus, Å. Cluster of *S. maltophilia* among patients with respiratory tract infections at an intensive care unit. *Infect. Prev. Pract.* **2020**, *2*, 100097. [CrossRef] [PubMed]

57. Rizek, C.F.; Jonas, D.; Garcia Paez, J.I.; Rosa, J.F.; Perdigão Neto, L.V.; Martins, R.R.; Moreno, L.Z.; Rossi Junior, A.; Levin, A.S.; Costa, S.F. Multidrug-resistant *Stenotrophomonas maltophilia*: Description of new MLST profiles and resistance and virulence genes using whole-genome sequencing. *J. Glob. Antimicrob. Resist.* **2018**, *15*, 212–214. [CrossRef]

58. Gallo, S.W.; Ramos, P.L.; Ferreira, C.A.S.; de Oliveira, S.D. A specific polymerase chain reaction method to identify *Stenotrophomonas maltophilia*. *Mem. Inst. Oswaldo Cruz.* **2013**, *108*, 390–391. [CrossRef]

59. Magiorakos, A.P.; Srinivasan, A.; Carey, R.B.; Carmeli, Y.; Falagas, M.E.; Giske, C.G.; Harbarth, S.; Hindler, J.F.; Kahlmeter, G.; Olsson-Liljequist, B.; et al. Multidrug-resistant, extensively drug-resistant and pandrug-resistant bacteria:An international expert proposal for interim standard definitions for acquired resistance. *Clin. Microbiol. Infect.* **2012**, *18*, 268–281. [CrossRef] [PubMed]

60. Wang, M.; Wei, H.; Zhao, Y.; Shang, L.; Di, L.; Lyu, C.; Liu, J. Analysis of multidrug-resistant bacteria in 3223 patients with hospital-acquired infections (HAI) from a tertiary general hospital in China. *Bosn. J. Basic Med. Sci.* **2019**, *19*, 86–93. [CrossRef]

61. Yang, Z.; Liu, W.; Cui, Q.; Niu, W.; Li, H.; Zhao, X.; Wei, X.; Wang, X.; Huang, S.; Dong, D.; et al. Prevalence and detection of *Stenotrophomonas maltophilia* carrying metallo-β-lactamase bla_{L1} in Beijing, China. *Front. Microbiol.* **2014**, *9*, 692. [CrossRef] [PubMed]

62. Azimi, A.; Aslanimehr, M.; Yaseri, M.; Shadkam, M.; Douraghi, M. Distribution of *smf-1*, *rmlA*, *spgM* and *rpfF* genes among *Stenotrophomonas maltophilia* isolates in relation to biofilm-forming capacity. *J. Glob. Antimicrob. Resist.* **2020**, *23*, 321–326. [CrossRef]

63. Toleman, M.A.; Bennett, P.M.; Walsh, T.R. Common regions e.g. orf513 and antibiotic resistance: IS91-like elements evolving complex class 1 integrons. *J. Antimicrob. Chemother.* **2006**, *58*, 1–6. [CrossRef]

64. Toleman, M.A.; Bennett, P.M.; Bennett, D.M.; Jones, R.N.; Walsh, T.R. Global emergence of trimethoprim/sulfamethoxazole resistance in *Stenotrophomonas maltophilia* mediated by acquisition of *sul* genes. *Emerg. Infect. Dis.* **2007**, *13*, 559–565. [CrossRef] [PubMed]

65. Vattanaviboon, P.; Dulyayangkul, P.; Mongkolsuk, S.; Charoenlap, N. Overexpression of *Stenotrophomonas maltophilia* major facilitator superfamily protein MfsA increases resistance to fluoroquinolone antibiotics. *J. Antimicrob. Chemother.* **2018**, *73*, 1263–1266. [CrossRef] [PubMed]

66. Madi, H.; Lukić, J.; Vasiljević, Z.; Biočanin, M.; Kojić, M.; Jovčić, B.; Lozo, J. Genotypic and phenotypic characterization of *Stenotrophomonas maltophilia* strains from a Pediatric Tertiary Care Hospital in Serbia. *PLoS ONE* **2016**, *11*, e0165660. [CrossRef]

67. Cruz-Córdova, A.; Mancilla-Rojano, J.; Luna-Pineda, V.M.; Escalona-Venegas, G.; Cázares-Domínguez, V.; Ormsby, C.; Franco-Hernández, I.; Zavala-Vega, S.; Hernández, M.A.; Medina-Pelcastre, M. Molecular epidemiology, antibiotic resistance, and virulence traits of *Stenotrophomonas maltophilia* strains associated with an outbreak in a Mexican tertiary care hospital. *Front. Cell Infect. Microbiol.* **2020**, *18*, 50. [CrossRef] [PubMed]

68. Thomas, R.; Hamat, R.A.; Neela, V. Extracellular enzyme profiling of *Stenotrophomonas maltophilia* clinical isolates. *Virulence* **2014**, *5*, 326–330. [CrossRef] [PubMed]

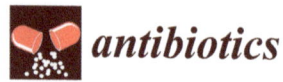

MDPI

Article

The Occurrence and Characteristics of Methicillin-Resistant Staphylococcal Isolates from Foods and Containers

Rada Kansaen [1], Parichart Boueroy [1], Rujirat Hatrongjit [2], Watcharaporn Kamjumphol [3], Anusak Kerdsin [1] and Peechanika Chopjitt [1,*]

[1] Faculty of Public Health, Chalermphrakiat Sakon Nakhon Province Campus, Kasetsart University, Sakon Nakhon 47000, Thailand; rada.kan@ku.th (R.K.); parichart.bou@ku.th (P.B.); anusak.ke@ku.th (A.K.)
[2] Faculty of Science and Engineering, Chalermphrakiat Sakon Nakhon Province Campus, Kasetsart University, Sakon Nakhon 47000, Thailand; rujirat.ha@ku.th
[3] National Institute of Health, Department of Medical Sciences, Ministry of Public Health, Nonthaburi 11000, Thailand; watcharaporn.k@dmsc.mail.go.th
* Correspondence: peechanika.c@ku.th

Abstract: Antimicrobial resistance (AMR) has emerged as an urgent global public health issue that requires immediate attention. Methicillin-resistant staphylococci (MRS) is a major problem, as it may cause serious human and animal infections, eventually resulting in death. This study determined the proportional distribution, genetic characteristics, and antimicrobial susceptibility of *mec*A- or *mec*C-carrying staphylococci isolated from food chain products. A total of 230 samples were taken from meat, food, fermented food, and food containers. Overall, 13.9% (32/230) of the samples were identified to have *Staphylococcus aureus* isolates; of those, 3.9% (9/230) were MRS, with eight mecA-positive and one mecC-positive samples, and 1.3% (3/230) methicillin-resistant *Staphylococcus aureus* (MRSA). MRSA strains belonging to three sequence types (ST9, ST22, and a newly identified ST), three different *spa* types (T005, t526, and a newly identified type), and three different SCC*mec* types (IV, V, and an unidentified SCC*mec*) were detected. Additionally, eight *mec*A-positive staphylococcal isolates were identified as *S. haemolyticus*, *S. sciuri*, *S. simulans*, and *S. warneri*, while the *mec*C-harboring isolate was *S. xylosus*. The enterotoxin gene, *SEm*, was detected at 1.56% in *S. aureus*, whereas *SEq* was detected at 0.31%, and *SEi* was also found in MRSA. Our study emphasizes the importance of enhanced hygiene standards in reducing the risk of occupational and foodborne MRSA infections associated with the handling or consumption of meat, food, and preserved food products.

Keywords: foods; methicillin-resistant *Staphylococcus* spp.; SCC*mec* type; multilocus sequencing typing; *spa* type; staphylococcal enterotoxins (SEs)

Citation: Kansaen, R.; Boueroy, P.; Hatrongjit, R.; Kamjumphol, W.; Kerdsin, A.; Chopjitt, P. The Occurrence and Characteristics of Methicillin-Resistant Staphylococcal Isolates from Foods and Containers. *Antibiotics* **2023**, *12*, 1287. https://doi.org/10.3390/antibiotics12081287

Academic Editors: Brian Wilkinson and Juhee Ahn

Received: 12 June 2023
Revised: 14 July 2023
Accepted: 31 July 2023
Published: 4 August 2023

1. Introduction

Staphylococci are natural inhabitants of the skin and mucous membranes in both humans and various animals. They are typically classified into two groups based on their ability to produce coagulase: coagulase-positive (CoPS) and coagulase-negative staphylococci (CoNS) [1]. *Staphylococcus aureus* (*S. aureus*), a CoPS member, is widely recognized as a major causative agent of food poisoning and infections in both clinical and community settings [2–5]. The production of coagulase by *S. aureus* promotes blood clotting, and the resulting fibrin coat on the bacterial surface may facilitate the evasion of the immune system. CoNS consist of numerous species, including opportunistic pathogens such as *S. epidermidis*, *S. capitis*, *S. hominis*, *S. haemolyticus*, *S. saccharolyticus*, *S. warneri*, *S. lugdunensis*, *S. saprophyticus*, and *S. cohnii*. Although CoNS lack the ability to produce coagulase, they possess species and strain-specific virulence factors that contribute to their role as notorious opportunistic pathogens. One significant pathogenicity mechanism employed by CoNS is their ability to form biofilms, allowing them to colonize both abiotic surfaces of medical devices and biotic surfaces such as host tissues coated with host factors [6].

This opportunistic pathogen is capable of infecting both humans and other mammals, resulting in a broad spectrum of diseases. These include food poisoning, which manifests as abdominal pains, diarrhea, nausea, and vomiting, as well as more serious conditions such as endocarditis, pneumonia, osteomyelitis, toxic shock syndrome, septicemia, and soft tissue and skin infections [7,8]. In addition, *S. aureus* is frequently found in animal-derived foods such as undercooked meat and dairy products [9–11]. Its ability to survive in a variety of environments and to cause such a wide range of diseases highlights the need for effective prevention and control measures concerning public health.

The pathogenicity of *S. aureus* is attributed to a combination of factors that contribute to its invasive nature, the production of extracellular factors, and its antibiotic resistance. In order to enhance the process of pathogenesis and facilitate udder infection, *S. aureus* has developed a range of virulence factors. These factors include various extracellular enzymes such as lipases, proteases, amylases, hyaluronidase, DNases, coagulase, lactamase, hemolysins, and capsules [12]. Additionally, *S. aureus* produces enterotoxins (SEs: SEA to SEE) and non-classical SE-like toxins (SEl: SEG to SEU) that are associated with food poisoning. Notably, these toxins are resistant to heat, proteolytic enzymes, and low pH conditions. Furthermore, *S. aureus* is known to produce toxic shock syndrome toxin 1 (TSST-1), a potent superantigenic toxin. The presence of TSST-1 can lead to severe symptoms such as high fever, rash, shock syndrome, hypotension, and the inflammation of the blood system, as well as to the Panton–Valentine leucocidin (PVL), which causes leukocytosis along with necrosis on the skin or mucosa surface, and TSST-1 is capable of inducing lysis of human neutrophils and enhances the adherence of *S. aureus* to the extracellular matrix [12–15].

The emergence of methicillin-resistant staphylococci (MRS) presents a significant and concerning threat, as these strains exhibit resistance to all beta-lactam antibiotics, thereby compromising treatment options and increasing the risk of life-threatening infections. It is important to recognize that other coagulase-positive (*S. aureus*, *S. schleiferi*, *S. delphini*, *S. intermedius*, *S pseudintermedius*, and *S. lutrae*) and coagulase-negative MRS species (*S. cohnii*, *S. epidermidis*, *S. haemolyticus*, *S. hominis*, *S. lentus*, *S. lugdunensis*, *S. sciuri*, and *S. xylosus*) have gained significance in recent years. These species have been implicated in a variety of opportunistic infections, particularly among immunocompromised patients [16]. The development of methicillin resistance is primarily attributed to the presence of the *mec*A gene, a pivotal genetic element located on the mobile genetic element known as the staphylococcal cassette chromosome mec (SCC*mec*). This genetic element encodes an altered penicillin-binding protein (PBP2a), which imparts resistance to methicillin and other beta-lactam antibiotics. In addition to *mec*A, the presence of other *mec* genes, including *mec*B and *mec*C, has also been recognized as being associated with beta-lactam resistance [1]. This gene is widespread in *S. aureus* and coagulase-negative staphylococci (CoNS) from both human and animal origin [17,18]. The widespread consumption of antibiotics in the livestock sector has led to their persistent release into the environment and increased antibiotic-resistant bacteria. Numerous studies have demonstrated the presence of *mec*A-positive methicillin-resistant *Staphylococcus aureus* (MRSA) in various food sources, such as retail meat, fish, poultry, pork, beef, ready-to-eat foods, and even vegetables [11,19–21]. Additionally, CoNS carrying *mec*A, which are known for their increasing rates of methicillin resistance, have been detected in milk at a rate of 0.6% in Brazil and 6.7% in Tunisia [22,23], in ready-to-eat foods at a rate of 16.4% in Poland [24], and in meat at a rate 2.3–8% in Egypt [25,26], which raises additional concerns about the spread of resistance. In Thailand, the prevalence of MRA was found to be 20.5% in the university environment and 52.3% in the hospital environment [27]. The prevalence of MRSA in meat has been reported as 44.8–50% [28,29]. However, a lower prevalence of MRSA (3.8%) in non-human isolates was reported [30].

The presence of staphylococci in meat is oftentimes because personnel participating in the production process engage in unhygienic behaviors during the processing, shipping, slicing, storage, and point-of-sale stages throughout the production process. By evaluating these factors, valuable insights into the potential transmission of antibiotic resistance and virulence factors through the food chain can be obtained. In light of these findings, the purpose of the present study was to investigate the distribution of methicillin-resistant staphylococci in various food types, with a concentration on characterizing their SCC*mec* types, spa types, and the presence of enterotoxin genes.

2. Results

2.1. Distribution of Methicillin-Resistant Staphylococci

From the 230 samples, 666 staphylococcal isolates were identified comprising 3 MRSA isolates from 3 samples (1 pork and 2 beef; 3/230, 1.30%); 8 MRS carrying *mec*A from 8 samples (8/230, 3.47%) consisting of pork (*n* = 4), beef (*n* = 2), and chicken (*n* = 2); 1 MRS harboring *mec*C from pork (1/230, 0.43%); and 70 *S. aureus* (methicillin-susceptible) isolates from 32 samples (32/230, 13.91%) consisting of pork (*n* = 6), beef (*n* = 5), chicken (*n* = 19), and fermented food (*n* = 2). (Table 1)

Table 1. The number of *mec*A- and *mec*C-positive strains, *S. aureus* and MRSA in different types in this study.

Category of Samples	No. of Sample	No. of Sample Positive for *mecA*	No. of Sample Positive for *mecC*	No. of Sample Positive for *S. aureus*	No. of Sample Positive for MRSA	Enterotoxin Genes (SEj, SEl, SEq, SEm, SEr)
Food container	80	-	-	-	-	-
Food samples	30	-	-	-	-	-
Pork	30	4 (1.74%)	1 (0.43%)	6 (2.6%)	2 (0.87%)	-
Chicken	30	2 (0.87%)	-	19 (8.26%)	-	2
Beef	30	2 (0.87%)	-	5 (2.17%)	1 (0.43%)	1
Fermented food	30	-	-	2 (0.87%)	-	2
Total	230	8 (3.47%)	1 (0.43%)	32 (13.91%)	3 (1.3%)	5 (2.17%)

The *mec*A-harboring MRS (n = 8) were identified as three *S. haemolyticus* strains, two *S. sciuri* strains, two *S. warneri* strains, and one *S. stimulans* strain. We identified one MRS harboring *mec*C as *S. xylosus* (n = 1). These are summarized in Table 2. The proportion of methicillin-resistant staphylococci (MRSA and MRS) present in foods was 12/320, 5.21% in the current study.

Table 2. Genetic characteristics and resistance profiles of MRSA and mecA- and mecC-positive isolates.

ID	Sample	mecA/C	Species	SCCmec Types	STs	Spa Types	Resistance Profiles **	
P(2)12.4	Pork	mecA	MRSA	* UN	ST9	t526	FOX-OX-E-DA-CN-AZM -TE-CIP-SXT-C- D+	MDR
B(3)1.2	Beef	mecA	MRSA	IV	ST22	t005	FOX-OX-E-DA-CN-AZM -CIP-D+	MDR
B22.5	Beef	mecA	MRSA	V	new	new	FOX-OX -E-CN-AZM-CIP	MDR
P3.5	Pork	mecA	S. sciuri	* UN.	-	-	FOX-OX-DA-AZM-TE -SXT	MDR
P(3) 1.2	Pork	mecA	S. haemolyticus	* UN.	-	-	FOX-OX-DA-AZM-TE	MDR
P(3) 1.3	Pork	mecA	S. sciuri	* UN.	-	-	FOX-OX -DA-TE	MDR
P(3) 1.5	Pork	mecA	S. haemolyticus	* UN.	-	-	FOX-OX -DA--TE	MDR
C49.2	Chicken	mecA	S. haemolyticus	III	-	-	FOX-OX	-
C49.4	Chicken	mecA	S. simulans	* UN.	-	-	FOX-OX -TE	MDR

Table 2. *Cont.*

ID	Sample	mecA/C	Species	SCCmec Types	STs	Spa Types	Resistance Profiles **	
B57.3	Beef	mecA	*S. warneri*	V	-	-	FOX-OX -E-DA- AZM -TE-C	MDR
B79.1	Beef	mecA	*S. warneri*	V	-	-	FOX-OX -E-DA-AZM-TE	MDR
P20.3	Pork	mecC	*S. xylosus*	* UN.	-	-	OX-TE	-

* UN = unidentified, ** FOX = cefoxitin, OX = oxacillin, TE = tetracycline, DA; clindamycin, E = erythromycin, AZM = azithromycin, C = chloramphenicol, CIP = ciprofloxacin, ST = strain, SXT = trimethoprim/sulfamethoxazole, CN = gentamycin, D$^+$ = induce clindamycin resistance. MDR; multidrug-resistant.

As shown in Table 2, MRSA strain no. B(3)1.2 belonged to SCC*mec* type IV, ST22, *spa* t005, and carried the pvl gene. MRSA strain no. P(2)12.4 showed unidentified SCC*mec* types, ST9, and *spa* t526, whereas MRSA strain no. B22.5 was SCC*mec* type V, a new *spa* type and a new ST; however, it is closely related to ST1455, which is isolated from the lung aspirate of a Chinese patient, as shown in Figure 1. Among the eight *mec*A-harboring MRS isolates, the most common SCC*mec* type was an unidentified SCCmec type (5/8, 62.5%), followed by SCCmec types V (2/8, 25%) and III (1/8, 12.5%), as shown in Table 2. Finally, the *mec*C-harboring *S. xylosus* carried an unidentified SCC*mec* type (Table 2).

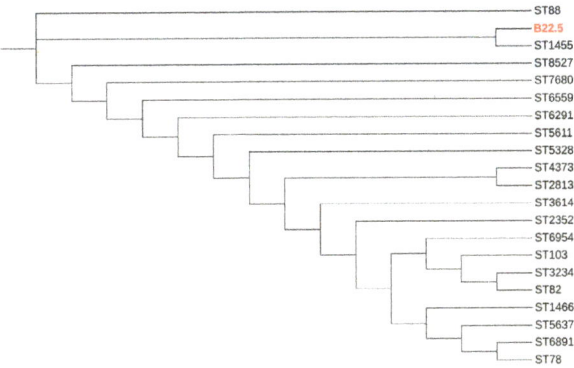

Figure 1. Dendrogram of concatenated sequences of seven MLST loci of MRSA strain B22.5 (red color), as a new ST isolate, and its related STs.

2.2. Antimicrobial Resistance

All three of the MRSA isolates were multidrug-resistant (MDR), with resistance to erythromycin, oxacillin, cefoxitin, gentamycin, azithromycin, and ciprofloxacin, while two isolates (strain no. P(2)12.4 and B(3)1.2) could induce clindamycin resistance. The *mec*A- and *mec*C-carrying staphylococci were classified as MDR in seven strains except for *S. haemolyticus* strain no.C49.2 and *S. xylosus* strain no P20.3, as shown in Table 2. However, all isolates were susceptible to vancomycin, linezolid, and rifampin.

2.3. Detection of Foodborne Staphylococcus Aureus Enterotoxin Genes

In total, 73 *S. aureus* isolates, including 3 MRSA, were detected with five enterotoxin genes (*SEj, SEl, Seq, Sem,* and *SEr*). The *SEm* gene was found in *S. aureus* (5/73, 6.85%), and the *SEq* and *SEj* genes were found in MRSA strain no B22.5 (1/73, 1.37%).

3. Discussion

Antibiotic resistance bacteria are a major global health problem, emerging in a variety of environmental samples. To better comprehend the dissemination of methicillin-resistant staphylococci in food product chains in northeast Thailand, we characterized staphylococcal isolates from foods, food containers, and meat. Our study showed that the proportion of *S. aureus* (10%) was lower than in other studies in Thailand, for example, 83% (87/105) of *S. aureus* present in ready-to-eat food samples in Songkhla Province [31] and 60% (36/60) in fermented pork sausage in Amnatcharoen Province [32]. In other countries, *S. aureus* has been found in retail raw meat samples: 21.23% (96/452) in Tukey [33], 21.81% (89/408) in India [34], 16.9–35% in China [35–37], 33.9% (165/487) in Chile [38], and 13.8% (22/160) in Greece [39]. In contrast, in the current study, the proportion of MRSA in food samples was also low (0.94%; 3/320), which was less than for the proportions reported in other regions of Thailand, such as 20% (2/10) [28] and 44.8% (55/116) [29], both in retail pork samples. However, some studies showed a low prevalence of MRSA in non-human samples, for example, 2.2% from retail food and food handlers' gloves, 1.7% in beef, 1.2–1.9% in pork, 0.3% in chicken, 3.5% in turkey, 1.86% in secondary school environments, and 1.58% from environmental contamination in railway stations and coach stations [30]. Differences in the sampling period, sample size, sampling site, sampling techniques, isolation method, single enrichment step, the frequency of MRSA in different samples, or geographical locations could partially explain the variation in prevalence. However, these results highlight the necessity to mitigate the risk of *S. aureus* and MRSA transmission via meat products to humans in the food supply chain.

The current study revealed that SCC*mec* types IV and V were detected concordant with several studies in retail meat products worldwide [40–44]. One MRSA in the current study was ST9, which is predominant in most Asian countries, including Taiwan, Hong Kong, Malaysia, and Thailand [45–49]. The ST9 strains are generally MDR, with >80% resistance to erythromycin, ciprofloxacin, gentamicin, tetracycline, and clindamycin [50], which was similar to our strain in the current study. Our MRSA ST22 strain is the epidemic clone EMRSA-15, and it is a hospital-associated pathogen, typically resistant to ciprofloxacin and erythromycin [51–53]. However, some studies have reported MRSA ST22 isolated from animals [54,55]. It is interesting that a novel ST of MRSA was identified from beef samples in the current study. This ST was closely related to ST 1455, which was isolated from a human patient's bronchoalveolar lavage [56]. Therefore, this novel ST should be subjected to monitoring and surveillance.

The *mec*A-carrying staphylococcal isolates other than MRSA in the current study belonged to five species of coagulase-negative staphylococci, namely *S. haemolyticus* (37.5%), *S. sciuri* (25%), *S. warneri* (25%), and *S. simulans* (12.5%), while the *mec*C-harboring isolate was *S. xylosus*. In Egypt, Osman et al. detected *S. hyicus* (30%), *S. intermedius* (15%), *S. epidermidis* (5%), *S. hemilyticus* (5%), *S. hominis* (5%), *S. lugdumenis* (15%), *S. simulants* (5%), and *S. scuri* (20%) in imported beef meat [25]. Boamah et al. identified *S. gallinarum* (32%); *S. saprophyticus* (20%); *S. chromogens* (20%); *S. warneri* (12%); *S. hominis* (8%); *S. caprae* and *S. epidermidis* (4%); *S. sciuri* (42.97%); *S. lentus* (35.94%); *S. xylosus* (4.30%); *S. haemolyticus* (3.91%); *S. saprophyticus* (1.95%); and *S. cohnii* (0.39%) in poultry in Ghana [57]. Pimenta et al. found *S. gallinarum* (35.2%); *S. simulans* (17%); *S. sciuri* (10.2%); *S. lentus* (4.5%); and *S. cohnii* and *S. xylosus* (2.2%) in broiler chicken products in Brazil [58]. Moreover, in Korea, *S. agnetis* (19.4%), *S. saprophyticus* (19%), *S. chromogens* (14.5%), S *hyicus* (12.9%), and *S. sciuri* (13.8%) were detected in retail chicken meat [1]. These findings suggest that the frequent occurrence of non-aureus staphylococci in meat may be a hazard associated with food and public health safety. Some of them can cause foodborne infections [59,60], contribute to antibiotic resistance transmission [61], and lead to zoonotic infections [62]. Therefore, close monitoring should be carefully considered.

Regarding the risk of foodborne intoxication, numerous surveys of staphylococcal enterotoxins (SEs) have been reported, which have identified five classical enterotoxin types, SEa to SEe [63], and many new types of SEs have been reported: SEg, SEh, SEi, SEk, SEl, SEm, SEn, SEo, SEp, SEq, SEr, and SEu [64]. One of the limitations of this study is that we did not detect the classical enterotoxin genes; therefore, these classical enterotoxin genes could not be ruled out in our *S. aureus* isolates. Hu et al. showed five new types of enterotoxin genes, namely SEj, SEl, SEq, SEm, and SEr. Of these, SEj and SEr were detected in 16.6% and 14.3%, respectively [65]. Additionally, SEi (97.2%) and SEm (86.1%) were frequently detected in retail foods in China [11]. In contrast, our study revealed SEm in *S. aureus* (6.1%, 5/82) and SEq and SEi in MRSA (1.2%, 1/82). There has been a rise in the number of foodborne staphylococcal isolates, especially MRSA, which is linked to novel enterotoxins; therefore, these data indicate that we should pay attention to both types of toxins. In addition, the five new enterotoxin genes were extensively present in proteins of animal origin compared with that from other origins. This is related to the animal characteristics and interaction with the living environment, operation environment for food processing, and storage environment for finished products [65].

4. Materials and Methods

4.1. Ethical Statement

Ethical review and approval were not required because this study did not involve human subjects.

4.2. Sample Collection, Isolation, and Presumptive Deification

From June to December 2019, a total of 230 samples were taken from various foods and storage containers located in rural northeastern Thailand. A variety of samples, including food containers, meat, pork, chicken, beef, and pickled food, were gathered. The samples included 80 food container samples, 30 food samples, 90 meat samples (30 pork, 30 chicken, and 30 beef), and 30 pickled food samples. The collection of samples was performed in sterile conditions. Storage containers were swabbed using sterile cotton that was immediately placed in 1 mL of Mannitol salt broth (MSB) (HiMedia Laboratories Pvt. Ltd.; Nashik, India). Food product samples were collected in accordance with Sorour et al. [26]. The samples were transferred to the laboratory in sterile plastic bags. A 10 g amount of each food sample was diluted with 90 mL of buffer peptone water (BPW) (HiMedia Laboratories Pvt. Ltd.; Nashik, India), incubated overnight at 37 °C under aerobic conditions, and then streaked on mannitol salt agar medium (MSA) (HiMedia Laboratories Pvt. Ltd.; Nashik, India) before incubating at 37 °C and examined after 24 h to 48 h. There was a presumption that the colonies on MSA, which were colored yellow and pink, were staphylococci. Following the preliminary fundamental phenotypic examination (which included a microscopic inspection, Gram staining, catalase production, and coagulase tube test utilizing rabbit plasma), these isolates were identified at the species level via either PCR or DNA sequencing, as will be detailed in subsequent sections.

4.3. Microbiology and Molecular Characterization of S. Aureus and MRSA

In accordance with the protocol provided by the manufacturer, total genomic DNA was extracted using a ZymoBIOMICsTM DNA Miniprep Kit (Zymo Research; Irvine, CA, USA). The quantity and purity of DNA were determined using a NanoDropTM 2000 Spectrometer (Thermo Fisher Scientific; Waltham, MA, USA), and the DNA sample was stored at −20 °C for further study.

Multiplex PCR was performed to detect *fem*A genes specific for *S. aureus* species, and the *mec*A, *mec*C, and *luk*S genes following a previously established protocol [66,67]. The sequence primers are shown in Table 3. DNA amplification was carried out in 25 µL of a PCR mixture that contained 12.5 µL of 2x JumpStart™ REDTaq® ReadyMix™ Reaction Mix (SIGMA; Saint Louis, MO, USA), 0.4 µM of each primer, 100 ng of the DNA sample, and sterile deionized water. PCR was carried out using the following thermal cyclic conditions: initial denaturation at 94 °C for 3 min, followed by 35 cycles of denaturation at 94 °C for 30 s, annealing at 55 °C for 30 s, an extension at 72 °C for 30 s, a final extension of 72 °C for 5 min, and cooling to 4 °C.

Table 3. Sequences primers of target genes in the current study.

Target Gene	Primer Sequence (5'-3')	Size (bp)	Reference
femA	F: CGATCCATATTTACATATCA R: ATAACGCTCTTCGTTTAGTT	450	
mecA	F: ACGAGTAGATGCTCAATATAA R: CTTAGTTCTTTAGCGATTGC	293	[66]
Luks	F: CAGGAGGTAATGGTTCATTT R: ATGTCCAGACATTTTACCTAA	151	
mecC	F: GAAAAAAAGGCTTAGAACGCCTC R: GAAGATCTTTTCCGTTTTCAGC	138	[67]
SEj	F: CACCAGAACTGTTGTTCTGCTAG R: CTGAATTTTACCATCAAAGGTAC	114	
SEl	F: TGGACATAACGGCACTAAAA R: TTGGTARCCCATCATCTCCT	145	
SEq	F: ATACCTATTAATCTCTGGGTCAATG R: AATGGAAAGTAATTTTTCCTTTG	222	[65]
SEm	F: AGTTTGTGTAAGAAGTCAAGTGTAGA R: ATCTTTAAATTCAGCAGATATTCCATCTAA	178	
SEr	F: TCCCATTCCTTATTTAGAATACA R: GGATATTCCAAACACATCTGAC	440	

4.4. Enterotoxin Genes and PVL Detection

S. aureus isolates were subjected to PCR for the identification of five enterotoxin genes, namely *SEj, SEl, SEq, SEm,* and *SEr,* as described elsewhere [65]. Briefly, the total reaction volume was 25 μL and included the following: 12.5 μL 2x Mytaq™ HS Red Mix (Bioline Reagents Ltd.; London, UK), sterile deionized water, 1 μM of each primer, and 100 ng DNA template. The PCR conditions were as follows: pre-denaturation at 94 °C, 40 s; annealing at 52 °C, 40 s; and extension at 72 °C, 1 min for a total of 35 cycles; and final extension for at 72 °C, 10 min. This procedure was used for all genes except *SEj,* for which the annealing temperature was 55 °C.

4.5. Sequencing of mecA-or mecC-Harboring Staphylococci

Sequencing was carried out as described by Poyart et al. [68]. The DNA samples were amplified for the *sod*A gene with the primer sodA-F (5' CCITAYICITAYGAYGCIYTIGARCC-3') and sodA-R (5'-ARRTARTAIGCRT GYTCCCAIACRTC-3'). Briefly, 50 μL of the reaction mixture was used, which contained 25 μL of 2x Mytaq™ HS Red Mix (Bioline Reagents Ltd.; London, UK), sterile deionized water, 0.75 μM of each primer, and 100 ng of bacterial DNA sample. Thermal cycling reaction conditions consisted of initial denaturing at 95 °C for 3 min and then being subjected to 35 cycles of amplification, denaturation at 95 °C for 30 s, annealing at 37 °C for 60 s, and elongation at 72 °C for 45 s. The PCR amplicons were purified using a GF-1 AmbiClean Kit (Vivantis Technologies Sdn Bhd; Kuala Lumpur, Malaysia) and then sequenced at 1st BASE products and services company, Malaysia. The Basic Local Alignment Search Tool (BLASTN) was used to identify species of staphylococci using a cut-off value of ≥97% [69].

4.6. Molecular Typing

To determine the Staphylococcal Chromosomal Cassette (SCC*mec*) type, a multiplex PCR (M-PCR) was performed according to the method described by Kondo et al. [68]. M-PCR 1, designed for the *ccr* type assignment, employed two primers for *mecA* detection and eight primers for the identification of five *ccr* genes. Within these eight primers, there were four primers that included a forward primer shared by *ccrB1-3* and three reverse primers specific to *ccrA1, ccrA2,* and *ccrA3.* This allowed for the identification of *ccr1-3* based on the differences in the *ccrA* genes. Additionally, two primers were utilized for identifying *ccr4* and two for identifying *ccr5*. In M-PCR 2, which aimed to assign *mec* classes, four primers were employed to identify the gene lineages of *mec*A-*mec*I (class A *mec*), *mec*A-IS1272 (class B *mec*), and *mec*A-IS431 (class C *mec*). The PCR reaction mixture for both M-PCR 1 and M-PCR 2 consisted of 100 ng of DNA extract in a total volume of 25 μL. This mixture included 12.5 μlx of 2× JumpStart™ REDTaq® ReadyMix™ PCR Reaction Mix (SIGMA; Saint Louis, MO, USA) and a concentration of 0.2 μM for each primer. The thermal cycling conditions involved an initial denaturation step at 94 °C for 2 min, followed by 35 cycles of denaturation at 94 °C for 2 min, annealing at 57 °C for 1 min, and extension at 72 °C for 2 min. The amplification process concluded with a final extension step at 72 °C for 2 min.

Multilocus sequence typing (MLST) was performed following the protocol described elsewhere [70]. Seven housekeeping genes (*arcC*, *aroE*, *glpF*, *gmk*, *pta*, *tpi*, and *yqiL*) were amplified using PCR. The PCRs were carried out with 50 μL reaction volumes containing 12.5 μL 2x Mytaq™ HS Red Mix (Bioline Reagents Ltd.; London, UK), 2.5 μM of each primer, 100 ng bacterial DNA sample, and sterile deionized water. PCR amplification was performed with thermal cycling reaction conditions consisting of initial denaturation at 95 °C for 5 min, followed by 35 cycles of denaturation at 95 °C for 1 min, annealing at 55 °C for 1 min, and extension at 72 °C for 1 min, and the cycle was completed with a single extension at 72 °C for 5 min. The PCR amplicons were purified using a GF-1 AmbiClean Kit (Vivantis Technologies Sdn Bhd; Kuala Lumpur, Malaysia) and then sequenced at 1st BASE products and services company, Malaysia. The alleles and sequence types (STs) were identified using the scheme published in multilocus sequence typing databases (https://pubmlst.org/organisms/staphylococcus-aureus, (accessed on 20 February 2023).

The *spa* typing was performed via the amplification of polymorphic X region of the *S. aureus* protein A gene (*spa*) using the standard primers spa-1095F (5′-AGACGATCCTT CGGTGAGC3′) and spa-1517R (5′-GCTTTTGCAATGTCATTTACTG3′) and a PCR program described elsewhere [71]. Briefly, 50 μL of the reaction mixture was used, which contained 25 μL 2X Mytaq™ HS Red Mix (Bioline Reagents Ltd., London, UK), sterile deionized water, and 100 ng of the bacterial DNA sample. Thermal cycling reaction conditions consisted of initial denaturation at 80 °C, 5 min; 35 cycles of denaturation at 94 °C, 45 s; annealing at 60 °C, 45 s; and extension at 72 °C, 90 s; and finally, a single extension at 72 °C, 10 min. The PCR amplicons were purified using a GF-1 AmbiClean Kit (Vivantis Technologies Sdn Bhd; Kuala Lumpur, Malaysia) and then sequenced at 1st BASE products and services company, Malaysia. Spa types were determined with the *Spa* Typer website http://spatyper.fortinbras.us, (accessed on 20 February 2023).

4.7. Electrophoretic Analysis of PCR Products

After amplification, 5 μL of PCR product was subjected to analysis on 2% agarose gel (Bioline Reagents Ltd., London, UK) in 0.5X TBE buffer (Omega BioTek, Inc; Norcross, Georgia) to determine the molecular weight of the amplified DNA fragment. The 5 μL GeneRuler 100 bp Plus DNA ladder (Thermo Scientific; Vilnius, Lithuania) was loaded onto the same agarose gel as a molecular weight standard. Subsequently, the gel was stained with ethidium bromide (Wako, Wako Pure Chemical Industries, Ltd.; Tokyo, Japan) and destained by soaking it in water. Electrophoresis was performed on horizontal electrophoresis equipment (Mupid-Exu; Chuo-ku, Japan) for 30 min at a constant 100 Volts. Subsequently, the gel was visualized using a UV Transilluminator (SynGene; Cambridge, UK), enabling a comparison between the migration patterns of the DNA ladder bands and the PCR products.

4.8. Analysis of New STs

The construction of the phylogenetic tree for STs that are closely related to strain B22.5, a new ST, was performed in this study via Phylogeny.fr [72]. The phylogenetic tree was visualized using the Interactive Tree of Life (iTOL) (http://itol.embl.de, (accessed on 7 July 2023) [73].

4.9. Antimicrobial Susceptibility Testing

The antimicrobial susceptibility test was performed using disk diffusion in Mueller–Hinton agar (Merck; Darmstadt, Germany) according to the 2023 Clinical and Laboratory Standards Institute guidelines, using 13 antimicrobials of different classes including cefoxitin (FOX, 30 μg), oxacillin (OX, 1 μg), tetracycline (TE, 30 μg), erythromycin (E, 15 μg), azithromycin (AZM, 15 μg), chloramphenicol (C, 30 μg), ciprofloxacin (CIP, 5 μg), trimethoprim/sulfamethoxazole (SXT, 25 μg), gentamycin (CN, 10 μg), rifampin (RA, 5 μg), linezolid (LZD, 30 μg), and clindamycin (DA, 2 μg) sourced from OXOID Ltd. (Hampshire, UK), while vancomycin was determined with minimum inhibitory concentrations (MICs). *S. aureus* ATCC 25,923 was used as a quality control strain for antimicrobial susceptibility testing. The plates were incubated at 37 °C for 18–24 h. After overnight incubation, the zone of inhibition was measured and interpreted as susceptible, intermediate, and resistant based on the recommendation of CLSI (2023) [74]. All antimicrobial susceptibility tests were repeated three times. Multi-drug resistance patterns of the isolates were identified according to the guideline described by Magiorakos et al. [75].

The D test method was carried out in accordance with Chavez-Bueno S et al. [76] in order to determine whether or not inducible resistance to clindamycin develops. In Brief, the bacterial isolates were plated on a Mueller–Hinton agar plate at a MacFarland concentration of 0.5 to evenly cover the agar surface. Clindamycin and erythromycin disks, containing 2 μg and 15 μg of each antibiotic, were placed in the middle of the plate separated by a distance of 1.5 cm between the edges. Plates were incubated at 37 °C for 24 h. Inducible resistance to clindamycin was defined as the blunting of the clear circular area of no growth surrounding the clindamycin disk on the side adjacent to the erythromycin disk, and a positive D test result indicated that this type of resistance had been induced. It was determined the D test was negative since there was no evidence of a blunted zone of inhibition, which demonstrates that the strain is in fact susceptible to clindamycin.

5. Conclusions

Through the course of our research, we were able to present a comprehensive analysis that shed light on the proportional distribution of *S. aureus*, methicillin-resistant *staphylococcus aureus* (MRSA), and coagulase-negative staphylococci carrying *mec*A or *mec*C genes in various food categories such as meat, general food items, and pickled foods, as well as in food containers across the rural landscape of northeastern Thailand. These findings bring to light possible concerns with regard to public health, more notably those concerning the environmental contamination of staphylococci that are present within the food chain. It is essential to understand that the existence of these bacteria in meat and other food products may serve as a possible source of antimicrobial resistance and enterotoxin genes, leading to cross-contamination between the population and livestock. As a result, it is necessary to give careful consideration to the control of these bacteria and take appropriate preventative actions in order to limit the risks associated with their presence.

Author Contributions: Conceptualization, A.K. and P.C.; formal analysis, R.K.; funding acquisition, P.C.; investigation, R.K., P.B. and R.H.; methodology, R.K., W.K. and P.C.; resources, A.K.; supervision, A.K.; validation, W.K. and P.C.; writing—original draft preparation, R.K. and P.C.; writing—review and editing, A.K. and P.C. All authors have read and agreed to the published version of the manuscript.

Funding: This research is supported in part by the Graduate Program Scholarship from The Graduate School, Kasetsart University, Bangkok, Thailand.

Institutional Review Board Statement: Not applicable.

Informed Consent Statement: Not applicable.

Data Availability Statement: Not applicable.

Acknowledgments: The Kasetsart University Research and Development Institute (KURDI), Bangkok, Thailand, provided English editing.

Conflicts of Interest: The authors declare no conflict of interest.

References

1. Lee, S.I.; Kim, S.D.; Park, J.H.; Yang, S.J. Species Distribution, Antimicrobial Resistance, and Enterotoxigenicity of Non- aureus Staphylococci in Retail Chicken Meat. *Antibiotics* **2020**, *9*, 809. [CrossRef]
2. Lakhundi, S.; Zhang, K. Methicillin-Resistant *Staphylococcus aureus*: Molecular Characterization, Evolution, and Epidemiology. *Clin. Microbiol. Rev.* **2018**, *31*, 10–1128. [CrossRef]
3. Khairullah, A.R.; Sudjarwo, S.A.; Effendi, M.H.; Ramandinianto, S.C.; Gelolodo, M.A.; Widodo, A.; Riwu, K.H.P.; Kurniawati, D.A. Pet animals as reservoirs for spreading methicillin-resistant *Staphylococcus aureus* to human health. *J. Adv. Vet. Anim. Res.* **2023**, *10*, 1–13. [CrossRef] [PubMed]
4. Campos, B.; Pickering, A.C.; Rocha, L.S.; Aguilar, A.P.; Fabres-Klein, M.H.; de Oliveira Mendes, T.A.; Fitzgerald, J.R.; de Oliveira Barros Ribon, A. Diversity and pathogenesis of *Staphylococcus aureus* from bovine mastitis: Current understanding and future perspectives. *BMC Vet. Res.* **2022**, *18*, 115. [CrossRef]
5. Ren, Q.; Liao, G.; Wu, Z.; Lv, J.; Chen, W. Prevalence and characterization of *Staphylococcus aureus* isolates from subclinical bovine mastitis in southern Xinjiang, China. *J. Dairy Sci.* **2020**, *103*, 3368–3380. [CrossRef]
6. Becker, K.; Both, A.; Weißelberg, S.; Heilmann, C.; Rohde, H. Emergence of coagulase-negative staphylococci. *Expert Rev. Anti-Infect. Ther.* **2020**, *18*, 349–366. [CrossRef] [PubMed]
7. Holden, M.T.G.; Feil, E.J.; Lindsay, J.A.; Peacock, S.J.; Day, N.P.J.; Enright, M.C.; Foster, T.J.; Moore, C.E.; Hurst, L.; Atkin, R.; et al. Complete genomes of two clinical *Staphylococcus aureus* strains: Evidence for the rapid evolution of virulence and drug resistance. *Proc. Natl. Acad. Sci. USA* **2004**, *101*, 9786–9791. [CrossRef] [PubMed]
8. Urmi, M.R.; Ansari, W.K.; Islam, M.S.; Sobur, M.A.; Rahman, M.; Rahman, M.T. Antibiotic resistance patterns of *Staphylococcus* spp. isolated from fast foods sold in different restaurants of Mymensingh, Bangladesh. *J. Adv. Vet. Anim. Res.* **2021**, *8*, 274–281. [CrossRef]
9. Sadat, A.; Shata, R.R.; Farag, A.M.M.; Ramadan, H.; Alkhedaide, A.; Soliman, M.M.; Elbadawy, M.; Abugomaa, A.; Awad, A. Prevalence and Characterization of PVL-Positive *Staphylococcus aureus* Isolated from Raw Cow's Milk. *Toxins* **2022**, *14*, 97. [CrossRef]
10. Al-Ashmawy, M.A.; Sallam, K.I.; Abd-Elghany, S.M.; Elhadidy, M.; Tamura, T. Prevalence, Molecular Characterization, and Antimicrobial Susceptibility of Methicillin-Resistant *Staphylococcus aureus* Isolated from Milk and Dairy Products. *Foodborne Pathog. Dis.* **2016**, *13*, 156–162. [CrossRef]
11. Wu, S.; Huang, J.; Zhang, F.; Wu, Q.; Zhang, J.; Pang, R.; Zeng, H.; Yang, X.; Chen, M.; Wang, J.; et al. Prevalence and Characterization of Food-Related Methicillin-Resistant *Staphylococcus aureus* (MRSA) in China. *Front. Microbiol.* **2019**, *10*, 304. [CrossRef] [PubMed]
12. Fernandes, A.; Ramos, C.; Monteiro, V.; Santos, J.; Fernandes, P. Virulence Potential and Antibiotic Susceptibility of S. aureus Strains Isolated from Food Handlers. *Microorganisms* **2022**, *10*, 2155. [CrossRef] [PubMed]
13. Papadopoulos, P.; Papadopoulos, T.; Angelidis, A.S.; Kotzamanidis, C.; Zdragas, A.; Papa, A.; Filioussis, G.; Sergelidis, D. Prevalence, antimicrobial susceptibility and characterization of *Staphylococcus aureus* and methicillin-resistant *Staphylococcus aureus* isolated from dairy industries in north-central and north-eastern Greece. *Int. J. Food Microbiol.* **2019**, *291*, 35–41. [CrossRef] [PubMed]
14. Poudel, B.; Zhang, Q.; Trongtorsak, A.; Pyakuryal, B.; Egoryan, G.; Sous, M.; Ahmed, R.; Trelles-Garcia, D.P.; Yanez-Bello, M.A.; Trelles-Garcia, V.P.; et al. An overlooked cause of septic shock: Staphylococcal Toxic Shock Syndrome secondary to an axillary abscess. *IDCases* **2020**, *23*, e01039. [CrossRef]
15. Schaumburg, F.; Ngoa, U.A.; Kösters, K.; Köck, R.; Adegnika, A.A.; Kremsner, P.G.; Lell, B.; Peters, G.; Mellmann, A.; Becker, K. Virulence factors and genotypes of *Staphylococcus aureus* from infection and carriage in Gabon. *Clin. Microbiol. Infect.* **2011**, *17*, 1507–1513. [CrossRef] [PubMed]
16. Buz On-Dur, L.; Capita, R.; Alonso-Calleja, C. Antibiotic susceptibility of methicillin-resistant staphylococci (MRS) of food origin: A comparison of agar disc diffusion method and a commercially available miniaturized test. *Food Microbiol.* **2017**, *72*, 220–224. [CrossRef]
17. Huber, H.; Ziegler, D.; Pflüger, V.; Vogel, G.; Zweifel, C.; Stephan, R. Prevalence and characteristics of methicillin-resistant coagulase-negative staphylococci from livestock, chicken carcasses, bulk tank milk, minced meat, and contact persons. *BMC Vet. Res.* **2011**, *7*, 6. [CrossRef]
18. Nemeghaire, S.; Vanderhaeghen, W.; Angeles Argudín, M.; Haesebrouck, F.; Butaye, P. Characterization of methicillin-resistant Staphylococcus sciuri isolates from industrially raised pigs, cattle and broiler chickens. *J. Antimicrob. Chemother.* **2014**, *69*, 2928–2934. [CrossRef]
19. Igbinosa, E.O.; Beshiru, A.; Igbinosa, I.H.; Ogofure, A.G.; Ekundayo, T.C.; Okoh, A.I. Prevalence, multiple antibiotic resistance and virulence profile of methicillin-resistant *Staphylococcus aureus* (MRSA) in retail poultry meat from Edo, Nigeria. *Front. Cell. Infect. Microbiol.* **2023**, *13*, 183. [CrossRef]
20. Bernier-Lachance, J.; Arsenault, J.; Usongo, V.; Parent, E.; Labrie, J.; Jacques, M.; Malouin, F.; Archambault, M. Prevalence and characteristics of Livestock-Associated Methicillin-Resistant *Staphylococcus aureus* (LA-MRSA) isolated from chicken meat in the province of Quebec, Canada. *PLoS ONE* **2020**, *15*, e0227183. [CrossRef]

21. Yang, X.; Zhang, J.; Yu, S.; Wu, Q.; Guo, W.; Huang, J.; Cai, S. Prevalence of *Staphylococcus aureus* and Methicillin-Resistant *Staphylococcus aureus* in Retail Ready-to-Eat Foods in China. *Front. Microbiol.* **2016**, *7*, 816. [CrossRef] [PubMed]

22. Klibi, A.; Maaroufi, A.; Torres, C.; Jouini, A. Detection and characterization of methicillin-resistant and susceptible coagulase-negative staphylococci in milk from cows with clinical mastitis in Tunisia. *Int. J. Antimicrob. Agents* **2018**, *52*, 930–935. [CrossRef] [PubMed]

23. Fernandes dos Santos, F.; Mendonça, L.C.; Reis, D.R.d.L.; Guimarães, A.d.S.; Lange, C.C.; Ribeiro, J.B.; Machado, M.A.; Brito, M.A.V.P. Presence of mecA-positive multidrug-resistant Staphylococcus epidermidis in bovine milk samples in Brazil. *J. Dairy Sci.* **2016**, *99*, 1374–1382. [CrossRef] [PubMed]

24. Chajecka-Wierzchowska, W.; Zadernowska, A.; Nalepa, B.; Sierpińska, M.; Laniewska-Trokenheim, L. Coagulase-negative staphylococci (CoNS) isolated from ready-to-eat food of animal origin--phenotypic and genotypic antibiotic resistance. *Food Microbiol.* **2015**, *46*, 222–226. [CrossRef]

25. Osman, K.; Alvarez-Ordóñez, A.; Ruiz, L.; Badr, J.; ElHofy, F.; Al-Maary, K.S.; Moussa, I.M.I.; Hessain, A.M.; Orabi, A.; Saad, A.; et al. Antimicrobial resistance and virulence characterization of *Staphylococcus aureus* and coagulase-negative staphylococci from imported beef meat. *Ann. Clin. Microbiol. Antimicrob.* **2017**, *16*, 35. [CrossRef]

26. Sorour, H.K.; Shalaby, A.G.; Abdelmagid, M.A.; Hosny, R.A. Characterization and pathogenicity of multidrug-resistant coagulase-negative Staphylococci isolates in chickens. *Int. Microbiol.* **2023**, 1–12. [CrossRef]

27. Seng, R.; Kitti, T.; Thummeepak, R.; Kongthai, P.; Leungtongkam, U.; Wannalerdsakun, S.; Sitthisak, S. Biofilm formation of methicillin-resistant coagulase negative staphylococci (MR-CoNS) isolated from community and hospital environments. *PLoS ONE* **2017**, *12*, e0184172. [CrossRef]

28. Vestergaard, M.; Cavaco, L.M.; Sirichote, P.; Unahalekhaka, A.; Dangsakul, W.; Svendsen, C.A.; Aarestrup, F.M.; Hendriksen, R.S. SCCmec Type IX Element in Methicillin Resistant Staphylococcusaureusspa Type t337 (CC9) Isolated from Pigs and Pork in Thailand. *Front. Microbiol.* **2012**, *3*, 103. [CrossRef]

29. Tanomsridachchai, W.; Changkaew, K.; Changkwanyeun, R.; Prapasawat, W.; Intarapuk, A.; Fukushima, Y.; Yamasamit, N.; Kapalamula, T.F.; Nakajima, C.; Suthienkul, O.; et al. Antimicrobial Resistance and Molecular Characterization of Methicillin-Resistant *Staphylococcus aureus* Isolated from Slaughtered Pigs and Pork in the Central Region of Thailand. *Antibiotics* **2021**, *10*, 206. [CrossRef]

30. Saenhom, N.; Kansan, R.; Chopjitt, P.; Boueroy, P.; Hatrongjit, R.; Kerdsin, A. Evaluation of in-house cefoxitin screening broth to determine methicillin-resistant staphylococci. *Heliyon* **2022**, *8*, ee08950. [CrossRef]

31. Sukhumungoon, P.; Bunnueang, N.; Kongpheng, S.; Singkhamanan, K.; Saengsuwan, P.; Rattanachuay, P.; Dangsriwan, S. Methicillin-Resistant *Staphylococcus aureus* from Ready-to-Eat Foods in a Hospital Canteen, Southern Thailand: Virulence Characterization And Genetic Relationship. *Southeast Asian J. Trop. Med. Public Health* **2015**, *46*, 86.

32. Sankomkai, W.; Boonyanugomol, W.; Kraisriwattana, K.; Nutchanon, J.; Boonsam, K.; Kaewbutra, S.; Wongboot, W. Characterisation of Classical Enterotoxins, Virulence Activity, and Antibiotic Susceptibility of *Staphylococcus aureus* Isolated from Thai Fermented Pork Sausages, Clinical Samples, and Healthy Carriers in Northeastern Thailand. *J. Vet. Res.* **2020**, *64*, 289–297. [CrossRef] [PubMed]

33. Şanlıbaba, P. Prevalence, antibiotic resistance, and enterotoxin production of *Staphylococcus aureus* isolated from retail raw beef, sheep, and lamb meat in Turkey. *Int. J. Food Microbiol.* **2022**, *361*, 109461. [CrossRef]

34. Zehra, A.; Gulzar, M.; Singh, R.; Kaur, S.; Gill, J.P.S. Prevalence, multidrug resistance and molecular typing of methicillin-resistant *Staphylococcus aureus* (MRSA) in retail meat from Punjab, India. *J. Glob. Antimicrob. Resist.* **2019**, *16*, 152–158. [CrossRef]

35. Wu, S.; Huang, J.; Wu, Q.; Zhang, J.; Zhang, F.; Yang, X.; Wu, H.; Zeng, H.; Chen, M.; Ding, Y.; et al. *Staphylococcus aureus* Isolated From Retail Meat and Meat Products in China: Incidence, Antibiotic Resistance and Genetic Diversity. *Front. Microbiol.* **2018**, *9*, 2767. [CrossRef]

36. Ou, C.; Shang, D.; Yang, J.; Chen, B.; Chang, J.; Jin, F.; Shi, C. Prevalence of multidrug-resistant *Staphylococcus aureus* isolates with strong biofilm formation ability among animal-based food in Shanghai. *Food Control* **2020**, *112*, 107106. [CrossRef]

37. Zhu, Z.; Liu, X.; Chen, X.; Zou, G.; Huang, Q.; Meng, X.; Pei, X.; Chen, Z.; Zhou, R.; Hu, D.; et al. Prevalence and Virulence Determinants of *Staphylococcus aureus* in Wholesale and Retail Pork in Wuhan, Central China. *Foods* **2022**, *11*, 4114. [CrossRef]

38. Velasco, V.; Vergara, J.L.; Bonilla, A.M.; Muñoz, J.; Mallea, A.; Vallejos, D.; Quezada-Aguiluz, M.; Campos, J.; Rojas-García, P. Prevalence and Characterization of *Staphylococcus aureus* Strains in the Pork Chain Supply in Chile. *Foodborne Pathog. Dis.* **2018**, *15*, 262–268. [CrossRef]

39. Komodromos, D.; Kotzamanidis, C.; Giantzi, V.; Pappa, S.; Papa, A.; Zdragas, A.; Angelidis, A.; Sergelidis, D. Prevalence, Infectious Characteristics and Genetic Diversity of *Staphylococcus aureus* and Methicillin-Resistant *Staphylococcus aureus* (MRSA) in Two Raw-Meat Processing Establishments in Northern Greece. *Pathog.* **2022**, *11*, 1370. [CrossRef]

40. Feßler, A.T.; Kadlec, K.; Hassel, M.; Hauschild, T.; Eidam, C.; Ehricht, R.; Monecke, S.; Schwarz, S. Characterization of methicillin-resistant *Staphylococcus aureus* isolates from food and food products of poultry origin in Germany. *Appl. Environ. Microbiol.* **2011**, *77*, 7151–7157. [CrossRef]

41. Boost, M.V.; Wong, A.; Ho, J.; O'Donoghue, M. Isolation of methicillin-resistant *Staphylococcus aureus* (MRSA) from retail meats in Hong Kong. *Foodborne Pathog. Dis.* **2013**, *10*, 705–710. [CrossRef] [PubMed]

42. Bhargava, K.; Wang, X.; Donabedian, S.; Zervos, M.; da Rocha, L.; Zhang, Y. Methicillin-resistant *Staphylococcus aureus* in retail meat, Detroit, Michigan, USA. *Emerg. Infect. Dis.* **2011**, *17*, 1135–1137. [CrossRef] [PubMed]

43. Hanson, B.M.; Dressler, A.E.; Harper, A.L.; Scheibel, R.P.; Wardyn, S.E.; Roberts, L.K.; Kroeger, J.S.; Smith, T.C. Prevalence of *Staphylococcus aureus* and methicillin-resistant *Staphylococcus aureus* (MRSA) on retail meat in Iowa. *J. Infect. Public Health* **2011**, *4*, 169–174. [CrossRef] [PubMed]

44. Benito, D.; Gómez, P.; Lozano, C.; Estepa, V.; Gómez-Sanz, E.; Zarazaga, M.; Torres, C. Genetic lineages, antimicrobial resistance, and virulence in *Staphylococcus aureus* of meat samples in Spain: Analysis of immune evasion cluster (IEC) genes. *Foodborne Pathog. Dis.* **2014**, *11*, 354–356. [CrossRef]

45. Lo, Y.P.; Wan, M.T.; Chen, M.M.; Su, H.Y.; Lauderdale, T.L.; Chou, C.C. Molecular characterization and clonal genetic diversity of methicillin-resistant *Staphylococcus aureus* of pig origin in Taiwan. *Comp. Immunol. Microbiol. Infect. Dis.* **2012**, *35*, 513–521. [CrossRef]

46. Guardabassi, L.; O'donoghue, M.; Moodley, A.; Ho, J.; Boost, M. Novel Lineage of Methicillin-Resistant *Staphylococcus aureus*, Hong Kong. *Emerg. Infect. Dis.* **2009**, *15*, 1998. [CrossRef]

47. Neela, V.; Zafrul, A.M.; Mariana, N.S.; Van Belkum, A.; Liew, Y.K.; Rad, E.G. Prevalence of ST9 methicillin-resistant *Staphylococcus aureus* among pigs and pig handlers in Malaysia. *J. Clin. Microbiol.* **2009**, *47*, 4138–4140. [CrossRef]

48. Anukool, U.; O'Neill, C.E.; Butr-Indr, B.; Hawkey, P.M.; Gaze, W.H.; Wellington, E.M.H. Meticillin-resistant *Staphylococcus aureus* in pigs from Thailand. *Int. J. Antimicrob. Agents* **2011**, *38*, 86–87. [CrossRef]

49. Larsen, J.; Imanishi, M.; Hinjoy, S.; Tharavichitkul, P.; Duangsong, K.; Davis, M.F.; Nelson, K.E.; Larsen, A.R.; Skov, R.L. Methicillin-resistant *Staphylococcus aureus* ST9 in pigs in Thailand. *PLoS ONE* **2012**, *7*, e31245. [CrossRef]

50. Chuang, Y.Y.; Huang, Y.C. Livestock-associated meticillin-resistant *Staphylococcus aureus* in Asia: An emerging issue? *Int. J. Antimicrob. Agents* **2015**, *45*, 334–340. [CrossRef]

51. Silva, V.; Almeida, F.; Carvalho, J.A.; Castro, A.P.; Ferreira, E.; Manageiro, V.; Tejedor-Junco, M.T.; Caniça, M.; Igrejas, G.; Poeta, P. Emergence of community-acquired methicillin-resistant *Staphylococcus aureus* EMRSA-15 clone as the predominant cause of diabetic foot ulcer infections in Portugal. *Eur. J. Clin. Microbiol. Infect. Dis.* **2020**, *39*, 179–186. [CrossRef] [PubMed]

52. Bonura, C.; Plano, M.R.A.; Di Carlo, P.; Calà, C.; Cipolla, D.; Corsello, G.; Mammina, C. MRSA ST22-IVa (EMRSA-15 clone) in Palermo, Italy. *J. Infect. Public Health* **2010**, *3*, 188–191. [CrossRef] [PubMed]

53. Niek, W.K.; Teh, C.S.J.; Idris, N.; Thong, K.L.; Ponnampalavanar, S. Predominance of ST22-MRSA-IV Clone and Emergence of Clones for Methicillin-Resistant *Staphylococcus aureus* Clinical Isolates Collected from a Tertiary Teaching Hospital Over a Two-Year Period. *Jpn. J. Infect. Dis.* **2019**, *72*, 228–236. [CrossRef]

54. Coelho, C.; Torres, C.; Radhouani, H.; Pinto, L.; Lozano, C.; Gómez-Sanz, E.; Zaragaza, M.; Igrejas, G.; Poeta, P. Molecular detection and characterization of methicillin-resistant *Staphylococcus aureus* (MRSA) isolates from dogs in Portugal. *Microb. Drug Resist.* **2011**, *17*, 333–337. [CrossRef]

55. Costa, S.S.; Ribeiro, R.; Serrano, M.; Oliveira, K.; Ferreira, C.; Leal, M.; Pomba, C.; Couto, I. *Staphylococcus aureus* Causing Skin and Soft Tissue Infections in Companion Animals: Antimicrobial Resistance Profiles and Clonal Lineages. *Antibiotics* **2022**, *11*, 599. [CrossRef] [PubMed]

56. Li, D.Z.; Chen, Y.S.; Yang, J.P.; Zhang, W.; Hu, C.P.; Li, J.S.; Mu, L.; Hu, Y.H.; Geng, R.; Hu, K.; et al. Preliminary molecular epidemiology of the *Staphylococcus aureus* in lower respiratory tract infections: A multicenter study in China. *Chin. Med. J.* **2011**, *124*, 687–692. [CrossRef]

57. Boamah, V.E.; Agyare, C.; Odoi, H.; Adu, F.; Gbedema, S.Y.; Dalsgaard, A. Prevalence and antibiotic resistance of coagulase-negative Staphylococci isolated from poultry farms in three regions of Ghana. *Infect. Drug Resist.* **2017**, *10*, 175–183. [CrossRef]

58. Pimenta, R.L.; de Melo, D.A.; Bronzato, G.F.; de Salles Souza, V.R.; Holmström, T.C.N.; de Oliveira Coelho, S.D.M.; da Silva Coelho, I.; de Souza, M.M.S. Characterization of staphylococcus spp. isolates and β-lactam resistance in broiler chicken production. *Rev. Bras. Med. Vet.* **2021**, *43*, e00720. [CrossRef]

59. Rall, V.L.M.; Sforcin, J.M.; De Deus, M.F.R.; De Sousa, D.C.; Camargo, C.H.; Godinho, N.C.; Galindo, L.A.; Soares, T.C.S.; Araújo, J.P. Polymerase Chain Reaction Detection of Enterotoxins Genes in Coagulase-Negative Staphylococci Isolated from Brazilian Minas Cheese. *Foodborne Pathog. Dis.* **2010**, *7*, 1121–1123. [CrossRef]

60. Podkowik, M.; Park, J.Y.; Seo, K.S.; Bystroń, J.; Bania, J. Enterotoxigenic potential of coagulase-negative staphylococci. *Int. J. Food Microbiol.* **2013**, *163*, 34–40. [CrossRef]

61. Silva, V.; Caniça, M.; Ferreira, E.; Vieira-Pinto, M.; Saraiva, C.; Pereira, J.E.; Capelo, J.L.; Igrejas, G.; Poeta, P. Multidrug-Resistant Methicillin-Resistant Coagulase-Negative Staphylococci in Healthy Poultry Slaughtered for Human Consumption. *Antibiotics* **2022**, *11*, 365. [CrossRef]

62. El-Deeb, W.; Cave, R.; Fayez, M.; Alhumam, N.; Quadri, S.; Mkrtchyan, H.V. Methicillin Resistant Staphylococci Isolated from Goats and Their Farm Environments in Saudi Arabia Genotypically Linked to Known Human Clinical Isolates: A Pilot Study. *Microbiol. Spectr.* **2022**, *10*, e00387-22. [CrossRef]

63. Dinges, M.M.; Orwin, P.M.; Schlievert, P.M. Exotoxins of *Staphylococcus aureus*. *Clin. Microbiol. Rev.* **2000**, *13*, 16–34. [CrossRef]

64. Chiang, Y.C.; Liao, W.W.; Fan, C.M.; Pai, W.Y.; Chiou, C.S.; Tsen, H.Y. PCR detection of Staphylococcal enterotoxins (SEs) N, O, P, Q, R, U, and survey of SE types in *Staphylococcus aureus* isolates from food-poisoning cases in Taiwan. *Int. J. Food Microbiol.* **2008**, *121*, 66–73. [CrossRef]

65. Hu, W.D. Distribution of food-borne *Staphylococcus aureus* enterotoxin genes. *Genet. Mol. Res.* **2016**, *15*, 1–9. [CrossRef] [PubMed]

66. Al-Talib, H.; Yean, C.Y.; Al-Khateeb, A.; Hassan, H.; Singh, K.K.B.; Al-Jashamy, K.; Ravichandran, M. A pentaplex PCR assay for the rapid detection of methicillin-resistant *Staphylococcus aureus* and Panton-Valentine Leucocidin. *BMC Microbiol.* **2009**, *9*, 113. [CrossRef] [PubMed]

67. Stegger, M.; Andersen, P.S.; Kearns, A.; Pichon, B.; Holmes, M.A.; Edwards, G.; Laurent, F.; Teale, C.; Skov, R.; Larsen, A.R. Rapid detection, differentiation and typing of methicillin-resistant *Staphylococcus aureus* harbouring either mecA or the new mecA homologue mecA(LGA251). *Clin. Microbiol. Infect.* **2012**, *18*, 395–400. [CrossRef] [PubMed]

68. Kondo, Y.; Ito, T.; Ma, X.X.; Watanabe, S.; Kreiswirth, B.N.; Etienne, J.; Hiramatsu, K. Combination of multiplex PCRs for staphylococcal cassette chromosome mec type assignment: Rapid identification system for mec, ccr, and major differences in junkyard regions. *Antimicrob. Agents Chemother.* **2007**, *51*, 264–274. [CrossRef]

69. Petti, C.A.; Bosshard, P.P.; Brandt, M.E.; Clarridge, J.E.; Feldblyum, T.V.; Foxall, P.; Furtado, M.R.; Pace, N.; Procop, G. Interpretive Criteria for Identification of Bacteria and Fungi by DNA Target Sequencing; Approved Guideline. *Clin. Lab. Stand. Inst. (CLSI) Doc.* **2008**, *28*, 19087–19898.

70. Enright, M.C.; Day, N.P.J.; Davies, C.E.; Peacock, S.J.; Spratt, B.G. Multilocus sequence typing for characterization of methicillin-resistant and methicillin-susceptible clones of *Staphylococcus aureus*. *J. Clin. Microbiol.* **2000**, *38*, 1008–1015. [CrossRef]

71. Shopsin, B.; Gomez, M.; Waddington, M.; Riehman, M.; Kreiswirth, B.N. Use of coagulase gene (coa) repeat region nucleotide sequences for typing of methicillin-resistant *Staphylococcus aureus* strains. *J. Clin. Microbiol.* **2000**, *38*, 3453–3456. [CrossRef]

72. Dereeper, A.; Guignon, V.; Blanc, G.; Audic, S.; Buffet, S.; Chevenet, F.; Dufayard, J.-F.; Guindon, S.; Lefort, V.; Lescot, M.; et al. Phylogeny.fr: Robust phylogenetic analysis for the non-specialist. *Nucleic Acids Res.* **2008**, *36*, 465–469. [CrossRef]

73. Letunic, I.; Bork, P. Interactive Tree Of Life (iTOL) v5: An online tool for phylogenetic tree display and annotation. *Nucleic Acids Res.* **2021**, *49*, W293–W296. [CrossRef]

74. Clinical and Laboratory Standards Institute (CLSI). *Performance Standards for Antimicrobial Susceptibility Testing*, 32nd ed.; M100; Clinical Laboratory Standard Institute: Wayne, PA, USA, 2023.

75. Magiorakos, A.P.; Srinivasan, A.; Carey, R.B.; Carmeli, Y.; Falagas, M.E.; Giske, C.G.; Harbarth, S.; Hindler, J.F.; Kahlmeter, G.; Olsson-Liljequist, B.; et al. Multidrug-resistant, extensively drug-resistant and pandrug-resistant bacteria: An international expert proposal for interim standard definitions for acquired resistance. *Clin. Microbiol. Infect.* **2012**, *18*, 268–281. [CrossRef]

76. Chavez-Bueno, S.; Bozdogan, B.; Katz, K.; Bowlware, K.L.; Cushion, N.; Cavuoti, D.; Ahmad, N.; McCracken, G.H.; Appelbaum, P.C. Inducible clindamycin resistance and molecular epidemiologic trends of pediatric community-acquired methicillin-resistant *Staphylococcus aureus* in Dallas, Texas. *Antimicrob. Agents Chemother.* **2005**, *49*, 2283–2288. [CrossRef]

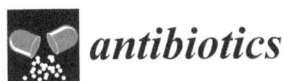 *antibiotics*

MDPI

Article

Isolation, Identification and Genetic Characterization of Antibiotic Resistant *Escherichia coli* from Frozen Chicken Meat Obtained from Supermarkets at Dhaka City in Bangladesh

Mridha. Md. Kamal Hossain [1], Md. Sharifull Islam [1,2], Md. Salah Uddin [1,3], A. T. M. Mijanur Rahman [3], Asad Ud-Daula [3], Md. Ariful Islam [1,3], Rubaya Rubaya [1], Anjuman Ara Bhuiya [1], Md. Abdul Alim [1], Nusrat Jahan [1], Jinquan Li [4,*] and Jahangir Alam [1,*]

[1] Animal Biotechnology Division, National Institute of Biotechnology, Savar 1349, Bangladesh
[2] Center for Cancer Immunology, Institute of Biomedicine and Biotechnology, Shenzhen Institutes of Advanced Technology, Chinese Academy of Sciences, Shenzhen 518055, China
[3] Department of Applied Nutrition and Food Technology, Islamic University, Kushtia 7003, Bangladesh
[4] State Key Laboratory of Agricultural Microbiology, Huazhong Agricultural University, Wuhan 430070, China
* Correspondence: lijinquan@mail.hzau.edu.cn (J.L.); alamjahan2003@yahoo.com (J.A.)

Citation: Hossain, M.M.K.; Islam, M.S.; Uddin, M.S.; Rahman, A.T.M.M.; Ud-Daula, A.; Islam, M.A.; Rubaya, R.; Bhuiya, A.A.; Alim, M.A.; Jahan, N.; et al. Isolation, Identification and Genetic Characterization of Antibiotic Resistant *Escherichia coli* from Frozen Chicken Meat Obtained from Supermarkets at Dhaka City in Bangladesh. *Antibiotics* **2023**, *12*, 41. https://doi.org/10.3390/antibiotics12010041

Academic Editor: Jesus Simal-Gandara

Received: 29 November 2022
Revised: 13 December 2022
Accepted: 22 December 2022
Published: 27 December 2022

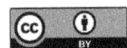

Abstract: Antimicrobials have been used to improve animal welfare, food security, and food safety that promote the emergence, selection, and dissemination of antimicrobial-resistant (AMR) bacteria. In this study, 50 *E. coli* were isolated from frozen chicken meat samples in Dhaka city. Antibiotic sensitivity patterns were assessed through the disk diffusion method and finally screened for the presence of antimicrobial resistance genes (ARG) using the polymerase chain reaction (PCR). Among the 160 samples, the prevalence of *E. coli* was observed in fifty samples (31.25%). All of these isolates were found resistant to at least one antimicrobial agent, and 52.0% of the isolates were resistant against 4–7 different antimicrobials. High resistance was shown to tetracycline (66.0%), followed by resistance to erythromycin (42.0%), ampicillin and streptomycin (38.0%), and sulfonamide (28.0%). In addition, the most prevalent ARGs were *tet(A)* (66.0%), *ereA* (64.0%), *tet(B)* (60.0%), *aadA1* and *sulI* (56.0%), *blaCITM* (48.0%) and *blaSHV* (40.0%). About 90.0% of isolates were multidrug resistant. This study reveals for the first time the current situation of *E. coli* AMR in broilers, which is helpful for the clinical control of disease as well as for the development of policies and guidelines to reduce AMR in broilers production in Bangladesh.

Keywords: frozen chicken meat; *E. coli*; Antimicrobials; Antimicrobial resistance genes; Dhaka city

1. Introduction

Antimicrobial agents have been used in humans, veterinary medicine, food security, and food safety since their discovery in the 1920s. However, due to inadequate selection, overuse, and misuse of antimicrobials have been responsible for the selection of resistant isolates, known as antimicrobial resistance (AMR) [1]. Over the past decade, AMR has become a global threat to human and animal health. Development of resistance can be the result of both chromosomal mutations and the acquisition of mobile genetic elements (MGEs), harboring AMR gene mutations [2,3]. It has been reported that, antibiotics are no longer effective against infection-causing bacteria due to increased AMR rate, as a result, every 10 min a patient dies in the USA or Europe [4,5]. However, a substantially higher prevalence of increased AMR is likely to be found in developing countries especially in Africa and Asia due to limited diagnosis facilities, unauthorized antibiotics sale, poor patient education, the inappropriate function of drug regulatory action, inappropriate prescription practices, and non-human practice of antibiotics in livestock sectors [6,7]. Due to the magnitude of the threat, the World Health Organization (WHO) recommended global surveillance programs for animal and human populations.

According to WHO, the first-ever list of antibiotic-resistant "priority pathogens", *Escherichia coli* is included in the most critical group of all twelve families of bacteria that carriage the greatest threat to human and animal health [8]. The level of antimicrobial resistance in *E. coli* has been used as an indicator of resistance dissemination in bacterial populations, and of selective pressure imposed by antimicrobials used in food animals and humans [9–12]. However, the frequency of AMR in *E. coli* depends on the source of the isolates. Animal origin has been reported to be the cause of drug-resistant *E. coli* infections in humans, and that these agents harbored the same mobile resistance genes found in diverse bacterial species from a variety of animal sources [13–17]. However, a high prevalence of AMR *E. coli* was isolated from chicken compared with other animals' origins [18]. Additionally, AMR *E. coli* isolated from humans is similar to *E. coli* from poultry [19]. It has been reported that commensal *E. coli*, can serve as a good reservoir of resistance genes with the ability to transfer these genes to pathogens in the hosts as well as in the human intestinal tract after the consumption of contaminated foods of animal origin [20]. Furthermore, a number of studies have established the transfer of AMR between commensal bacteria and zoonotic pathogens in various ecological environments [21–23].

Poultry meat production has been increased and doubled over the past 20 years. Poultry is traded at live bird markets, and products are sold unprocessed with bigger clusters of them in city areas which presents significant public and poultry health challenges. A number of companies have already integrated their operations. Poultry and meat processing is a very new movement in the food processing industry in Bangladesh. It has been said that frozen chickens are mostly obtainable through high-end supermarkets charging premium prices and this market is growing every year. Another market segment is food preparation for the main fast-food chains. The local frozen food market is also growing, at a rate of almost 30% in 2011–2012 over the preceding year. City dwellers, are progressively becoming more conscious of their accessibility and the lifestyle they permit, as they desire to go to supermarket instead of to wet markets to buy their everyday stuff, including frozen chicken meat [24]. Tenants in the city becoming more conscious of their accessibility to safe food. Nonetheless, warranting the microbiological safety of frozen chicken meat evolves as a challenge.

Few studies have already reported bacterial contamination in frozen chicken meat from different cities in Bangladesh. Customers in cities have a habit of buying frozen chicken meat along with other frozen and ready-to-cook foodstuffs as these frozen items need slight processing for cooking and, thus, they can save time [25–27]. Two of these studies were bacteriological along with AMR phenotype. Another study includes a few genes related to extended spectrum beta-lactamase (ESBL) and non- ESBL producing *E. coli*. However, recent reviews reported the uses of nineteen and ten different types of antibiotics in the broiler and layer farms, respectively in Bangladesh [28]. Therefore, further study is needed for genotyping which shows higher diversity than phenotypes and consequently allows for more accurate comparisons between resistant bacterial populations [29,30]. The aim of this study was to determine the prevalence of *E. coli* in frozen chicken and phenotypic AMR profile as well as the detection of ARG.

2. Results

2.1. Prevalence of E. coli in Frozen Chicken Meat

E. coli was isolated and identified in fifty samples out of 160 samples with an overall prevalence of 31.25%. However, the prevalence of *E. coli* was found to range from 20.0–40.0% in the tested samples (Table 1). The highest prevalence (40.0%) was found in chickens purchased from supermarkets in the Mirpur region while the lowest prevalence (20.0%) was in samples of the Gulshan region.

Table 1. Prevalence of *E. coli* in frozen chicken meat collected from different supermarkets located in Dhaka city.

Location	Number of Supermarkets	No. of Chicken Sample	Sources of Chicken	No. of Positive Sample	Prevalence (%)
Gulshan	4	40	Contract farmers	8	20.0
Dhanmondi	4	40	Contract farmers	14	35.0
Mirpur	4	40	Contract farmers	16	40.0
Uttara	4	40	Contract farmers	12	30.0
Overall		160		50	31.25

2.2. Antimicrobial Resistance Profiles of E. coli

Antimicrobial resistance among *E. coli* isolates was determined by the disc diffusion method using seven different antibiotics spanning six different classes. The distribution of AMR patterns is presented in Table 2 and Figure 1.

Table 2. Antimicrobial resistance profile of *E. coli* isolated from frozen chicken meat (*n* = 50).

Antimicrobial Class	Antimicrobial Agent (Conc.)	No. of *E. coli* Tested	No. of Isolates (%)		
			Resistance	Intermediate	Sensitive
Aminoglycosides	Streptomycin (10 µg)	50	19 (38.0)	10 (20.0)	21 (42.0)
	Gentamicin (10 µg)	50	8 (16.0)	14 (28.0)	28 (56.0)
Tetracyclines	Tetracycline (30 µg)	50	33 (66.0)	0 (0.0)	17 (34.0)
Beta-lactams	Ampicillin (10 µg)	50	19 (38.0)	3 (6.0)	28 (56.0)
Macrolides	Erythromycin (15 µg)	50	21 (42.0)	10 (20.0)	19 (38.0)
Phenicols	Chloramphenicol (30 µg)	50	11 (22.0)	4 (8.0)	35 (70.0)
Sulfonamides	Sulfonamide (300 µg)	50	14 (28.0)	15 (30.0)	21 (42.0)
Overall		350	125 (35.7)	56 (16.0)	169 (48.3)

Overall, 35.7, 16.0 and 48.3% of the isolates were found resistant, intermediate, and sensitive, respectively to all the antibiotics used in this study. About 2.0% of isolates showed resistance to seven antibiotics spanning six classes of antimicrobial agents (Str-Gen-Tet-Amp-Ery-Chl-Sul) (Supplementary Table S1).

About 90.0% of the isolates were found to MDR and about 52.0% of the isolates showed resistance against 4–7 different antimicrobials (Table 3).

Table 3. Distribution of resistance profiles of *E. coli* (*n* = 50).

Antibiotic Class	No. of Antimicrobials	No. of Isolate Resistant (%)	MDR [a] No. of Isolate (%)
1	1	3 (6.00)	No
2	2	2 (4.00)	
	3	3 (6.00)	
3	3	16 (32.00)	Yes
	4	4 (8.00)	45 (90.00)
4	4	13 (26.00)	
	5	3 (6.00)	
5	5	3 (6.00)	
	6	2 (4.00)	
6	7	1 (2.00)	

[a] Isolate is defined as multidrug-resistant when it shows resistance to >3 classes of antimicrobial agents.

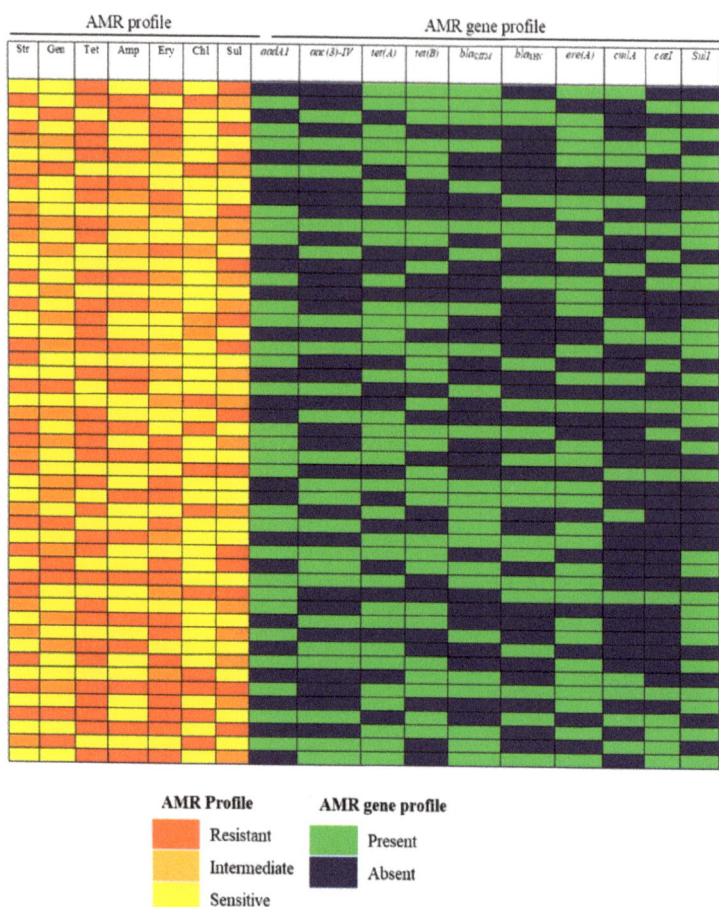

Figure 1. Distribution of antimicrobial resistance phenotype and antimicrobial resistance genes of *E. coli* isolated from chicken meat from supermarkets of Dhaka city. Str: streptomycin, Gen: gentamicin, Tet: tetracycline, Amp: ampicillin, erythromycin, Chl: chloramphenicol, Sul: sulfonamide.

2.3. Antimicrobial Resistance Genes (ARGs) in E. coli

Ten ARGs were detected using PCR in all isolated *E. coli* and the results are presented in Table 5. Tetracycline efflux genes *tet(A)* and *tet(B)* were found in 66.0 % and 60.0 % of the total isolates in this study, respectively. Both *tet(A)* and *tet(B)* genes were found in 60.0% of the isolates. About 64.0% of the isolates harbored the erythromycin esterase (*ereA*) gene. Besides, 56.0 %, 56.0 %, 44.0% of the isolates were found to carrying *aadA1*, *sul1*, *aac(3)-IV* genes, respectively. The presence of the AmpC beta-lactamase-producing gene (*bla$_{CITM}$*) was observed in 48.0% of chicken *E. coli* isolates. Moreover, about 40.0% of chicken *E. coli* isolates carried genes coding for extended-spectrum SHV (*bla$_{SHV}$*) beta-lactamases (Table 4).

Table 4. Distribution of antimicrobial resistance genes (ARGs) in *E. coli* isolates (*n* = 50).

Antimicrobial Class	Antimicrobial Agent	ARGs	No. of *E. coli* Positive (%)	No. of *E. coli* Negative (%)
Aminoglycosides	Streptomycin	*aadA1*	28 (56.0)	22 (44.0)
	Gentamicin	*aac(3)-IV*	22 (44.0)	28 (56.0)
Tetracyclines	Tetracycline	*tet(A)*	33 (66.0)	17 (34.0)
		tet(B)	30 (60.0)	20 (40.0)
Beta-lactams	Ampicillin	bla_{CITM}	24 (48.0)	26 (52.0)
		bla_{SHV}	20 (40.0)	30 (60.0)
Macrolides	Erythromycin	*ereA*	32 (64.0)	18 (36.0)
Phenicols	Chloramphenicol	*cmlA*	17 (34.0)	33 (66.0)
		cat1	18 (36.0)	32 (64.0)
Sulfonamides	Sulfonamide	*sul1*	28 (56.0)	22 (44.0)

Antimicrobial resistance genes (3-9) were detected in 84.0% of the isolates. While 70.0% of the isolates were found to carry 5–9 of the ten ARGs investigated in this study (Figure 2).

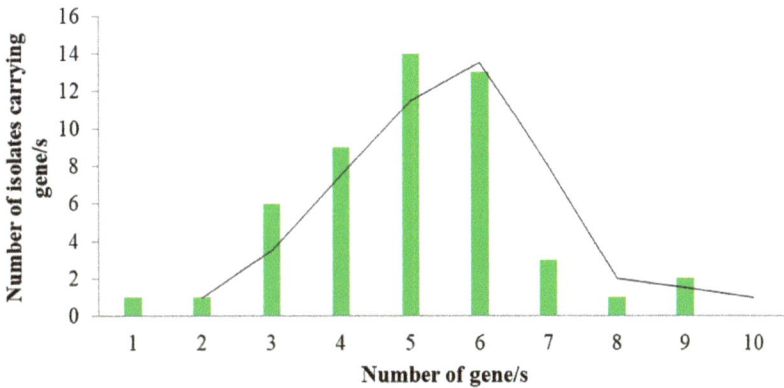

Figure 2. A number of antimicrobial resistance genes (ARGs) detected in isolated *E. coli* from chicken meat from supermarkets in Dhaka city (*n* = 50).

2.4. Antimicrobial Resistance Phenotype and Genotype Association

Strong positive associations were found among AMR phenotypes and the corresponding resistance genes except for tetracycline-*tet(B)* (OR: 1.33, 95% CI 0.41–4.31, *p* = 0.63) (Table 5). The observed strongest associations were between the following pairs of antibiotics and corresponding genes: tetracycline-*tet(A)* (OR: 512.0, 95% CI: 30.03–8728.99, *p* ≤ 0.0001), streptomycin-*aadA1* (OD: 270.0, 95% CI: 22.86–3189.39, *p* < 0.0001), erythromycin-*ere(A)* (OD: 255, 95% CI: 21.50–3024.21, *p* ≤ 0.0001), sulfonamide-*sulI* (OD: 82.33, 95% CI: 12.51–542.00, *p* ≤ 0.0001), gentamicin-*aac(3)-IV* (OD: 52.0, 95% CI: 9.57–291.19, *p* ≤ 0.0001). Positive associations were also observed for other antibiotics and corresponding genes analyzed in this study. By pairwise association analysis, non-significant positive and negative associations were found within AMR phenotypes and genotypes (Supplementary Tables S2 and S3).

Table 5. Comparison of AMR in *E. coli* isolates according to phenotypic and genotypic results.

Antimicrobial	NP	ARG	NG	P+/G+	P+/G-	P-/G+	P-/G-	Odds Ratio	95% CI	p
Streptomycin	29	*aadA1*	28	27	2	1	20	270.00	22.86–3189.39	<0.0001
Gentamycin	22	*aac(3)-IV*	22	19	3	3	25	52.78	9.57–291.19	<0.0001
Tetracycline	33	*tet(A)*	33	32	1	1	16	512.00	30.03–8728.99	<0.0001
		tet(B)	30	20	12	10	8	1.33	0.41–4.31	0.63
Ampicillin	22	*bla*$_{CITM}$	24	15	7	9	19	4.52	1.37–14.98	0.01
		bla$_{SHV}$	20	13	9	7	21	4.33	1.30–14.47	0.02
Erythromycin	31	*ereA*	32	30	1	2	17	255.00	21.50–3024.21	<0.0001
Chloramphenicol	15	*cmlA*	17	11	4	6	29	13.29	3.14–56.27	0.0004
		cat1	18	12	3	6	29	19.33	4.14–90.24	0.0002
Sulfonamide	29	*sulI*	28	26	3	2	19	82.33	12.51–542.00	<0.0001

NP: number of *E. coli* isolates expressing phenotypic resistance; ARG: antibiotic resistance gene; NG: number of *E. coli* isolates carrying the indicated resistance gene; P+/G+: number of phenotypically resistant *E. coli* isolates (P+) with resistance gene (G+) for the drug identified; P+/G-: number of phenotypically resistant *E. coli* isolates (P+) with no resistance gene (G-) for the drug identified; P-/G+: number of phenotypically susceptible *E. coli* isolates (P-) with resistance gene (G-) for the drug identified; P-/G-: number of phenotypically susceptible *E. coli* isolates (P-) with no resistance gene (G-) for the drug identified; CI: confidence interval.

3. Discussion

E. coli is recognized as a common inhabitant of the vertebrate intestinal tract which frequently causes contamination in retail meat products. It is one of the most common food-borne pathogens associated with mortality in commercial poultry as well as condemning the carcasses in slaughterhouses and has been considered a significant public health threat and economic burden [31]. It has been reported that resistant strains from the gut readily contaminate poultry carcasses at slaughter, and consequently, poultry meats are often contaminated with resistant *E. coli* [32]. Antibiotics have been widely used for preventing economic losses caused by *E. coli* and increasing production efficiency [33]. However, with increased consumption of these drugs may lead to scattering them into manure and other poultry wastes and transferring them to humans by their residues in carcasses and can be the origin of bacterial resistance, mortality, and increase in human hospitalization [34]. In this study, the overall prevalence of *E. coli* in frozen chicken was found 31.25% which is lower than the prevalence (76.1%) reported from frozen chicken [25]. Our findings are also lower than the findings of the previous study [35]. It has been reported about a 63.5% prevalence of *E. coli* in raw chicken meat covering both layer and broiler swab samples. We have taken about 10 g of meat from the surface of the breast and thigh muscles of each of the broilers. However, processed meat samples for *E. coli* isolation from various parts of the body of layer, broiler and cockerel has been examined [25,35]. On the other hand, the present study was limited only to Dhaka city. Moreover, sampling time, season, etc. were also different. All of these factors may contribute to the differences of *E. coli* prevalence in frozen meat samples. Moreover, broilers sold in supermarkets especially come from contract farms that manage their farms more hygienically than the general farmers may also contribute to lower occurrences of *E. coli*. A contract farm is defined as a farm where farmers have a contract with the company (supermarket authority) that the company provides the chicks, the feed, veterinary care, and technical advice, etc. while the farmers provide the day-to-day care of the birds, land, and housing, as well as utilities/maintenance of the housing and finally share benefits as per contract [25]. Additionally, the prevalence may not show actual prevalence as we have examined a portion of muscle sample from the surface of the frozen chicken. The source of *E. coli* may be the chicken itself or it comes from contamination during the dressing and packing of chicken. It is to be mentioned that we have ensured the aseptic handling of samples in the laboratory to avoid laboratory-acquired contamination.

From Bangladesh, many studies have been reported on AMR and the majority of them concentrate on the isolation and investigation of the antibiotic resistance patterns of *E. coli* by disc diffusion technique [36,37]. Although the conventional method is most widely used for determining AMR because of convenience, efficiency, and cost; it has some limitations.

Results may be unexpected or borderline in addition to some other limitations such as its inapplicability to many fastidious organisms and anaerobes [38], unable to obtain minimal inhibitory concentration (MIC) values [39], labor-intensive and time-consuming [40]. In this study, we have used both phenotypic detection of AMR as well as detection of ARGs from the same isolates. It has been reported that tetracycline resistance *E. coli* was found more frequently [28]. Besides, resistances were also found against almost all antibiotics used in this study. ESBL *E. coli* isolates from frozen meat displayed resistance to oxytetracycline and amoxicillin (91.9%), ampicillin and trimethoprim–sulfamethoxazole (89.2%), pefloxacin (87.8%), cefepime (81.1%), piperacillin–tazobactam (73.0%), and doxycycline (70.3%) [25]. A recent review [28] reported that nineteen and ten different types of antibiotics are used in the broiler and layer farms, respectively in Bangladesh. The most commonly used antibiotics included ciprofloxacin, ampicillin, amoxicillin, trimethoprim, oxytetracycline, tylosin tartrate, tiamulin, norfloxacin, enrofloxacin, doxycycline, and colistin sulfate. Information regarding the use of antimicrobials in broiler was not available to the research team to draw further insights.

MDR bacteria are an emerging clinical challenge in the poultry sector as well as the livestock sector. In this study, about 90.0% of the *E. coli* isolates were found MDR, and 52% of the isolates showed resistance against 4–7 different antimicrobials. Our findings are within the findings of recent reports regarding MDR phenotypes of *E. coli*. It has been reported eighty-six *E. coli* isolates from frozen chicken meat against sixteen antimicrobials and found that all the isolates are MDR [25] and as suggested by other literature reported 49.23 and 51.09% MDR *E. coli* isolates from broiler and layer meat samples [35]. AMR pattern (streptomycin-gentamicin-tetracycline-ampicillin-erythromycin-chloramphenicol-sulfonamide) of one *E. coli* isolates (Supplementary Table S1) indicates the necessity of prudent use of antibiotics. AmpC beta-lactamase-producing gene (bla_{CITM}) and the gene coding for extended-spectrum SHV beta-lactamases (bla_{SHV}) were detected in broiler chicken *E. coli* isolates in the present study. It has been also reported that 12.8% of broiler chicken *E. coli* isolates carried bla_{SHV} and 4.56% of isolates possess bla_{CITM} genes [35]. Differences in findings might reflect the sources and number of samples etc. In Bangladesh, $blaCTX$-M-1 (94.4%) and bla_{TEM} (50–91.3%) ESBL-producing *E. coli* were reported in the droppings of chickens [41,42]. Strong correlations between most of the antimicrobial-resistant phenotypes and genotypes were observed among the investigated *E. coli* isolates that the similar findings are reported earlier [35].

In *E. coli*, the AMR phenotypic-genotypic agreement of 33–85% [29] has been reported for different antimicrobial agents and related genes. In the present study, it was found that few isolates with resistance phenotypes lacked the corresponding ARGs tested, indicating the occurrence of multi-gene mediated AMR. On the other hand, some isolates carry the resistance genes but phenotypically not resistant to the corresponding antibiotics used in this study. The occurrence of similar AMR phenomena was also reported previously [29]. Sometimes, the phenotype or the genotype alone is unable to accurately predict the outcome of the other, as molecular mechanisms of AMR are multifaceted. Thus, the presence or absence of a specific gene corresponding to a particular phenotype does not necessarily infer that the particular strain is resistant or susceptible [43]. The differences between the genotype and phenotype observed in this study might be due to not testing for all possible resistance genes, or genes not being turned on, or the presence of 'silent gene cassettes' in certain isolates.

It is established that the use of a specific antibiotic can result in its own resistance. It can also play a role as a co-selection marker for other antibiotics. This may happen in completely unrelated drug classes [44,45]. The use of chloramphenicol in the poultry sector is very rare. However, about 22.0% of the isolates showed resistance to chloramphenicol. Moreover, chloramphenicol resistance genes viz. *catA1* and *cmlA* were detected in 36.0 and 34.0% of the *E. coli* isolates, respectively. Resistance to chloramphenicol might be due to the co-selection dynamics among chloramphenicol, oxytetracycline, and sulfonamide [30,44]. A non-significant poor association between *tet(A)* and *tet(B)* resistance genes among *E. coli* isolates (Supplementary Table S3) was observed which may be due to the incompatibility of plasmids carrying the tetracycline resistance determinants [30]. However, further study is required to enumerate the relationships among the resistance gene(s) and the probable link to antimicrobial exposure.

The findings of this study indicated that more caution are required for personnel hygiene in the processing and handling of poultry and poultry products to prevent the transfer of AMR *E. coli* from frozen poultry sold in supermarkets in Bangladesh. Present findings also highlighted the necessity of cautious use of antimicrobials in chickens to minimize the development of antibiotic-resistant bacterial strains. The study has limitations and these include a small sample size and fewer antibiotic-resistance genes tested. Further detailed investigation using a large number of samples, targeting more antibiotics including latest antibiotics as well as more ARGs, etc. would provide broader insights into the AMR patterns, prevalent ARGs, etc. among clinically important pathogens from food producing animals.

4. Materials and Methods

4.1. Collection of Whole Frozen Chicken

This cross-sectional study was conducted in Dhaka district in Bangladesh. A total of 160 frozen chicken meat were purchased from different supermarkets located in Gulshan, Dhanmondi, Mirpur, and Uttara regions in Dhaka city (Figure 3) during the period of July 2018 to June 2019 for the isolation and identification of *E. coli*. After purchase chicken samples were individually placed in a sterile zipper bag, kept in an ice box, and immediately brought to the laboratory of the Animal Biotechnology Division, National Institute of Biotechnology. Samples were either shortly stored in the refrigerator (4 °C) in case of immediate processing or at −20 °C in case of processing after 1–2 days of purchase.

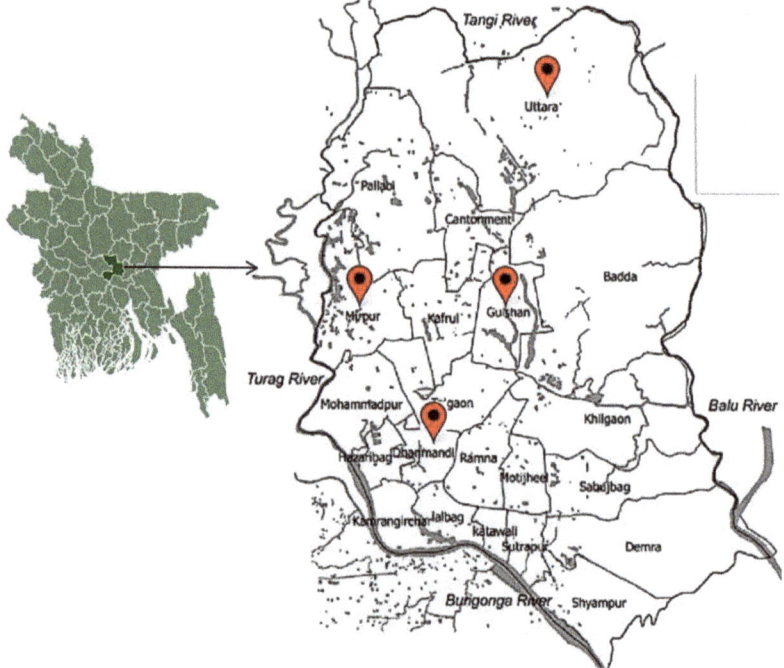

Figure 3. Sample collection from supermarkets of four different locations in Dhaka city, Bangladesh.

4.2. Sample Processing and Isolation of E. coli

The preparation of the meat samples was based on the slight modification of the European standard ISO-16654:2001 [46] About 10 g of meat sample, thigh and breast muscles each 5 g, was obtained from the surface of each of the chickens, cut into small pieces, added with 90 ml of sterile 1% peptone and mixed well. Enrichment was performed for 16 to 24 h at 150 rpm at 37 °C in a shaking incubator. A portion of enriched samples (25 µL) were plated on MacConkey's agar (MCA; Difco) and incubated at 37 °C for 24 h. Typical colonies of *E. coli* were randomly picked, mixed with 100 µL phosphate-buffer saline, inoculated onto eosine methyline blue (EMB) agar, and incubated at 37 °C for 18–24 h. After incubation, the selected bacterial colonies from EMB agar were inoculated into 5 mL of sterile Luria Bertani (LB) broth and placed into a shaking incubator at 37 °C for overnight. This culture was used for further analysis.

4.3. Identification of E. coli by Polymerase Chain Reaction (PCR)

Genomic DNA was isolated from selected bacteria cultured in LB broth by using a mixture of phenol: chloroform: isoamyl alcohol (25:24:1) [47], followed by precipitation with isopropanol. Finally, the DNA was dissolved in 50 µL of Tris-EDTA buffer. The concentration (ng/µL) and absorbance ratio (260 nm/280 nm) was determined by spectrophotometry (NanoDrop 2000, Thermo Scientific). PCR amplification was performed using primers (16E1-F: 5′-GGGAGTAAAGTTAATCCTTTGCTC-3′ and 16E2-R: 5′-TTCCCGAAGGCACATTCT-3′) targeting 584 bp fragment of 16S rRNA gene as reported earlier [48]. PCR amplification was performed on 25 µL scale, containing 1.5 mM MgCl$_2$, 50 mM KCl, 10 mM Tris-HCl (pH 9.0), 0.1% Triton X-100, 200 µM of each dNTP, 1 µM primers, 1 unit of Taq DNA polymerase, and 5 µL (~50 ng/µL) of genomic DNA in Gene Atlas thermocycler (ASTEC Gene Atlas, G02, Japan). The thermal condition included an initial denaturation for 5 m at 95 °C, followed by 35 cycles consisting of denaturation at 94 °C for 1 m, annealing at 55 °C for 90 s and extension at 72 °C for 1 m, and a final extension of 10 m at 72 °C. Amplified DNA was separated on 1.5% agarose gel and visualized under ultraviolet light in an Axygen™ Gel documentation system (Corning Inc., Corning, NY, USA).

4.4. Antimicrobial Resistance Profiling (ARP) of the Isolates

AMR profiling of the *E. coli* was performed by disc diffusion method according to Clinical and Laboratory Standards Institute (CLSI) guidelines, 2018 [49]. A total of seven antimicrobials from six different classes were used in the AMR profile test. These included (i) aminoglycosides: gentamicin (10 µg) and streptomycin (10 µg), (ii) tetracyclines: tetracycline (30 µg), (iii) β-lactam: ampicillin (10 µg), (iv) macrolides: erythromycin (15 µg) (v) phenicols: chloramphenicol (30 µg), and (vi) sulfonamides: sulfonamide (300 µg) (oxoid™). *E. coli* (ATCC 25922) strain was used as a reference strain for interpretations of the antimicrobial susceptibility test results. The isolates were categorized as resistant, intermediate, or sensitive based on the diameter of the zone of inhibition according to CLSI guidelines. As there is no standard zone of inhibition mentioned for erythromycin with *Enterobacteriaceae*, the interpretation was performed based on the zone of inhibition for *Staphylococcus* spp. *E. coli* showed resistance to three or more than three different classes of antimicrobials, which was defined as multidrug-resistance (MDR) [50].

4.5. Detection of Antimicrobial Resistance Genes (ARGs) in the Isolates

All the isolates were tested for the presence of *aadA1*, *aac(3)-IV*, *tet(A)*, *tet(B)*, *bla*$_{SHV}$, *bla*$_{CITM}$, *ereA*, *catA1*, *cmlA*, and *sulI* ARGs by PCR as described [51–53]. Details of the primer sequences, annealing temperature, PCR product size, etc. are presented in Table 6. Basic thermal conditions were initial denaturation for 5 m at 95 °C, 35 cycles consisting of denaturation for 1 m at 94 °C, annealing for 40 s at the temperature of each respective gene and extension for 1 m at 72 °C, followed by a final extension step of 10 m at 72 °C. The annealing temperature varied for each gene (Table 6).

Antibiotics **2023**, 12, 41

Table 6. Primers used for amplification of antimicrobial resistance genes (ARGs) from *E. coli.*

Antimicrobial Agent	Resistance Gene	Sequence (5"-3")	Size (bp)	Annealing Temp (°C)	References
Streptomycin	Adenylyl transferases (*aadA1*)	F- TATCCAGCTAAGCGCGAACT R- ATTTGCCGACTACCTTGGTC	447	58	[51]
Gentamicin	Aminoglycoside acetyltransferases (*aac(3)-IV*)	F- CTTCAGGATGGCAAGTTGGT R- TCATCTCGTTCTCCGCTCAT	286	55	[52]
Tetracycline	Efflux pump resistance (*tet(A)*)	F- GGTTCACTCGAACGACGTCA R- CTGTCCGACAAGTTGCATGA	577	57	
	Efflux pump resistance (*tet(B)*)	F- CCTCAGCTTCTCAACGCGTG R- GCACCTTGCTGATGACTCTT	634	56	[51]
Ampicillin	β-lactamase encoding penicillin resistance (*Bla$_{SHV}$*)	F- TCGCCTGTGTATTATCTCCC R- CGCAGATAAATCACCACAATG	768	52	
	β-lactamase encoding cephalosporin resistance (*Bla$_{CITM}$*)	F- TGGCCAGAACTGACAGGCAAA R- TTTCTCCTGAACGTGGCTGGC	462	47	
Erythromycin	Erythromycin esterase (*ereA*)	F- GCCGGTGCTCATGAACTTGAG R- CGACTCTATTCGATCAGAGGC	419	60	[52]
Chloramphenicol	Acetyltransferases (*catA1*)	F-AGTTGCTCAATGTACCTATAACC R- TTGTAATTCATTAAGCATTCTGCC	547	55	
	Transporter resistance (*cmlA*)	F- CCGCCACGGTGTTGTTGTTATC R- CACCTTGCCTGCCCATCATTAG	698	33	[53]
Sulfonamide	Dihydropteroate synthase (*sul1*)	F- TTCGGCATTCTGAATCTCAC R- ATGATCTAACCCTCGGTCTC	822	47	

4.6. Statistical Analysis

Descriptive and association-based statistical analyses were conducted using Microsoft Excel v.13.0 and GraphPad Prism v.8.0 statistical tools, respectively. The association between specific AMR phenotype and the ARG was calculated and an association was considered significant at a p-value of <0.05 and was reported as an odds ratio (OR) with 95% confidence intervals (CI). An OR of > 1 was considered a positive association or the increasing probability of the co-occurrence of the genotype or phenotype, while an OR of <1 was considered a negative association or the decreasing probability of the co-occurrence of the genotype or phenotype. The degree of agreement between phenotypic and genotypic relations was assessed by Kappa coefficients (κ) [54].

5. Conclusions

The results of the present study indicate that a good percentage of frozen chicken sold in supermarkets in Dhaka city carries *E. coli* and they are resistant to commonly used antibiotics and the majority of them are MDR. Furthermore, more cautions are necessary for choosing a drug for the treatment of clinical cases of poultry because the transfer of drug resistant gene from one bacterium to other may be hazardous for human being too. Therefore, careful use of antimicrobials in poultry production is recommended.

Supplementary Materials: The following supporting information can be downloaded at: https://www.mdpi.com/article/10.3390/antibiotics12010041/s1, Table S1: Antimicrobial resistance patterns of *E. coli* (*n* = 50), Table S2: Pairwise association analysis of phenotypic antimicrobial resistance patterns, Table S3: Pairwise association analysis antimicrobial resistance genes (ARGs).

Author Contributions: Author Contributions: This work was carried out in collaboration with all authors. Conceptualization, M.M.K.H. and J.A.; Methodology, M.M.K.H., M.S.U., R.R., A.A.B. and J.A.; Software, M.M.K.H., M.A.I., M.A.A. and J.A.; Validation, M.M.K.H., M.S.U., M.A.I., M.S.I., J.A. and J.L.; Formal Analysis, M.M.K.H., M.S.U., M.S.I. and J.A.; Investigation, M.M.K.H., M.S.U., R.R. and A.A.B.; Resources, M.M.K.H. and J.A.; Data Curation, M.M.K.H., M.S.U., N.J. and R.R.; Writing—Original Draft Preparation, M.M.K.H., M.S.U., A.A.B. and M.S.I.; Writing—Review and Editing, A.T.M.M.R., A.U.-D., M.A.A., J.A. and J.L.; Visualization, M.M.K.H., R.R., N.J. and J.A.; Supervision, M.A.A. and J.A.; Project Administration, M.M.K.H.; Funding Acquisition, J.A. All authors have read and agreed to the published version of the manuscript.

Funding: This work was supported by the Ministry of Science and Technology (MoST, R&D: BMN-124), Bangladesh through a R&D project.

Institutional Review Board Statement: Not applicable.

Informed Consent Statement: Not applicable.

Data Availability Statement: Not applicable.

Acknowledgments: Authors would like to acknowledge to MoST, Bangladesh for the funding this research.

References

1. Kolár, M.; Urbánek, K.; Látal, T. Antibiotic selective pressure and development of bacterial resistance. *Int. J. Antimicrob. Agents* **2001**, *17*, 357–363. [CrossRef] [PubMed]
2. Zhang, L.; Kinkelaar, D.; Huang, Y.; Li, Y.; Li, X.; Wang, H.H. Acquired antibiotic resistance: Are we born with it? *Appl. Environ. Microbiol.* **2011**, *77*, 7134–7141. [CrossRef] [PubMed]
3. Fu, Y.; Zhang, W.; Wang, H. Specific patterns of gyrA mutations determine the resistance difference to ciprofloxacin and levofloxacin in *Klebsiella pneumoniae* and *Escherichia coli*. *BMC Infect. Dis.* **2013**, *13*, 8. [CrossRef]
4. Centers for Disease Control and Prevention. Antimicrobial Resistance Threat Report. 2013. Available online: http://www.cdc.gov/drugresistance/threat-report-2013 (accessed on 21 October 2015).

5. European Commission. Action Plan against the Rising Threats from Antimicrobial Resistance. Communication from the Commission to the European Parliament and the Council. COM (2011) 748. Available online: http://ec.europa.eu/dgs/health_food-safety/docs/communication_amr_2011_748_en.pdf (accessed on 21 October 2015).
6. Byarugaba, D.K. A view on antimicrobial resistance in developing countries and responsible risk factors. *Int. J. Antimicrob. Agents* **2004**, *24*, 105–110. [CrossRef]
7. Ayukekbong, J.A.; Ntemgwa, M.; Atabe, A.N. The threat of antimicrobial resistance in developing countries: Causes and control strategies. *Antimicrob. Resist. Infect. Control.* **2017**, *6*, 47. [CrossRef] [PubMed]
8. WHO. List of Bacteria for Which New Antibiotics Are Urgently Needed. Available online: http://www.who.int/mediacentre/news/releases/2017/bacteria-antibiotics-needed/en/ (accessed on 27 February 2017).
9. Alhaj, N.; Mariana, N.; Raha, A.; Ishak, Z. Prevalence of antimicrobial resistance among *Escherichia coli* from different sources in Malaysia. *Int. J. Poultry Sci.* **2007**, *6*, 293–297. [CrossRef]
10. Saenz, Y.; Zarazaga, M.; Brinas, L.; Lantero, M.; Ruiz-Larrea, F.; Torres, C. Antibiotic resistance in *Escherichia coli* isolates obtained from animals, foods and humans in Spain. *Int. J. Antimicrob. Agents* **2001**, *18*, 353–358. [CrossRef]
11. Scott, H.M.; Campbell, L.D.; Harvey, R.B.; Bischoff, K.M.; Alali, W.Q.; Barling, K.S.; Anderson, R.C. Patterns of antimicrobial resistance among commensal *Escherichia coli* isolated from integrated multi-site housing and worker cohorts of humans and swine. *Foodborne Pathog. Dis.* **2005**, *2*, 24–37. [CrossRef]
12. Sorum, H.; Sunde, M. Resistance to antibiotics in the normal flora of animals. *Vet. Res.* **2001**, *32*, 227–241. [CrossRef]
13. Pereira, J.G.; Fernandes, J.; Duarte, A.R.; Fernandes, S.M. β-Lactam Dosing in Critical Patients: A Narrative Review of Optimal Efficacy and the Prevention of Resistance and Toxicity. *Antibiotics.* **2022**, *11*, 1839. [CrossRef]
14. Hammerum, A.M.; Heuer, O.E. Human health hazards from antimicrobial-resistant *Escherichia coli* of animal origin. *Clin. Infect. Dis.* **2009**, *48*, 916–921. [CrossRef] [PubMed]
15. Johnson, J.R.; McCabe, J.S.; White, D.G.; Johnston, B.; Kuskowski, M.A.; McDermott, P. Molecular Analysis of *Escherichia coli* from retail meats (2002–2004) from the United States National Antimicrobial Resistance Monitoring System. *Clin. Infect. Dis.* **2009**, *49*, 195–201. [CrossRef] [PubMed]
16. Johnson, J.R.; Sannes, M.R.; Croy, C.; Johnston, B.; Clabots, C.; Kuskowski, M.A.; Bender, J.; Smith, K.E.; Winokur, P.L.; Belongia, E.A. Antimicrobial drug-resistant *Escherichia coli* from humans and poultry products, Minnesota and Wisconsin, 2002-2004. *Emerg. Infect. Dis.* **2007**, *13*, 838–846. [CrossRef] [PubMed]
17. Von, B.; Marre, R. Antimicrobial resistance of *Escherichia coli* and therapeutic implications. *Int. J. Med. Microbiol.* **2005**, *295*, 503–511.
18. Kikuvi, G.M.; Schwarz, S.; Ombui, J.N.; Mitema, E.S.; Kehrenberg, C. Streptomycin and chloramphenicol resistance genes in *Escherichia coli* isolates from cattle, pigs, and chicken in Kenya. *Microb. Drug Resist.* **2007**, *1*, 62–68. [CrossRef]
19. Vieira, A.R. Association between antimicrobial resistance in *Escherichia coli* isolates from food animals and blood stream isolates from humans in Europe: An ecological study. *Foodborne Pathog. Dis.* **2011**, *8*, 1295–1301. [CrossRef]
20. Blake, D.P.; Hillman, K.; Fenlon, D.R.; Low, J.C. Transfer of antibiotic resistance between commensal and pathogenic members of the Enterobacteriaceae under ideal conditions. *J. Appl. Microbiol.* **2003**, *95*, 428–436. [CrossRef]
21. Mathew, A.G.; Liamthong, S.; Lin, J.; Hong, Y. Evidence of class 1 integron transfer between *Escherichia coli* and *Salmonella* spp. on livestock farms. *Foodborne Pathog. Dis.* **2009**, *6*, 959–964. [CrossRef] [PubMed]
22. Walsh, C.; Duffy, G.; Nally, P.; O'Mahoney, R.; McDowell, D.A.; Fanning, S. Transfer of ampicillin resistance from Salmonella Typhimurium DT104 to *Escherichia coli* K12 in food. *Lett. Appl. Microbiol.* **2008**, *46*, 210–215. [CrossRef]
23. Poppe, C.; Martin, L.C.; Gyles, C.L.; Reid-Smith, R.; Boerlin, P.; McEwen, S.A.; Prescott, J.F.; Forward, K.R. Acquisition of resistance to extended-spectrum cephalosporins by Salmonella Newport and *Escherichia coli* in the intestinal tract of turkey poults. *Appl. Environ. Microbiol.* **2005**, *71*, 1184–1192. [CrossRef]
24. Rahman, M.S.; Jang, D.H.; Yu, C.J. Poultry industry of Bangladesh: Entering a new phase. *Korean J. Agric. Sci.* **2017**, *44*, 272–282.
25. Parvin, M.S.; Talukder, S.; Ali, M.Y.; Chowdhury, E.H.; Rahman, M.T.; Islam, M.T. Antimicrobial resistance pattern of *Escherichia coli* isolated from frozen chicken meat in Bangladesh. *Pathogens* **2020**, *9*, 420. [CrossRef]
26. Uddin, J.; Hossain, K.; Hossain, S.; Saha, K.; Jubyda, F.T.; Haque, R.; Billah, B.; Talukder, A.A.; Parvez, A.K.; Dey, S.K. Bacteriological assessments of foodborne pathogens in poultry meat at different super shops in Dhaka, Bangladesh. *Ital. J. Food Saf.* **2019**, *8*, 6720. [CrossRef]
27. Alam, S.T.; Howard, M.; Fatema, K.; Haque, K.M.F. Antibiogram of pre-processed raw chicken meat from different super shops of Dhaka city, Bangladesh. *J. Allied Health Sci.* **2015**, *2*, 45–52.
28. Al-Amin, M.; Hoque, M.N.; Siddiki, A.Z.; Saha, S.; Kamal, M.M. Antimicrobial resistance situation in animal health of Bangladesh. *Vet. World.* **2020**, *13*, 2713–2727. [CrossRef]
29. Rosengren, L.B.; Waldner, C.L.; Reid-Smith, R.J. Associations between antimicrobial resistance phenotypes, antimicrobial resistance genes, and virulence genes of fecal *E. coli* isolates from healthy grow-finish pigs. *Appl. Environ. Microbiol.* **2009**, *75*, 1373–1380. [CrossRef]
30. Gow, S.P.; Waldner, C.L.; Harel, J.; Boerlin, P. Associations between antimicrobial resistance genes in fecal generic *E. coli* isolates from cow-calf herds in western Canada. *Appl. Environ. Microbiol.* **2008**, *74*, 3658–3666. [CrossRef]
31. Ewers, C.; Janßen, T.; Kießling, S.; Philipp, H.-C.; Wieler, L.H. Molecular epidemiology of avian pathogenic *Escherichia coli* (APEC) isolated from colisepticemia in poultry. *Vet. Microbiol.* **2004**, *104*, 91–101. [CrossRef]

32. Turtura, G.C.; Massa, S.; Chazvinizadeh, H. Antibiotic resistance among coliform bacteria isolated from carcasses of commercially slaughtered chickens. *Int. J. Food Microbiol.* **1990**, *11*, 351–354. [CrossRef]
33. Angulo, F.J.; Johnson, K.R.; Tauxe, R.V.; Cohen, M.L. Origins and consequences of antimicrobial-resistant nontyphoidal *Salmonella*: Implications for the use of fluoroquinolones in food animals. *Microb. Drug Resist.* **2000**, *6*, 77–83. [CrossRef]
34. Miles, T.D.; McLaughlin, W.; Brown, P.D. Antimicrobial resistance of *Escherichia coli* isolates from broiler chickens and humans. *BMC Vet. Res.* **2006**, *2*, 1–9. [CrossRef]
35. Rahman, M.M.; Husna, A.; Elshabrawy, H.A.; Alam, J.; Runa, N.Y.; Badruzzaman, A.T.M.; Banu, N.A.; Al Mamun, M.; Paul, B.; Das, S.; et al. Isolation and molecular characterization of multidrug-resistant *Escherichia coli* from chicken meat. *Sci. Rep.* **2020**, *10*, 21999. [CrossRef]
36. Akond, M.A.; Hassan, S.M.R.; Alam, S.; Shirin, M. Antibiotic Resistance of *Escherichia Coli* Isolated From Poultry and Poultry Environment of Bangladesh. *Am. J. Environ. Sci.* **2009**, *5*, 47–52.
37. Hasan, B.; Faruque, R.; Drobni, M.; Waldenström, J.; Sadique, A.; Ahmed, K.U.; Islam, Z.; Parvez, M.B.; Olsen, B.; Alam, M. High prevalence of antibiotic resistance in pathogenic *Escherichia coli* from large- and small-scale poultry farms in Bangladesh. *Avian Dis.* **2011**, *55*, 689–692. [CrossRef]
38. Sader, H.S.; Pignatari, A.C.C. E Test: A novel technique for antimicrobial susceptibility testing. *Sao Paulo Med. J.* **1994**, *112*, 635–638. [CrossRef]
39. Dickert, H.; Machka, K.; Braveny, I. The uses and limitations of disc diffusion in the antibiotic sensitivity testing of bacteria. *Infection* **1981**, *9*, 18–24. [CrossRef]
40. Klancnik, A.; Piskernik, S.; Jersek, B.; Mozina, S.S. Evaluation of diffusion and dilution methods to determine the antibacterial activity of plant extracts. *J. Microbiol. Methods* **2010**, *81*, 121–126. [CrossRef]
41. Al Azad, M.; Rahman, A.; Rahman, M.; Amin, R.; Begum, M.; Ara, I.; Fries, R.; Husna, A.; Khairalla, A.S.; Badruzzaman, A. Susceptibility and multidrug resistance patterns of *Escherichia coli* isolated from cloacal swabs of live broiler chickens in Bangladesh. *Pathogens* **2019**, *8*, 118. [CrossRef]
42. Parvez, M.A.K.; Marzan, M.; Liza, S.M.; Mou, T.J.; Azmi, I.J.; Rahman, M.S.; Mahmud, Z.H. Prevalence of inhibitor resistant beta lactamase producing *E. coli* in human and poultry origin of Bangladesh. *J. Bacteriol. Parasitol.* **2016**, *7*, 1–3.
43. Aarts, H.J.M.; Guerra, B.; Malorny, B. Molecular methods for detection of antimicrobial resistance. In *Aarestrup (ed) Antimicrobial Resistance in Bacteria of Animal Origin*; ASM Press: Washington, DC, USA, 2006.
44. O'Connor, A.M.; Poppe, C.; McEwen, S.A. Changes in the prevalence of resistant *E. coli* in cattle receiving subcutaneously injectable oxytetracycline in addition to in-feed chlortetracycline comparing with cattle receiving only in-feed chlortetracycline. *Can. J. Vet. Res.* **2002**, *66*, 145–150.
45. Yang, Y.; Du, H.; Zou, G.; Song, Z.; Zhou, Y.; Li, H.; Tan, C.; Chen, H.; Fischetti, V.A.; Li, J. Encapsulation and delivery of phage as a novel method for gut flora manipulation in situ: A review. *J. Control. Release* **2022**, *1*, S0168–S3659. [CrossRef]
46. WHO. Laboratory protocol. In *Isolation of Salmonella spp. From Food and Animal Faeces*, 5th ed.; WHO: Geneva, Switzerland, 2010; Volume 13, pp. 4–8.
47. Sambrook, J.; Russell, D.W. *Molecular Cloning: A Laboratory Manual*, 3rd ed.; Cold Spring Harbor Laboratory Press: Cold Spring Harbor, NY, USA, 2001.
48. Tsen, H.Y.; Lin, C.K.; Chi, W.R. Development and use of 16S rRNA gene targeted PCR primers for the identification of *Escherichia coli* cells in water. *J. Appl. Microbiol.* **1998**, *85*, 554–560. [CrossRef]
49. CLSI. *Performance Standards for Antimicrobial Susceptibility Testing*, 28th ed.; CLSI supplement M100; Clinical and Laboratory Standards Institute: Wayne, PA, USA, 2018.
50. Magiorakos, A.P.; Srinivasan, A.; Carey, R.B.; Carmeli, Y.; Falagas, M.E.; Giske, C.G.; Harbarth, S.; Hindler, J.F.; Kahlmeter, G.; Olsson-Liljequist, B.; et al. Multidrug-resistant, extensively drug-resistant and pandrug-resistant bacteria: An international expert proposal for interim standard definitions for acquired resistance. *Clin. Microbiol. Infect.* **2012**, *18*, 268–281. [CrossRef]
51. Randall, L.P.; Cooles, S.W.; Osborn, M.K.; Piddock, L.J.V.; Woodward, M.J. Antibiotic resistance genes, integrons and multiple antibiotic resistance in thirty-five serotypes of Salmonella enterica isolated from humans and animals in the UK. *J. Antimicrob. Chemother.* **2004**, *53*, 208–216. [CrossRef]
52. Van, T.T.; Chin, J.; Chapman, T.; Tran, L.T.; Coloe, P.J. Safety of raw meat and shellfish in Vietnam: An analysis of *Escherichia coli* isolations for antibiotic resistance and virulence genes. *Int. J. Food. Microbiol.* **2008**, *124*, 217–223. [CrossRef]
53. Toro, C.; Farfán, M.; Contreras, I.; Flores, O.; Navarro, N.; Mora, G.; Prado, V. Genetic analysis of antibiotic-resistance determinants in multidrug-resistant *Shigella* strains isolated from Chilean children. *Epidemiol. Infect.* **2005**, *133*, 81–86. [CrossRef]
54. Landis, J.R.; Koch, G.G. The measurement of observer agreement for categorical data. *Biometrics* **1977**, *33*, 159–174. [CrossRef]

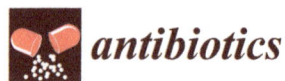

Article

Occurrence and Characterization of NDM-1-Producing *Shewanella* spp. and *Acinetobacter portensis* Co-Harboring *tet*(X3) in a Chinese Dairy Farm

Ruichao Li [1,2,†], **Lifei Zhang** [1,†], **Xiaoyu Lu** [1], **Kai Peng** [1], **Yuan Liu** [1,2], **Xia Xiao** [1], **Hongqin Song** [1,*] **and Zhiqiang Wang** [1,3,*]

[1] Jiangsu Co-Innovation Center for Prevention and Control of Important Animal Infectious Diseases and Zoonoses, College of Veterinary Medicine, Yangzhou University, Yangzhou 225009, China
[2] Institute of Comparative Medicine, Yangzhou University, Yangzhou 225009, China
[3] Joint International Research Laboratory of Agriculture and Agri-Product Safety, The Ministry of Education of China, Yangzhou University, Yangzhou 225009, China
* Correspondence: hqsong@yzu.edu.cn (H.S.); zqwang@yzu.edu.cn (Z.W.)
† These authors contributed equally to this work.

Citation: Li, R.; Zhang, L.; Lu, X.; Peng, K.; Liu, Y.; Xiao, X.; Song, H.; Wang, Z. Occurrence and Characterization of NDM-1-Producing *Shewanella* spp. and *Acinetobacter portensis* Co-Harboring *tet*(X3) in a Chinese Dairy Farm. *Antibiotics* 2022, 11, 1422. https://doi.org/10.3390/antibiotics11101422

Academic Editors: Anusak Kerdsin, Jinquan Li and Jonathan Frye

Received: 8 September 2022
Accepted: 14 October 2022
Published: 17 October 2022

Publisher's Note: MDPI stays neutral with regard to jurisdictional claims in published maps and institutional affiliations.

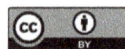
Abstract: Bacteria with carbapenem or tigecycline resistance have been spreading widely among humans, animals and the environment globally, being great threats to public health. However, bacteria co-carrying drug resistance genes of carbapenem and tigecycline in *Shewanella* and *Acinetobacter* species remain to be investigated. Here, we detected nine bla_{NDM-1}-carrying *Shewanella* spp. isolates as well as three *A. portensis* isolates co-harboring *tet*(X3) and bla_{NDM-1} from seventy-two samples collected from a dairy farm in China. To explore their genomic characteristic and transmission mechanism, we utilized various methods, including PCR, antimicrobial susceptibility testing, conjugation experiment, whole-genome sequencing, circular intermediate identification and bioinformatics analysis. Clonal dissemination was found among three *A. portensis*, of which *tet*(X3) and bla_{NDM-1} were located on a novel non-conjugative plasmid pJNE5-X3_NDM-1 (333,311 bp), and the circular intermediate ΔISCR2-*tet*(X3)-bla_{NDM-1} was identified. Moreover, there was another copy of *tet*(X3) on the chromosome of *A. portensis*. It was verified that bla_{NDM-1} could be transferred to *Escherichia coli* C600 from *Shewanella* spp. by conjugation, and self-transmissible IncA/C$_2$ plasmids mediated the transmission of bla_{NDM-1} in *Shewanella* spp. strains. Stringent surveillance was warranted to curb the transmission of such vital resistance genes.

Keywords: *Acinetobacter portensis*; *Shewanella* spp.; *tet*(X3); bla_{NDM-1}; co-existence

1. Introduction

Carbapenems are essential treatment options for clinically significant, multidrug-resistant (MDR) Gram-negative bacteria infections because they have a broad antibacterial spectrum and high antibacterial activity [1]. On the other hand, the populations of carbapenem-resistant bacteria have been quickly growing worldwide in recent years, posing a severe threat to public health [2]. Diverse carbapenemases, which are typically encoded on transmissible plasmids, are the fundamental mechanism of carbapenem resistance. The New Delhi metallo-β-lactamase (NDM), *Klebsiella pneumoniae* carbapenemase (KPC) and OXA-48-type oxacillinase are the three most common carbapenemases [3]. The NDM-1 was initially discovered in India and has now spread throughout the world. It has the ability to hydrolyze practically all β-lactam antibiotics, resulting in the development of MDR bacteria [4]. Because of their excellent therapeutic action on extended-spectrum β-lactamases (ESBLs) and the AmpC enzyme-producing bacteria, meropenem and imipenem are frequently used to treat severe Gram-negative bacteria infections. However, due to the wide prevalence of carbapenem-resistant Gram-negative bacteria in recent years, effective antibiotics against drug-resistant bacteria remain scarce, with tigecycline serving as the last-resort option [5].

Tigecycline is used to treat a variety of clinical infections caused by Gram-positive and Gram-negative bacteria with multidrug resistance. However, the discoveries of plasmid-mediated *tet*(X3) and *tet*(X4) have limited its utility, owing to the capacity of *tet*(X) to catalyze the degradation of tigecycline [6,7]. According to previous retrospective screening, plasmid-borne *tet*(X) genes were present in bacteria of different settings, including food animals, migratory birds, clinical specimens and environmental samples in China [7,8]. Importantly, *tet*(X3) also had a high carriage rate in the gastrointestinal tract of cows [9]. Considering that there are many cow-related food products, antibiotic resistance genes could have been transmitted to humans through vocational contact and transfer among humans.

Known as environmental bacteria, *Shewanella* spp. was widely distributed in marine ecosystems and could also be recovered from food-producing animals and human active areas such as hospitals [10–12]. Although most of the human infections reported linked with *Shewanella* spp. were opportunistic and sporadic, disease syndromes and multidrug resistance have still increased in recent years [13]. Previous reports about *Shewanella* related to multidrug resistance were usually associated with bla_{OXA} rather than bla_{NDM}. A $bla_{OXA-416}$-carrying extensively resistant isolate of *Shewanella xiamenensis* was isolated in Algeria from hospital effluents [14], bla_{OXA-55}-carrying *Shewanella algae* was isolated from a patient in the hospital in Marseille, France [15] and several chromosome-based bla_{OXA-48}-like variants were found in *Shewanella* spp. from ornamental fish in the Netherlands [10]. In 2017, *Shewanella putrefaciens* with chromosomal $bla_{OXA-436}$ and plasmid-borne bla_{NDM-1} was isolated from a hospital in Pakistan [11].

Acinetobacter portensis was a novel *Acinetobacter* species originally identified from raw meat [16]. It is now further described as one MDR pathogen in this study for the first time. The emergence of *Acinetobacter* spp. co-harboring *tet*(X3) and bla_{NDM-1} from animal samples in China has already been reported, but *A. portensis* was not investigated [5,17].

In this study, we looked at the prevalence and molecular characteristics of MDR bacteria with resistance to carbapenem and tigecycline from a dairy farm in China in 2021, and we totally identified twelve NDM-1-producing isolates, including nine *Shewanella* spp. strains and three *A. portensis* strains carrying two copies of *tet*(X) simultaneously, all of which were collected from milking environment samples. The genomic epidemiology of drug-resistant strains and the characteristics of resistance plasmids were also analyzed, with the goal of learning about the molecular genetic characteristics of carbapenem-resistant and tigecycline-resistant bacteria of dairy farm origin to infer the underlying potential public health concerns.

2. Results and Discussion

2.1. Collection of Antimicrobial-Resistant Strains and Resistance Phenotypes

Thirteen meropenem-resistant strains were isolated from seventy-two non-duplicated samples collected from a dairy farm in China, including three *A. portensis* (23.08%), nine *Shewanella* spp. (69.23%) and one *Stenotrophomonas maltophilia* (7.69%). Except for the strain *Stenotrophomonas maltophilia* with inherent resistance to carbapenems collected from the shed environment, the remaining isolates were all identified from milking environment samples and demonstrated to be bla_{NDM}-positive by PCR, with three *A. portensis* strains positive for *tet*(X) as well.

The results of antimicrobial susceptibility testing show that all the carbapenem-resistant isolates conferred resistance to meropenem, ceftiofur and amoxicillin but were susceptible to enrofloxacin, tigecycline and colistin. Five isolates showed resistance to chloramphenicol (38.46%) and seven isolates showed resistance to tetracycline (53.85%). Due to inherent drug resistance in *Stenotrophomonas maltophilia*, we only incorporated this strain into antimicrobial susceptibility testing, but no more in-depth explorations were conducted.

Three *A. portensis* isolates exhibited highly similar antimicrobial susceptibility profiles, being resistant to meropenem, ceftiofur, tetracycline and amoxicillin but susceptible to other antibiotics tested (Table 1). *Acinetobacter* spp. carrying *tet*(X) but susceptible to tigecycline was reported previously [9,18]. This phenomenon confirmed it was always possible to detect *tet*(X) in strains without a tigecycline resistance phenotype, which highlighted that the traditional methods of bacterial isolation based on selective media supplemented with antibiotics may impair the recovery of bacteria harboring critical precursors of resistance genes, although they may not confer the resistance phenotype directly. For some reasons to be investigated, one possibility was the inhibition of *tet*(X) function within certain species, suggesting *tet*(X) still could express its resistance by transmitting to other hosts [9,18]. In a manner of speaking, the existence of this silent dissemination was even more dangerous.

Table 1. Antimicrobial susceptibility testing of carbapenem-resistant isolates collected from the dairy farm and their corresponding transconjugants.

Strain	Species	MICs (mg/L)							
		CHL	COL	MEM	TGC	ENR	CFF	TET	AMX
C600	*E. coli* (recipient)	4	≤0.25	≤0.25	≤0.25	≤0.25	≤0.25	1	2
JNE5	*Acinetobacter portensis*	1	≤0.25	32	≤0.25	≤0.25	128	16	>128
JNE3-2	*Acinetobacter portensis*	0.5	≤0.25	32	≤0.25	≤0.25	128	16	>128
JNE10-1	*Acinetobacter portensis*	1	≤0.25	32	≤0.25	≤0.25	128	32	>128
JNE10-2	*Shewanella* spp.	32	≤0.25	32	≤0.25	≤0.25	128	32	>128
JNE9-1	*Shewanella* spp.	64	≤0.25	64	0.5	≤0.25	128	32	>128
CJNE9-1	*E. coli* (transconjugant)	8	≤0.25	32	≤0.25	≤0.25	>128	1	>128
JNE8	*Shewanella* spp.	1	≤0.25	64	≤0.25	≤0.25	>128	1	>128
CJNE8	*E. coli* (transconjugant)	8	≤0.25	32	≤0.25	≤0.25	>128	1	>128
JNE3-1	*Shewanella* spp.	64	≤0.25	64	≤0.25	≤0.25	128	16	>128
CJNE3-1	*E. coli* (transconjugant)	4	≤0.25	32	≤0.25	≤0.25	>128	1	>128
JNE17	*Shewanella* spp.	2	≤0.25	128	≤0.25	≤0.25	128	1	>128
CJNE17	*E. coli* (transconjugant)	4	≤0.25	32	≤0.25	≤0.25	>128	2	>128
JNE2	*Shewanella* spp.	2	≤0.25	64	≤0.25	≤0.25	128	0.5	>128
CJNE2	*E. coli* (transconjugant)	4	≤0.25	32	≤0.25	≤0.25	>128	2	>128
JNE7	*Shewanella* spp.	32	≤0.25	16	≤0.25	≤0.25	64	8	>128
CJNE7	*E. coli* (transconjugant)	4	≤0.25	16	≤0.25	≤0.25	>128	1	>128
JNE4-1	*Shewanella* spp.	32	≤0.25	32	0.5	≤0.25	64	16	>128
JNE4-2	*Shewanella* spp.	1	≤0.25	64	0.5	≤0.25	>128	1	>128
CJNE4-2	*E. coli* (transconjugant)	4	≤0.25	32	≤0.25	≤0.25	>128	1	>128
PS ES	*Stenotrophomonas maltophilia*	8	≤0.25	64	0.5	≤0.25	128	8	>128

Abbreviations: CHL, chloramphenicol; COL, colistin; MEM, meropenem; TGC, tigecycline; ENR, enrofloxacin; CFF, ceftiofur; TET, tetracycline; AMX, amoxicillin.

All of the *Shewanella* spp. isolates were sensitive to colistin, tigecycline and enrofloxacin but resistant to meropenem, ceftiofur and amoxicillin. Five strains (55.6%) and four strains (44.4%) were resistant to chloramphenicol and tetracycline, respectively. The minimum inhibitory concentrations of *Shewanella* spp. isolates to meropenem were in the range from 16 to 128 μg/mL (Table 1). As previously reported, in *Shewanella*, bla_{OXA} could lead to a low-level resistance (8–16 μg/mL) to meropenem or was incapable of reducing susceptibility to carbapenems in different occasions [19–21]. By contrast, the production of NDM was more concerned in terms of meropenem resistance in these bacteria.

2.2. Transfer Ability of MDR Plasmids

Conjugation experiments by broth mating were conducted on twelve bla_{NDM}-positive strains. The results show that the bla_{NDM-1} of seven *Shewanella* strains (77.8%) could be transferred to the recipient strain *E. coli* C600. Antimicrobial susceptibility testing demonstrated that the corresponding transconjugants were resistant to amoxicillin, meropenem and ceftiofur, and MICs of meropenem ranged from 16 to 32 μg/mL (Table 1). The fact that the carbapenem resistance gene bla_{NDM-1} could spread among different species of bacteria suggested *Shewanella* spp. was likely to be the reservoir of antibiotic resistance genes, including *bla*NDM-1.

For three *A. portensis*, both *tet*(X3) and *bla*NDM-1 genes could not be transferred to three different recipient strains by broth mating. Subsequently, we performed electroporation experiments on these strains but also failed after three repeats. Recently, isolates bearing *tet*(X) without corresponding tigecycline resistance have been reported [9,18]. Plasmidscarrying *tet*(X3) could be transferred to *Acinetobacter baumannii* from *Acinetobacter towneri* susceptible to tigecycline, making a 128-fold increase in the MIC of tigecycline in transconjugant. This species-dependent peculiarity was likely to explain the different resistance phenotypes conferred by the same gene [18]. However, plasmids carrying *tet*(X3) and *bla*NDM-1 in the same *Acinetobacter* species were often non-conjugative in lab experiment conditions [9].

2.3. Characteristics of Nine Shewanella spp. Isolates

For better characterization, the genomic DNA of nine *Shewanella* spp. isolates were extracted then subjected to short-read and long-read sequencing. Species identification by whole-genome sequences based on PubMLST displayed that the nine *Shewanella* strains had the highest match with *Shewanella putrefaciens* (52~60%). Considering the matching degrees were not high enough, we thought conservatively that these nine *Shewanella* strains belonged to other subspecies rather than *Shewanella putrefaciens*. There were only small SNPs among the core genomes of JNE2, JNE17, JNE4-2 and JNE8 (Figure 1a) and highly similar antibiotic resistance gene distribution (Figure 1b), indicating these four strains from different samples had a close phylogenetic relationship and may derive from the same ancestor. Likewise, there were no obvious SNPs differences among JNE4-1, JNE9-1, JNE10-2, JNE3-1 and JNE7 (Figure 1a), which means the five strains were clonally related. However, significant differences lay between these two groups of strains (SNPs > 14,500) (Figure 1a). Not only did this suggest that these two groups of strains are clearly not from the same clone, but their subspecies were also likely to be different. Based on this, we tended to classify these nine strains into two new distinct subspecies of *Shewanella*.

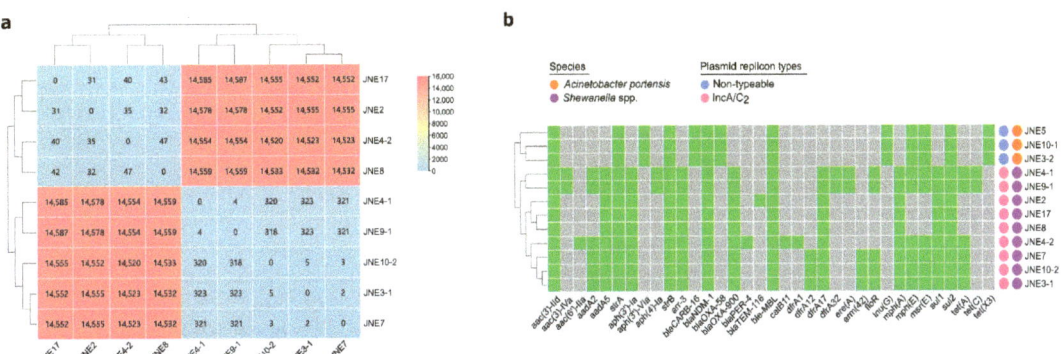

Figure 1. Characteristics of thirteen carbapenem-resistant isolates. (**a**) A heatmap of core genome SNPs analysis among nine *Shewanella* spp. strains carrying *bla*NDM-1. (**b**) A heatmap of antibiotic resistance genes, species and plasmid replicon types for thirteen carbapenem-resistant isolates. Resistance genes are marked positive by green and negative by gray. The species and plasmid replicon types are showed by different colored circles.

There were at least 14 resistance genes in every *Shewanella* strain, and a multicopy of *sul1* existed in these strains (Figure 1b). This further implied *Shewanella* spp. may well be the reservoir of significant antibiotic resistance genes, facilitating the wide spread of drug-resistant bacteria. Replicon analysis found that all of the *Shewanella* isolates carried plasmids of IncA/C2 type (Figure 1b). Over the years, the spread of *bla*NDM has been found associated with IncA/C plasmids [22,23].

In line with SNPs analysis, JNE7, JNE2, JNE4-2 and JNE10-2 were chosen as the representative strains to be sequenced with the MinION long-read platform. Results show that bla_{NDM-1} in four strains was located on IncA/C_2 plasmids, pJNE7-NDM (137,224 bp), pJNE2-NDM (152,348 bp), pJNE4-2-NDM (152,348 bp) and pJNE10-2-NDM (166,090 bp), respectively. Based on the WGS analysis, it was found that clonal dissemination existed among 9 *Shewanella* isolates, and it could be concluded that bla_{NDM-1} located on IncA/C_2 plasmids was prevalent in nine *Shewanella* isolates. The four plasmids showed high similarity, and pJNE2-NDM showed 100% sequence identity to the plasmid p1540-2 (94% coverage, CP019053) in *E. coli* and 99.98% sequence identity to the plasmid P2-NDM-1 (94% coverage, CP087671) in *K. pneumoniae* (Figure 2a), suggesting the dissemination of bla_{NDM-1} in milking environments was mediated by highly similar IncA/C_2 plasmids and highlighting the mobile nature of those resistance genes. We subsequently analyzed the detailed genetic contexts of bla_{NDM-1} by mapping the assembled sequences to the plasmid pSA70-3 in *Shewanella putrefaciens*, p1540-2 in *E. coli*, pCf75 in *Citrobacter freundii* and P2-NDM-1 in *K. pneumoniae* from the NCBI database (Figure 2b). Limited by the short-read data, complete accurate genetic structures were difficult to obtain. However, it could still be observed clearly that the genetic contexts of bla_{NDM-1} among strains in this study and those from the database were strikingly similar, revealing the wide spread of bla_{NDM-1} among different bacteria.

2.4. Characteristics of Three Acinetobacter Portensis Isolates

Three *A. portensis* strains co-carrying *tet*(X3) and bla_{NDM-1} were isolated from different milking environment samples, which were designated as JNE5, JNE3-2 and JNE10-1, respectively. The phylogenetic analysis based on SNPs of core genomes showed that three *A. portensis* strains had a high degree of similarity (Figure 3), and there were no more than 22 SNPs among core genomes of these strains, implying clonal dissemination was likely to occur in the dairy farm.

For better comparison, we gathered information of *Acinetobacter* isolates co-harboring *tet*(X3) and bla_{NDM-1} in recent years from an online database (Figure 3). According to the information collected, including the data of this study, *Acinetobacter indicus* carrying both *tet*(X3) and bla_{NDM-1} had been isolated as early as 2017 in China. However, the locations of *tet*(X3) and bla_{NDM-1} were not conserved, either on the same plasmid, on different plasmids, or on chromosome and plasmid separately (Figure 3). Such co-existing isolates were concentrated in China and sporadically distributed; they were diverse in species, with the majority of them belonging to *A. indicus* (Figure 3). Additionally, these isolates came from a wide range of sources, including dairy cows and their environments, ducks and gooses. *A. portensis* was a newly isolated species of *Acinetobacter* that harbored both *tet*(X3) and bla_{NDM-1}; this was the first time that such drug-resistant bacteria had been collected from the milking environment of dairy cows. In the *A. portensis* in this study, *tet*(X3) and bla_{NDM-1} were located on the same plasmid, similar to the majority of such co-existing stains collected in recent years (Figure 3). Considering the diverse sources and wide distribution of strains in China carrying both *tet*(X3) and bla_{NDM-1}, and the situation that there was probably clonal dissemination in this study, measures must be implemented to avoid their further dissemination and contamination.

Interestingly, each *A. portensis* isolate carried 13 identically acquired antibiotic resistance genes (Figure 1b), conferring resistance to aminoglycosides (*aac(3)-IId*, *aph(3')-Via*, *strA*, *strB*), sulphonamide (*sul2*), glycopeptides (ble_{MBL}), macrolide (*mph*(E), *msr*(E)), lincosamides (*lnu*(G)), carbapenems (bla_{NDM-1}, $bla_{CARB-16}$ and bla_{OXA-58}) and tetracyclines (*tet*(X3)), further supporting the aforementioned clonal dissemination.

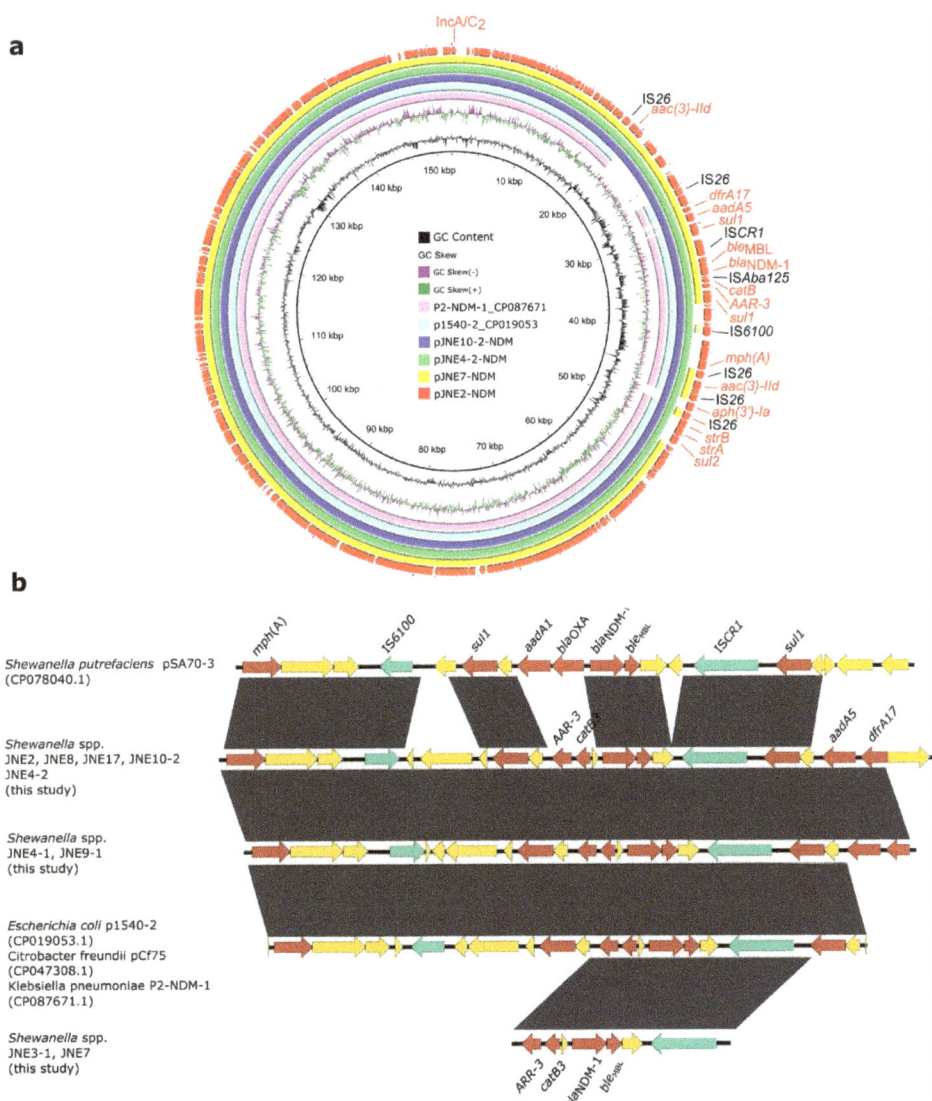

Figure 2. Genetic features of $bla_{\mathrm{NDM-1}}$ in *Shewanella* strains. (**a**) Circular comparison of $bla_{\mathrm{NDM-1}}$-carrying plasmids pJNE2-NDM, pJNE7-NDM, pJNE4-2-NDM and pJNE10-2-NDM. (**b**) Linear sequence comparison of genetic context of $bla_{\mathrm{NDM-1}}$ in the nine *Shewanella* spp. isolates in this study with pSA70-3 (CP078040.1), p1540-2 (CP019053.1), pCf75 (CP047308.1) and P2-NDM-1 (CP087671.1) from the NCBI database. Regions with >99% sequence identity are marked by gray shading, and red arrows denote antibiotic resistance genes. Green arrows denote insertion sequences, and yellow arrows represent other genes.

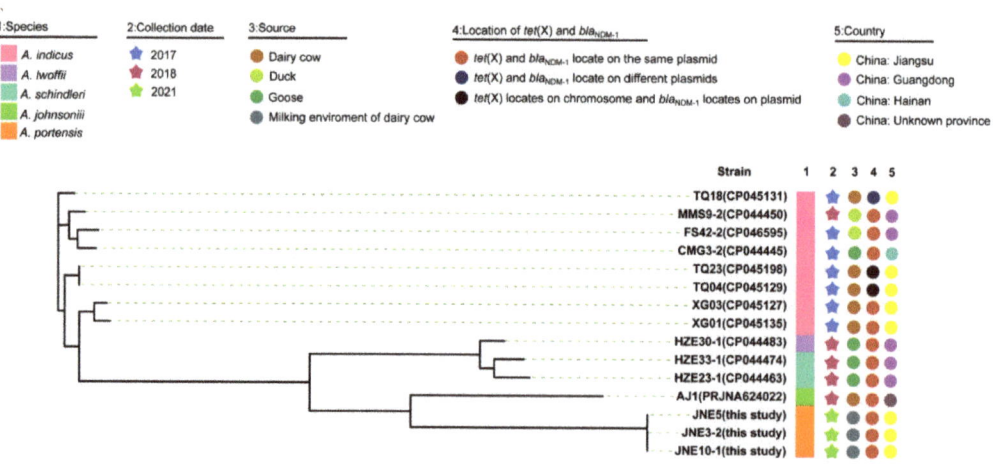

Figure 3. Phylogenetic analysis and genetic characteristics of *Acinetobacter* isolates co-harboring *tet*(X) and *bla*NDM-1 from this study and the NCBI database. The strain species, collection date, source, country and location of *tet*(X) and *bla*NDM-1 in the genomes are showed by subsequent color blocks.

2.5. Genetic Contexts of bla_{NDM-1} and tet(X3)

In the same way, we performed short-read sequencing of three *A. portensis*. According to the linear comparison of sequences, it was obvious that the genetic contexts of *bla*NDM-1 and *tet*(X3) in JNE5, JNE3-2 and JNE10-1 were identical (Figure 4). On account of the clonal dissemination among three *A. portensis* strains revealed by phylogenetic analysis, we chose the JNE5 strain as the representative strain to be sequenced with the MinION long-read platform to obtain the complete circular genome sequences. Analysis displayed that the genome of JNE5 was comprised of a chromosome (2,568,515 bp) and five non-typeable plasmids, pJNE5-X3_NDM-1 (333,311 bp), pJNE5-64k (64,629 bp), pJNE5-OXA-58 (59,583 bp), pJNE5-3k (3617 bp) and pJNE5-1k (1416 bp). Most of the drug resistance genes were located on plasmid pJNE5-X3_NDM-1. In addition, it should be noted that *tet*(X3) had two copies, one was located on the chromosome, and the other one was located on the plasmid pJNE5-X3_NDM-1 with *bla*NDM-1. Moreover, there was one *bla*OXA-58 existing in pJNE5-OXA-58.

The genetic context of chromosomal *tet*(X) had high coverage with that of the *A. indicus* TQ23 chromosome (CP045198.1). Similarly, genetic contexts of *bla*OXA-58 on plasmid pJNE5-OXA-58 and *A. indicus* p18TQ-X3 (CP045132.1) separately also had a large number of consistencies (Figure 5a,b). Plasmid comparison revealed that the plasmid pJNE5-X3_NDM-1 shared a low degree of genetic identity with two previously reported plasmids co-harboring *tet*(X3) and *bla*NDM-1 (pXG01-X3 and pHZE30-1-1). Although pOXA58_010030 showed the highest sequence identity to pJNE5-X3_NDM-1, it lacked the most important multidrug resistance region (Figure 6). The typical genetic context, IS*Aba125-bla*NDM-1-*ble*MBL-*trpF*-*dsbC*, appeared in plasmid pJNE5-X3_NDM-1 [24]. Additionally, *tet*(X3) was located within a 5200 bp region with the gene arrangement ISCR2-*xerD*-*tet*(X3)-*res*-ORF1-ΔISCR2, with one intact ISCR2 element located on the upstream of *tet*(X3) and another ΔISCR2 (83 bp) with the same orientation lay in the downstream (Figure 4).

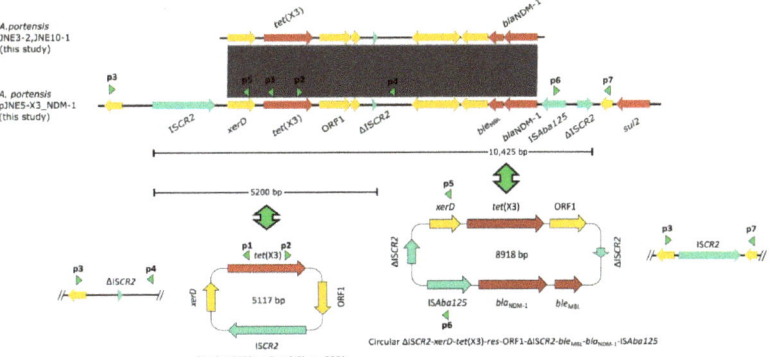

Figure 4. Linear sequence comparison of genetic context of *tet*(X3) and *bla*_{NDM-1} in three *Acinetobacter portensis* isolates. Regions of >99% homology are marked by gray shading, red arrows denote antibiotic resistance genes and arrows indicate the direction of transcription of the genes. Green arrowheads p1, p2, p3 and p4 indicate the positions of primers used for amplification of the IS*CR2*-*xerD*-*tet*(X3)-*res*-ORF1 circular intermediate, arrowheads p3, p5, p6 and p7 are used for amplification of the ΔIS*CR2*-*xerD*-*tet*(X3)-*res*-ORF1-ΔIS*CR2*-*ble*_{MBL}-*bla*_{NDM-1}-IS*Aba125* circular intermediate.

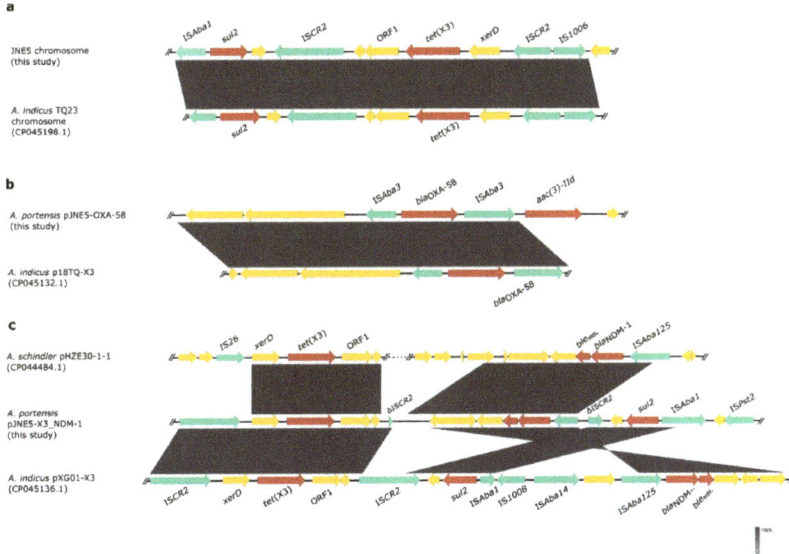

Figure 5. Genetic features of *bla*_{NDM-1}, *tet*(X) and *bla*_{OXA-48} in JNE5 strain. (**a**) Linear alignment of the *tet*(X3)-carrying chromosome in JNE5 with chromosome from *A. indicus* TQ23 (CP045198.1). (**b**) Linear alignment of the *bla*_{OXA-48}-positive plasmid pJNE5-OXA-58 with p18TQ-X3. (**c**), Linear sequence comparison of genetic context of *bla*_{NDM-1} and *tet*(X3) in plasmid pJNE5-X3_NDM-1 with that of pHZE30-1 (CP044484.1) and pXG01-X3 (CP045136.1). Regions of homology are marked by shading; red arrows denote antibiotic resistance genes. Green arrows denote insertion sequences, and yellow arrows represent other genes.

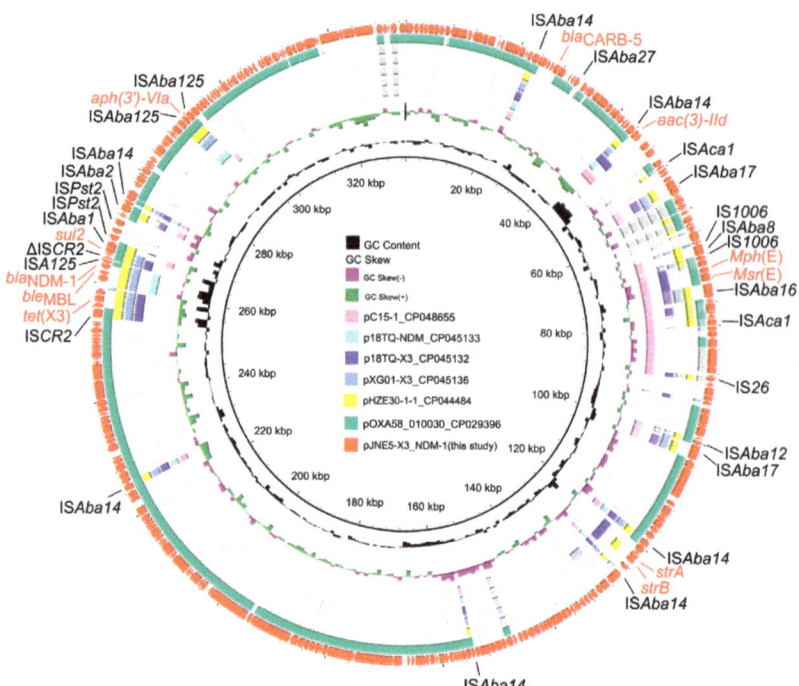

Figure 6. Circular comparison of the plasmid pJNE5-X3_NDM-1 co-harbouring *tet*(X3) and *bla*_{NDM-1} in *Acinetobacter portensis* JNE5 strain with similar plasmids from the NCBI database. The outmost circle denotes the reference plasmid pJNE5-X3_NDM-1.

Inverse PCR was carried out to examine whether the minicircle ISCR2-*tet*(X3) could take shape. Finally, we obtained a fragment of 4245 bp in length, and sequence analysis revealed that it included only one intact copy of ISCR2 element (ISCR2-*xerD*-*tet*(X3)-*res*-*orf1*) (Figure 4), which was the same as previously reported [9]. To reconfirm the above situation, we used inward-facing primers and then obtained a 1664 bp PCR amplicon, which included only one ΔISCR2 (83 bp) element (Figure 4). Compared with other reported plasmids co-harboring *tet*(X3) and *bla*_{NDM-1}, the significant difference in plasmid pJNE5-X3_NDM-1 was that *tet*(X3) and *bla*_{NDM-1} stood exceptionally close to each other (Figure 5c). What was noteworthy was that one ΔISCR2 (389 bp) element lay in the downstream of *bla*_{NDM-1}; since it was in the same direction as the intact ISCR2 element located on the upstream of *tet*(X3), outward-facing primers were designed to examine whether this MDR region could also be excised and mobilizable. A 1875 bp amplicon was generated and sequence analysis revealed that it included only one copy of the ΔISCR2 (389 bp) element. The results of PCR using inward-facing primers showed a 2933 bp amplicon, including one intact copy of the ISCR2 element, which verified the instability of circular intermediate ΔISCR2-*tet*(X3)-*bla*_{NDM-1} by excision (Figure 4). The generation of circular intermediate containing *tet*(X3) and *bla*_{NDM-1} was a warning that the two important antibiotic resistance genes were likely to transmit together, which warranted further investigations. Although conjugation experiments failed, the potential hazard of the MDR plasmids still could not be neglected.

3. Materials and Methods

3.1. Bacterial Isolation and Identification

In total, 72 non-duplicated samples were collected from a dairy farm in Xuzhou, Jiangsu Province in May 2021, including 14 milk samples from cows with mastitis, 31 stool samples, 15 milking environment samples and 12 shed environment samples. To enrich the microbiota, solid and liquid samples, as well as cotton swabs (surface samples), were incubated in a 5 mL LB broth without antimicrobials for 6 h. These enrichment broth suspensions were streaked onto MacConkey agar plates containing meropenem (2 mg/L) using a sterile loop to isolate carbapenem-resistant colonies. The boiling method was used to extract bacterial genome DNA, which was subsequently screened for carbapenem resistance genes (bla_{NDM}, bla_{VIM}, bla_{KPC}, bla_{IMP}, bla_{SIM}, bla_{DIM}, bla_{AIM}, bla_{BIC}, bla_{SPM}, bla_{OXA} and bla_{GIM}) using the previously reported primers [25]. The carbapenem-resistant bacteria were screened again for $tet(X)$ genes using primers described earlier [6]. 16S rRNA gene sequencing was conducted to further identify their species using the forward primer 5′-AGAGTTTGATCATGGCTCAG-3′ and the reverse primer 5′-GTGTGACGGGCGG TGTGTAC-3′.

3.2. Antimicrobial Susceptibility Testing

Fresh CAMH broth was prepared for antimicrobial susceptibility testing, and the minimal inhibitory concentrations (MICs) of chloramphenicol, colistin, meropenem, tigecycline, enrofloxacin, ceftiofur, tetracycline and amoxicillin were determined by the broth microdilution method. The results are interpreted according to the guidelines of the Clinical and Laboratory Standards Institute [26] and the European Committee on Antimicrobial Susceptibility Testing (EUCAST, v12.0) (http://www.eucast.org/clinical_breakpoints/ (accessed on 1 January 2022)) with *E. coli* ATCC 25922 as a quality control strain.

3.3. Conjugation and Electroporation Experiments

Conjugation experiments by broth mating were carried out using bla_{NDM}-positive strains as donors, with strains *E. coli* C600 (rifampicin resistant), *E. coli* J53 (sodium azide resistant) and *A. baumannii* ATCC19606 (chloramphenicol resistant) as recipients. Only *E. coli* C600 was used as the recipient of nine *Shewanella* spp. isolates, while all recipients mentioned above were used for *A. portensis*. Transconjugants were separately selected on LB agar plates containing rifampicin (300 mg/L) with meropenem (2 mg/L), sodium azide (300 mg/L) with meropenem (2 mg/L), or chloramphenicol (64 mg/L) together with meropenem (2 mg/L) and then confirmed by PCR. The broth microdilution method was used to determine the MICs of a range of antimicrobials for the transconjugants. For *A. portensis* isolates that meropenem resistance phenotype failed to transfer by conjugation, electroporation experiment was performed, in which *A. baumannii* ATCC19606 was prepared as the receipt strain.

3.4. Whole-Genome Sequencing and Bioinformatics Analysis

Genomic DNA of all bla_{NDM}-positive isolates from overnight cultures was extracted using the FastPure® Bacteria DNA Isolation Mini Kit (Vazyme, Nanjing, China). The genomic DNA was subjected to short-read sequencing (2×150 bp) with the Illumina HiSeq 2500 platform (Illumina, San Diego, CA, USA). Short-read Illumina raw reads were de novo assembled using SPAdes [27] with default parameters, and contigs less than 200 bp were discarded. To obtain the complete sequences, we selected several representative strains and extracted their genomic DNA to perform Oxford Nanopore Technologies MinION long-read sequencing [28,29]. The complete genome sequences were modified manually and automatically annotated using RAST (http://rast.nmpdr.org/ (accessed on 1 January 2022)). The BRIG tool was used to perform circular comparison of the plasmids in this study and the homologous plasmids available from the NCBI database [30]. A pairwise SNP distance matrix was generated using snp-dists 0.6.3 (https://github.com/tseemann/snp-dists (accessed on 1 January 2022)). Roary [31] and FastTree [32] based on the SNPs of core genomes were used to construct phylogenetic trees, which were visualized by iTOL v5 [33]. Easyfig was used to generate linear comparison in order to visualize the sequence comparison features of genetic contexts [34].

3.5. Identification of Circular Intermediates

To determine whether the recombination of ISCR2 and ΔISCR2 (83 bp) elements could form the *tet*(X3)-carrying circular intermediate, all plasmids, including the *tet*(X3)-carrying plasmid pJNE5-X3_NDM-1 from the JNE5 strain, were extracted for inverse PCR assays, using outward-facing primers p1 5′-TCGGTCGTTGTCTCTTTCGT-3′ and p2 5′-TTGATGTCGCCTTTTGCAGG-3′ for detection of minicircle ISCR2-*tet*(X3). When the band of target fragment was detected through agarose gel electrophoresis, the same primers were used to sequence the amplified minicircle product. Then inward-facing primers p3 5′-CGCAGCGTTTCGTACATCAG-3′ and p4 5′-AGGTCAATCAGACTGGGCGTT-3′ were used to verify the excision result. In the same way, to see if the recombination of ISCR2 and ΔISCR2 (389 bp) could lead to the formation of circular intermediate co-carrying *tet*(X3) and *bla*$_{NDM-1}$, outward-facing primers p5 5′-TGTTCCATTCCCTTGGTGGT-3′ and p6 5′-ATGTGCCTTTTTGCCAGGGT-3′ were used for detecting minicircle ΔISCR2-*tet*(X3)-*bla*$_{NDM-1}$. Inward-facing primers p3 and p7 5′-GACGGTATTCGTGGCAAAGC-3′ were used to confirm the excision result.

4. Conclusions

In this work, we detected nine NDM-1-producing *Shewanella* spp. strains and three *A. portensis* strains co-harboring *tet*(X3) and *bla*$_{NDM-1}$. Clonal dissemination existed among three *A. portensis* isolates, in which *tet*(X3) and *bla*$_{NDM-1}$ co-located on a novel non-conjugative plasmid, and there was another *tet*(X3) located on the chromosome. Additionally, we confirmed that the circular intermediate ΔISCR2-*tet*(X3)-*bla*$_{NDM-1}$ could be generated. The emergence of *tet*(X3) and *bla*$_{NDM-1}$-bearing plasmids in different bacteria among dairy cow farming environments constitutes a potential public health concern. Continuous monitoring and surveillance of critical resistance genes in such environments are necessary to ensure good farming standards.

Author Contributions: Conceptualization, Z.W., H.S. and R.L.; methodology, R.L., K.P. and X.L.; validation, R.L., L.Z. and X.L.; formal analysis, R.L., X.X., Y.L. and L.Z.; data curation, L.Z. and X.L.; writing—original draft preparation, L.Z. and X.L.; writing—review and editing, R.L., L.Z. and X.L.; visualization, R.L., L.Z. and K.P. All authors have read and agreed to the published version of the manuscript.

Funding: This work was supported by the National Natural Science Foundation of China (31872526 and 32161133005), the China Postdoctoral Science Foundation (no. 2020M671632) and the Priority Academic Program Development of Jiangsu Higher Education Institutions (PAPD).

Institutional Review Board Statement: Not applicable.

Informed Consent Statement: Not applicable.

Data Availability Statement: The draft genome sequences were submitted to NCBI with the Bio-Project number PRJNA828415. Complete genome sequences of four representative strains JNE5 (PRJNA828443), JNE10-2 (PRJNA829047), JNE2 (PRJNA829244) and JNE7 (PRJNA829126) were also deposited. The complete sequence of pJNE4-2-NDM was also submitted for reference (ON391944).

Conflicts of Interest: The authors declare no conflict of interest.

References

1. Papp-Wallace, K.M.; Endimiani, A.; Taracila, M.A.; Bonomo, R.A. Carbapenems: Past, Present, and Future. *Antimicrob. Agents Chemother.* **2011**, *55*, 4943–4960. [CrossRef]
2. Wang, H.; Li, X.; Liu, B.T. Occurrence and characterization of KPC-2-producing ST11 Klebsiella pneumoniae isolate and NDM-5-producing Escherichia coli isolate from the same horse of equestrian clubs in China. *Transbound. Emerg. Dis.* **2021**, *68*, 224–232. [CrossRef] [PubMed]
3. Kelly, A.M.; Mathema, B.; Larson, E.L. Carbapenem-resistant Enterobacteriaceae in the community: A scoping review. *Int. J. Antimicrob. Agents* **2017**, *50*, 127–134. [CrossRef] [PubMed]
4. Wang, T.; Xu, K.; Zhao, L.; Tong, R.; Xiong, L.; Shi, J. Recent research and development of NDM-1 inhibitors. *Eur. J. Med. Chem.* **2021**, *223*, 113667. [CrossRef]

5. Cui, C.Y.; Chen, C.; Liu, B.T.; He, Q.; Wu, X.T.; Sun, R.Y.; Zhang, Y.; Cui, Z.H.; Guo, W.Y.; Jia, Q.L.; et al. Co-occurrence of Plasmid-Mediated Tigecycline and Carbapenem Resistance in Acinetobacter spp. from Waterfowls and Their Neighboring Environment. *Antimicrob. Agents Chemother.* **2020**, *64*, e02502-19. [CrossRef]
6. He, T.; Wang, R.; Liu, D.; Walsh, T.; Zhang, R.; Lv, Y.; Ke, Y.; Ji, Q.; Wei, R.; Liu, Z.; et al. Emergence of plasmid-mediated high-level tigecycline resistance genes in animals and humans. *Nat. Microbiol.* **2019**, *4*, 1450–1456. [CrossRef]
7. Sun, J.; Chen, C.; Cui, C.Y.; Zhang, Y.; Liu, Y.H. Plasmid-encoded *tet*(X) genes that confer high-level tigecycline resistance in *Escherichia coli*. *Nat. Microbiol.* **2019**, *4*, 1457–1464. [CrossRef]
8. Cao, J.; Wang, J.; Wang, Y.; Wang, L.; Gao, G.F. Tigecycline resistance *tet*(X3) gene is going wild. *Biosaf. Health* **2020**, *2*, 9–11. [CrossRef]
9. Zhang, R.; Dong, N.; Zeng, Y.; Shen, Z.; Lu, J.; Liu, C.; Huang, Z.A.; Sun, Q.; Cheng, Q.; Shu, L.; et al. Chromosomal and Plasmid-Borne Tigecycline Resistance Genes *tet*(X3) and *tet*(X4) in Dairy Cows on a Chinese Farm. *Antimicrob. Agents Chemother.* **2020**, *64*, e00674-20. [CrossRef]
10. Ceccarelli, D.; Essen-Zandbergen, A.v.; Veldman, K.T.; Tafro, N.; Haenen, O.; Mevius, D.J. Chromosome-Based blaOXA-48-Like Variants in Shewanella Species Isolates from Food-Producing Animals, Fish, and the Aquatic Environment. *Antimicrob. Agents Chemother.* **2017**, *61*, e01013-16. [CrossRef] [PubMed]
11. Potter, R.F.; D'Souza, A.W.; Wallace, M.A.; Shupe, A.; Patel, S.; Gul, D.; Kwon, J.H.; Andleeb, S.; Burnham, C.-A.D.; Draft, G.D. Genome Sequence of the blaOXA-436 and blaNDM-1-Harboring Shewanella putrefaciens SA70 Isolate. *Genome Announc.* **2017**, *5*, e00644-17. [CrossRef] [PubMed]
12. Janda, J.M.; Abbott, S.L. The genus Shewanella: From the briny depths below to human pathogen. *Crit. Rev. Microbiol.* **2014**, *40*, 293–312. [CrossRef]
13. Yousfi, K.; Bekal, S.; Usongo, V.; Touati, A. Current trends in human infections and antibiotic resistance of the genus Shewanella. *Eur. J. Clin. Microbiol. Infect. Dis.* **2017**, *36*, 1353–1362. [CrossRef] [PubMed]
14. Yousfi, K.; Touati, A.; Lefebvre, B.; Fournier, É.; Côté, J.; Soualhine, H.; Walker, M.; Bougdour, D.; Tremblay, C.; Bekal, S. A Novel Plasmid, pSx1, Harboring a New Tn1696 Derivative from Extensively Drug-Resistant Shewanella xiamenensis Encoding OXA-416. *Microb. Drug Resist.* **2017**, *23*, 429–436. [CrossRef] [PubMed]
15. Cimmino, T.; Olaitan, A.; Rolain, J. Whole genome sequence to decipher the resistome of Shewanella algae, a multidrug-resistant bacterium responsible for pneumonia, Marseille, France. *Expert Rev. Anti-Infect. Ther.* **2016**, *14*, 269–275. [CrossRef]
16. Carvalheira, A.; Gonzales-Siles, L.; Salvà-Serra, F.; Lindgren, S.; Moore, E.R.B. *Acinetobacter portensis* sp. nov. and *Acinetobacter guerrae* sp. nov., isolated from raw meat. *Int. J. Syst. Evol. Microbiol.* **2020**, *70*, 4544–4554. [CrossRef]
17. He, T.; Li, R.; Wei, R.; Liu, D.; Bai, L.; Zhang, L.; Gu, J.; Wang, R.; Wang, Y. Characterization of Acinetobacter indicus co-harbouring *tet*(X3) and blaNDM-1 of dairy cow origin. *J. Antimicrob. Chemother.* **2020**, *75*, 2693–2696. [CrossRef] [PubMed]
18. Cheng, Y.-Y.; Liu, Y.; Chen, Y.; Huang, F.-M.; Chen, R.-C.; Xiao, Y.-H.; Zhou, K.; Downing, T.; Cevallos, M.; Siddavattam, D.; et al. Sporadic Dissemination of *tet*(X3) and *tet*(X6) Mediated by Highly Diverse Plasmidomes among Livestock-Associated Acinetobacter. *Microbiol. Spectr.* **2021**, *9*, e01141-21. [CrossRef]
19. Tacão, M.; Araújo, S.; Vendas, M.; Alves, A.; Henriques, I. Shewanella species as the origin of bla genes: Insights into gene diversity, associated phenotypes and possible transfer mechanisms. *Int. J. Antimicrob. Agents* **2018**, *51*, 340–348. [CrossRef] [PubMed]
20. Antonelli, A.; Di Palo, D.M.; Galano, A.; Becciani, S.; Montagnani, C.; Pecile, P.; Galli, L.; Rossolini, G.M. Intestinal carriage of Shewanella xiamenensis simulating carriage of OXA-48–producing Enterobacteriaceae. *Diagn. Microbiol. Infect. Dis.* **2015**, *82*, 1–3. [CrossRef] [PubMed]
21. Tacão, M.; Correia, A.; Henriques, I. Environmental Shewanella xiamenensis strains that carry bla OXA-48 or bla OXA-204 genes: Additional proof for bla OXA-48-like gene origin. *Antimicrob. Agents Chemother.* **2013**, *57*, 6399–6400. [CrossRef] [PubMed]
22. Kumarasamy, K.K.; Toleman, M.A.; Walsh, T.R.; Bagaria, J.; Woodford, N. Emergence of a new antibiotic resistance mechanism in India, Pakistan, and the UK: A molecular, biological, and epidemiological study. *Lancet Infect. Dis.* **2010**, *10*, 578–579. [CrossRef]
23. Marta, A.; Manuel, O.; Luísa, G.; Augusto, C.; Patrice, N.; Laurent, P. Occurrence of NDM-1-producing Morganella morganii and Proteus mirabilis in a single patient in Portugal: Probable in vivo transfer by conjugation. *J. Antimicrob. Chemother.* **2020**, *75*, 903–906.
24. Fu, Y.; Du, X.; Ji, J.; Chen, Y.; Jiang, Y.; Yu, Y. Epidemiological characteristics and genetic structure of blaNDM-1 in non-baumannii Acinetobacter spp. in China. *J. Antimicrob. Chemother.* **2012**, *67*, 2114–2122. [CrossRef]
25. Poirel, L.; Walsh, T.R.; Cuvillier, V.; Nordmann, P. Multiplex PCR for detection of acquired carbapenemase genes. *Diagn. Microbiol. Infect. Dis.* **2011**, *70*, 119–123. [CrossRef]
26. CLSI. *Performance Standards for Antimicrobial Susceptibility Testing*, 30th ed.; CLSI Supplement M100; CLSI: Wayne, PA, USA, 2020.
27. Bankevich, A.; Nurk, S.; Antipov, D.; Gurevich, A.A.; Dvorkin, M.; Kulikov, A.S.; Lesin, V.M.; Nikolenko, S.I.; Pham, S.; Prjibelski, A.D.; et al. SPAdes: A New Genome Assembly Algorithm and Its Applications to Single-Cell Sequencing. *J. Comput. Biol.* **2012**, *19*, 455–477. [CrossRef]
28. Li, R.; Xie, M.; Dong, N.; Lin, D.; Yang, X.; Yin, W.; Wai-Chi, C.E.; Chen, S. Efficient generation of complete sequences of MDR-encoding plasmids by rapid assembly of MinION barcoding sequencing data. *Gigascience* **2018**, *7*, gix132. [CrossRef]
29. Wick, R.R.; Judd, L.M.; Gorrie, C.L.; Holt, K.E. Unicycler: Resolving bacterial genome assemblies from short and long sequencing reads. *PLoS Comput. Biol.* **2017**, *13*, e1005595. [CrossRef] [PubMed]

30. Alikhan, N.F.; Petty, N.K.; Zakour, N.L.B.; Beatson, S.A.A. BLAST Ring Image Generator (BRIG): Simple prokaryote genome comparisons. *Bmc Genom.* **2011**, *12*, 402. [CrossRef]
31. Page, A.J.; Cummins, C.A.; Hunt, M.; Wong, V.K.; Parkhill, J. Roary: Rapid large-scale prokaryote pan genome analysis. *Bioinformatics* **2015**, *31*, 3691–3693. [CrossRef]
32. Price, M.; Dehal, P.; Arkin, A. FastTree: Computing large minimum evolution trees with profiles instead of a distance matrix. *Mol. Biol. Evol.* **2009**, *26*, 1641–1650. [CrossRef] [PubMed]
33. Letunic, I.; Bork, P. Interactive Tree Of Life (iTOL) v5: An online tool for phylogenetic tree display and annotation. *Nucleic Acids Res.* **2021**, *49*, W293–W296. [CrossRef] [PubMed]
34. Beatson, S.A. Easyfig: A genome comparison visualizer. *Bioinformatics* **2011**, *27*, 1009–1010.

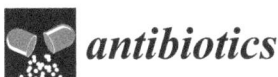

MDPI

Article

The Distribution of Mobile Colistin-Resistant Genes, Carbapenemase-Encoding Genes, and Fluoroquinolone-Resistant Genes in *Escherichia coli* Isolated from Natural Water Sources in Upper Northeast Thailand

Pongthep Tabut, Rapeepan Yongyod *, Ratchadaporn Ungcharoen and Anusak Kerdsin

The Faculty of Public Health, Kasetsart University Chalermphrakiat Sakon Nakhon Province Campus, Thailand. 59 Moo 1, Chiang Khruea Subdistrict, Mueang Sakon Nakhon District, Sakon Nakhon 47000, Thailand
* Correspondence: rapeepan.y@ku.th

Citation: Tabut, P.; Yongyod, R.; Ungcharoen, R.; Kerdsin, A. The Distribution of Mobile Colistin-Resistant Genes, Carbapenemase-Encoding Genes, and Fluoroquinolone-Resistant Genes in *Escherichia coli* Isolated from Natural Water Sources in Upper Northeast Thailand. *Antibiotics* **2022**, *11*, 1760. https://doi.org/10.3390/antibiotics11121760

Academic Editor: Xuxiang Zhang

Received: 1 November 2022
Accepted: 4 December 2022
Published: 6 December 2022

Publisher's Note: MDPI stays neutral with regard to jurisdictional claims in published maps and institutional affiliations.

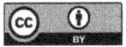
Abstract: Antimicrobial resistance (AMR) is considered a serious problem in many countries, including Thailand. AMR and antibiotic resistance genes (ARGs) could transfer between humans, animals, and the environment causing a threat to human health. This study described the antibiotic resistance of *Escherichia coli* (*E. coli*) from surface water, wastewater, and discharge water in the Namsuay watershed in upper northeast Thailand. The water samples were collected in the dry and wet seasons. The 113 *E. coli* isolates were confirmed using a polymerase chain reaction and examined for their antibiotic susceptibility, ARGs, and genetic relationship. The results indicated that *E. coli* was resistant to the following classes of antibiotics: fluoroquinolone, third-generation cephalosporin, polymyxin, and carbapenem. The isolates carried the *mcr-1*, *mcr-8*, *mcr-9*, *bla*$_{\text{oxa-48-like}}$, *aac(6')-bl-cr*, *qepA*, and *oqxAB* genes. Phylogroup B1 was a predominant group among the *E. coli* in the study. In addition, the *E. coli* isolates from the discharge water (a hospital and a fish farm) had a higher prevalence of antibiotic resistance and harboured more ARGs than the other water sample sources. The presence of antibiotic-resistant *E. coli* and ARG contamination in the natural water source reflected an AMR management issue that could drive strategic policy regarding the active surveillance and prevention of AMR contamination.

Keywords: *mcr*; PMQR; carbapenemase; *Escherichia coli*; natural water; Namsuay watershed; antibiotic resistance; antimicrobial resistance

1. Introduction

Antimicrobial resistance (AMR) is an increasing issue of global concern as it leads to antibiotic treatment failure that places a burden on public health, the economy, and the environment [1]. Human activities, such as agriculture, animal husbandry, and daily body hygiene, could cause wastewater, sewage contamination with chemicals, and faecal pollution, including causing antibiotics and antibiotic resistance genes (ARGs) to leak into the environment [2]. If wastewater management is not properly and effectively carried out, there may be adverse effects on the ecosystem and human health [3]. The identification of microorganisms in water is important to assess the safety and sanitation of water use from water sources. Among these organisms, *E. coli* is an indicator bacterium to measure the microbiological quality of water supplies. It is found in the intestines of humans and warm-blooded animals [4]. Furthermore, it is an important pathogen in both intra-intestinal tract and extra-intestinal tract infections in humans [5].

The inappropriate or overuse of antibiotics in both humans and animals is one action that could lead to AMR. Antibiotic contamination in the environment would encourage antibiotic-susceptible bacteria to become non-susceptible or resistant, as a consequence of selective pressures [6]. Mutations and evolution within selection due to antibiotic pressures or natural mechanism factors have resulted in the emergence of ARGs that could transfer antibiotic-resistance abilities to other bacteria via plasmids, transposons, chromosomal cassettes, and prophages [7]. ARGs, transferred by the mechanism of a horizontal gene, were found in bacteria from environmental samples, such as mobile colistin-resistant (*mcr*) genes [8,9], carbapenemase-encoding genes (CEG) [10], and plasmid-mediated-quinolone-resistance (PMQR) genes [11,12]. Therefore, areas with high use of antibiotics, such as hospitals, animal husbandries, and communities that do not control the use of antibiotics, are high-risk areas for AMR. These antibiotic resistance (AR) bacteria could contaminate water pollution sources, including hospital wastewater, community wastewater, livestock and fishery wastewater, and agricultural wastewater, by transmission mechanisms and many pathways. Humans acquire and emit AR bacteria through interactions between humans and the environment [13,14].

Herein, we described the contamination of antibiotic-resistant *E. coli* carrying important ARGs, consisting of *mcr*, CEG, and PMQR genes, from a natural water source in upper northeast Thailand. The water sources consisted of surface water above the ground in the Namsuay River and Mekong River; wastewater in this study was defined as untreated, used water affected by domestic, agricultural, and poultry areas, whereas discharge water was defined as used treated water affected by hospitals and catfish farms, as shown the examples in Figure 1. This information could drive strategic policies for the active surveillance and prevention of AR bacterial contamination in natural water sources throughout the country.

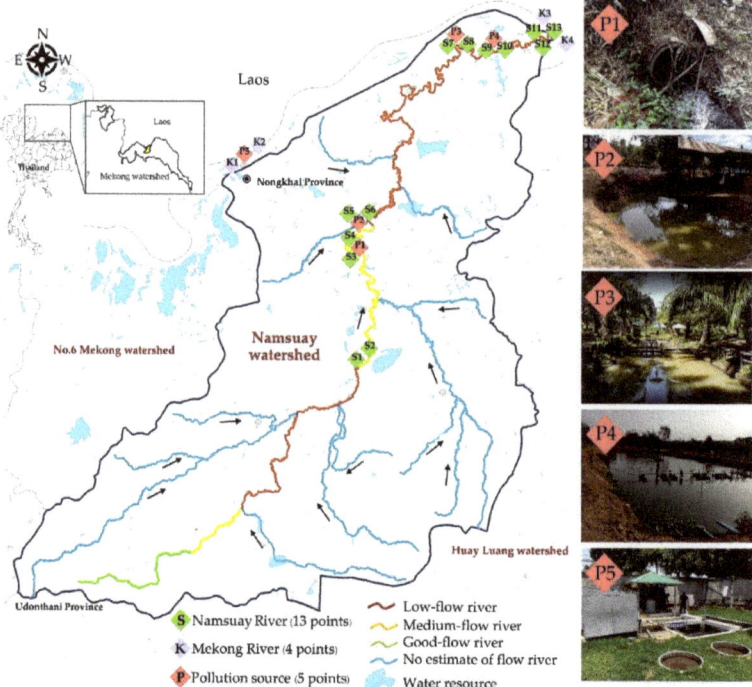

Figure 1. Study area and sampling sites. In total, 44 water samples were collected from 22 sites in the Nongkhai Province, northeast Thailand. The types of water sampling sites were: surface water (S1–S13 and K1–K4), wastewater (P1–P3), and discharge water (P4–P5).

2. Results

2.1. Microbiological Quality

As shown in Table 1, The most probable number (MPN) levels of the total coliforms and faecal coliforms in all samples were high. The surface water samples were highly contaminated with faecal coliform bacteria (43/44, 97.79%), except for the surface water samples from point K1 (Figure 1), which was less than 2 MPN/100 mL. The wastewater samples contained more faecal coliform bacteria than the other sources in the dry season (350 to >1600 MPN/100 mL) and the wet season (>1600 MPN/100 mL). It was clear that the faecal coliform bacteria count from the wastewater had a higher density than the other sampling types because the wastewater sources were untreated.

Table 1. Total coliform bacteria and faecal coliform bacteria.

Season	Sample Type	Number of Samples	Total Coliform Bacteria (MPN/100 mL, Number of Samples)		Faecal Coliform Bacteria (MPN/100 mL, Number of Samples)	
			Maximum (N)	Minimum (N)	Maximum (N)	Minimum (N)
Dry	Surface water	17	>1600.00, (1)	22.00, (1)	350.00, (1)	2.00, (2)
	Wastewater	3	>1600.00, (3)	-	>1600.00, (2)	350.00, (1)
	Discharge water	2	>1600.00, (2)	-	>1600.00, (1)	79.00, (1)
Wet	Surface water	17	>1600.00, (7)	41.00, (1)	>1600.00, (4)	79.00, (4)
	Wastewater	3	>1600.00, (2)	350.00, (1)	>1600.00, (3)	-
	Discharge water	2	>1600.00, (1)	79.00, (1)	>1600.00, (1)	0.00, (1)

2.2. Distribution of the Antibiotic Resistance Gene Profiles of the E. coli Isolates

The current study focused on three types of ARGs of public health concern: the CEGs, *mcr*, and PMQR in 113 *E. coli* isolates from 44 water samples that consisted of surface water (*n* = 89), wastewater (*n* = 17), and discharge water (*n* = 7). The most common ARG patterns in *E. coli* were for *oqxAB* alone, followed by *mcr-9* alone, and *mcr-8+mcr-9+ bla*$_{oxa-48-like}$. The *oqxAB* gene had a high prevalence in the wastewater and surface water samples, while the *mcr-9* gene had a high prevalence in only the surface water. The highest co-occurrences of the ARGs in *E. coli* were for *mcr-8+mcr-9+ bla*$_{oxa-48-like}$ (Table 2).

Table 2. Prevalence of the genotypic and phenotypic patterns of the *E. coli* isolates from each water source during the dry and wet seasons.

Genotypic and Phenotypic Patterns	Dry Season (*n* = 21)			Wet Season (*n* = 92)			Total (*n* = 113)		
	Surface Water (*n* = 16)	Waste-water (*n* = 3)	Discharge Water (*n* = 2)	Surface Water (*n* = 73)	Waste-water (*n* = 14)	Discharge Water (*n* = 5)	Surface Water (*n* = 89)	Waste-water (*n* = 17)	Discharge Water (*n* = 7)
ARG	13 (81.25)	2 (66.67)	2 (100.00)	27 (36.99)	6 (42.86)	2 (40.00)	40 (44.94)	8 (47.06)	4 (57.14)
mcr-8	1 (6.25)						1 (1.12)		
mcr-9	4 (25.00)			4 (5.48)			8 (8.99)		
oqxAB				20 (27.4)	5 (35.71)	1 (20.00)	20 (22.47)	5 (29.41)	1 (14.29)
qepA				1 (1.37)		1 (20.00)	1 (1.12)		1 (14.29)
bla$_{oxa-48-like}$	1 (6.25)						1 (1.12)		
mcr-8,mcr-9	2 (12.5)						2 (2.25)		
oqxAB, qepA				2 (2.74)			2 (2.25)		
mcr-1, oqxAB					1 (7.14)			1 (5.88)	
mcr-8,bla$_{oxa-48-like}$	1 (6.25)						1 (1.12)		
mcr-9, bla$_{oxa-48-like}$	1 (6.25)	1 (33.33)					1 (1.12)	1 (5.88)	
aac(6′)-Ib-cr, bla$_{oxa-48-like}$			1 (50.00)						1 (14.29)
mcr-8,mcr-9, bla$_{oxa-48-like}$	3 (18.75)		1 (50.00)				3 (3.37)		1 (14.29)

Table 2. *Cont.*

Genotypic and Phenotypic Patterns	Dry Season (*n* = 21)			Wet Season (*n* = 92)			Total (*n* = 113)		
	Surface Water (*n* = 16)	Waste-water (*n* = 3)	Discharge Water (*n* = 2)	Surface Water (*n* = 73)	Waste-water (*n* = 14)	Discharge Water (*n* = 5)	Surface Water (*n* = 89)	Waste-water (*n* = 17)	Discharge Water (*n* = 7)
Not detect ARGs	3 (18.75)	1 (33.33)		46 (63.01)	8 (57.14)	3 (60)	49 (55.06)	9 (52.94)	3 (42.86)
AR	10 (62.50)	3 (100.00)	2 (100.00)	17 (23.29)	6 (42.86)	3 (60.00)	27 (30.34)	9 (52.94)	5 (71.43)
mcr-9, oqxAB, *bla*$_{\text{oxa-48-like}}$		1 (33.33)						1 (5.88)	
CIP	3 (18.75)	1 (33.33)	1 (50.00)	12 (16.44)	4 (28.57)	3 (60.00)	15 (16.85)	5 (29.41)	4 (57.14)
COL	5 (31.25)	1 (33.33)					5 (5.62)	1 (5.88)	
IMP				2 (2.74)			2 (2.25)		
CTX + COL	1 (6.25)						1 (1.12)		
IMP + COL	1 (6.25)						1 (1.12)		
CIP + COL		1 (33.33)						1 (5.88)	
CIP + CTX				1 (1.37)			1 (1.12)		
IMP + CTX				1 (1.37)			1 (1.12)		
CIP + CTZ + CTX			1 (50.00)	1 (1.37)	2 (14.29)		1 (1.12)	2 (11.76)	1 (14.29)
Susceptibility	6 (37.5)			56 (76.71)	8 (57.14)	2 (40)	62 (69.66)	8 (47.06)	2 (28.57)

ARG, antibiotic resistance gene; AR, antibiotic resistance; CIP, ciprofloxacin; COL, colistin; IMP, imipenem; CTX, cefotaxime; CTZ, ceftazidime.

As shown in Table 2, in the dry season, the prevalence levels of the ARGs were 81.25% (13/16) in the *E. coli* from the surface water samples and 66.67% (2/3) in the *E. coli* from the wastewater samples. A predominant ARG pattern in the *E. coli* was *mcr-9* and *mcr-8+mcr-9+ bla*$_{\text{oxa-48-like}}$. In the wet season, the ARGs in the *E. coli* isolates from the wastewater samples (42.86%, 6/14) were higher than from the discharge water samples (40.00%, 2/5) and surface water samples (36.99%, 27/73). A predominant ARG pattern in *E. coli* was *oqxAB*.

2.3. Antibiotic Resistance Phenotypes of the E. coli Isolates

The antibiotic-resistant *E. coli* are shown in Table 2. *E. coli* from each water sample type had high resistance to ciprofloxacin, with 57.14% (4/7) in the discharge water samples, 29.41% (5/17) in the wastewater samples, and 16.85% (15/89) in the surface water samples.

In the dry season, the prevalence of antibiotic-resistant *E. coli* was detected in 100.00% of the wastewater (3/3) and discharge water (2/2) samples, while it was in 62.50% (10/16) of the surface water samples. The colistin resistance at 28.57% (6/21) was higher in *E. coli* compared to another antibiotic (Table 2).

In the wet season, the antibiotic resistance profiles of the *E. coli* isolates against the tested antibiotics in each water sample type were: discharge water, 60.00% (3/5), wastewater, 42.86% (6/14), and surface water, 23.39% (17/73). The most prevalent AR pattern was ciprofloxacin in 20.65% (19/92) (Table 2).

Table 3 shows the high distribution of antibiotic resistance in *E. coli* for ciprofloxacin (26.55%, 30/113), followed by colistin (7.96%, 9/113), cefotaxime (6.19%, 7/113), ceftazidime (3.54%, 4/113), and imipenem (3.54%, 4/113). The most prevalent ARG in antibiotic-resistant *E. coli* was *oqxAB* (7.08%, 8/113). In addition, all colistin-resistant *E. coli* harboured ARGs.

2.4. Phylogenetic Group of the E. coli Isolates

As shown in Table 4, the 113 *E. coli* isolates could be divided into phylogenetic groups, with 42.48% (43/113) in group B1, 10.62% (12/113) in group C, 9.73% (11/113) in groups A and E, 3.54% (4/113) in groups B2 and clade I or II, and 1.77% (2/113) in group F, while 18.58% (21/113) were unclassified into a phylogenetic group. The *E. coli* harbouring the *oqxAB* gene belonged to phylogroup B1 in this study. The *E. coli* harbouring co-ARGs were classified in phylogroups B1, B2, E, and clade I or II. Additionally, phylogroup B1 contained *E. coli*-harbouring ARGs (15.93%, 18/113) and antibiotic-resistant ones (7.08%, 8/113). However, the *oqxAB* gene was the most prevalent in phylogroup B1 (7.96%, 9/113). The *E. coli* resistance to ciprofloxacin demonstrated a relatively high prevalence in phylogroup

C (5.31%, 6/113). In this study, the *E. coli* in phylogroup B2 (3.54%, 4/113) had a lower prevalence than the other phylogroups (A, B1, C, E, F, clade I or II, and unknown); however, all isolates harboured ARGs, as shown in Table 4.

Table 3. Relationships between the antibiotic resistance of the *E. coli* isolates ($n = 113$) and the resistance genes.

Antibiotic Resistance Gene Patterns	Fluoroquinolone	Carbapenem	3rd Generation of Cephalosporins		Polymyxin
	Ciprofloxacin	Imipenem	Ceftazidime	Cefotaxime	Colistin
ARGs not detected	15 (13.27)	2 (1.77)	2 (1.77)	4 (3.54)	
mcr-8					1 (0.88)
mcr-9					3 (2.65)
oqxAB	8 (7.08)		1 (0.88)	1 (0.88)	
qepA	1 (0.88)	1 (0.88)			
bla$_{oxa-48-like}$	1 (0.88)				
mcr-8 + mcr-9					1 (0.88)
oqxAB + qepA	1 (0.88)				
mcr-1+ oqxAB	1 (0.88)				
mcr-8+ bla$_{oxa-48-like}$					
mcr-9+ bla$_{oxa-48-like}$					1 (0.88)
aac(6′)-Ib-cr + bla$_{oxa-48-like}$	1 (0.88)		1 (0.88)	1 (0.88)	
mcr-8 + mcr-9 + bla$_{oxa-48-like}$	1 (0.88)	1 (0.88)		1 (0.88)	2 (1.77)
mcr-9 + oqxAB + bla$_{oxa-48-like}$	1 (0.88)				1 (0.88)
Total	30 (26.55)	4 (3.54)	4 (3.54)	7 (6.19)	9 (7.96)

ARGs, antibiotic resistance genes.

Table 4. Profiles of the antibiotic resistance genes and the antibiotic resistance of *E. coli* according to the phylogenetic group.

Profile	A	B1	B2	C	E	F	Clade I or II	Unknown	Total
Number of isolates	11 (9.73)	48 (42.48)	4 (3.54)	12 (10.62)	4 (3.54)	11 (9.73)	2 (1.77)	21 (18.58)	113 (100.00)
Antibiotic resistance genes	5 (4.42)	18 (15.93)	4 (3.54)	5 (4.42)	2 (1.77)	8 (7.08)	1 (0.88)	9 (7.96)	52 (46.02)
mcr-8		1 (0.88)							1 (0.88)
mcr-9		3 (2.65)			2 (1.77)			3 (2.65)	8 (7.08)
oqxAB	4 (3.54)	9 (7.96)		4 (3.54)	4 (3.54)	1 (0.88)		4 (3.54)	26 (23.01)
qepA	1 (0.88)			1 (0.88)					2 (1.77)
bla$_{oxa-48-like}$		1 (0.88)							1 (0.88)
mcr-8 + mcr-9			2 (1.77)						2 (1.77)
oqxAB + qepA		2 (1.77)							2 (1.77)
mcr-1 + oqxAB						1 (0.88)			1 (0.88)
mcr-8 + bla$_{oxa-48-like}$								1 (0.88)	1 (0.88)
mcr-9 + bla$_{oxa-48-like}$		1 (0.88)						1 (0.88)	2 (1.77)
aac(6′)-Ib-cr + bla$_{oxa-48-like}$				1 (0.88)					1 (0.88)
mcr-8 + mcr-9 + bla$_{oxa-48-like}$		1 (0.88)	1 (0.88)				2 (1.77)		4 (3.54)
mcr-9 + oqxAB + bla$_{oxa-48-like}$				1 (0.88)					1 (0.88)
Undetectable ARGs	6 (5.31)	30 (26.55)		7 (6.19)	3 (2.65)	1 (0.88)	2 (1.77)	12 (10.62)	61 (53.98)

Table 4. *Cont.*

Profile	A	B1	B2	C	E	F	Clade I or II	Unknown	Total
Antibiotic resistance	3 (2.65)	8 (7.08)	3 (2.65)	6 (5.31)	4 (3.54)	6 (5.31)	1 (0.88)	10 (8.85)	41 (36.28)
CIP	1 (0.88)	4 (3.54)		6 (5.31)	3 (2.65)	5 (4.42)	1 (0.88)	4 (3.54)	24 (21.24)
COL			2 (1.77)	1 (0.88)				3 (2.65)	6 (5.31)
IMP	2 (1.77)								2 (1.77)
CTX + COL					1 (0.88)				1 (0.88)
IMP + COL			1 (0.88)						1 (0.88)
CIP + COL						1 (0.88)			1 (0.88)
CIP + CTX								1 (0.88)	1 (0.88)
IMP + CTX		1 (0.88)							1 (0.88)
CIP + CTZ + CTX		1 (0.88)	1 (0.88)					2 (1.77)	4 (3.54)
Susceptibility	8 (7.08)	40 (35.4)	1 (0.88)	6 (5.31)		5 (4.42)	1 (0.88)	11 (9.73)	72 (63.72)

ARGs, antibiotic resistance genes; AR, antibiotic resistance; CIP, ciprofloxacin; COL, colistin; IMP, imipenem; CTX, cefotaxime; CTZ, ceftazidime.

2.5. Location of the Antibiotic-Resistant E. coli Isolates

The location of the antibiotic-resistant *E. coli* isolates was based on the water sampling points. Almost all sampling points had *E. coli* harbouring ARGs, except for two sampling points, namely the surface water from the Namsuay River (K1) in the dry season and the discharge water from a hospital (P5) in the wet season. Almost all water samples in the study were from agricultural areas, with a high prevalence of *mcr* genes in the dry season and a high prevalence of PMQR genes in the wet season, as shown in Figure 2.

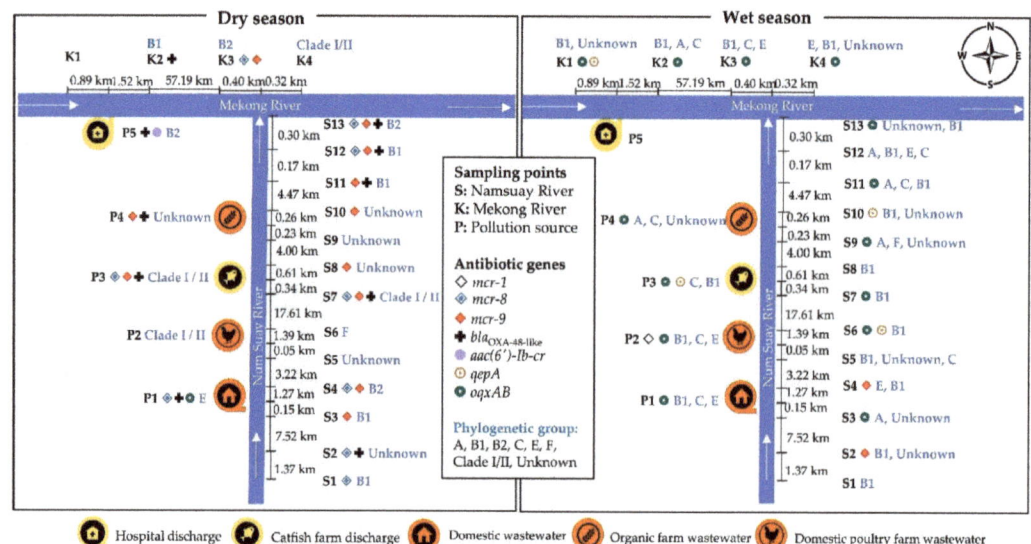

Figure 2. Distribution of the phylogenetic groups and antibiotic resistance genes, *mcr* (diamond symbol), CEGs (plus symbol) and PMQR (circle symbol) of *E. coli* at the water sample points.

In the dry season, *E. coli* was isolated from the water samples that carried the *mcr-8* gene from the surface water (S1, S2, S4, S7, S12, S13, and K3), domestic wastewater (P1), and fish farm discharge (P3), the *mcr-9* gene from surface water (S3, S4, S7, S8, S10, S11, S12, S13, and K3), fish farm (P3), and agricultural wastewater (P4), the *bla*$_{oxa-48-like}$ gene from surface water (S2, S7, S11, S12, S13, and K2), domestic wastewater (P1), fish farm discharge (P3), agricultural wastewater (P4), and hospital discharge (P5), the *aac(6′)-bl-cr* gene from hospital discharge (P5), and the *oqxAB* gene from domestic wastewater (P1).

In the wet season, *E. coli* carried the *mcr-1* gene from a poultry farm (P2), the *mcr-9* gene from surface water (S2 and S4), the *qepA* gene from surface water (S6, S10, and K1) and fish farm discharge (P3), and the *oqxAB* gene from surface water (S3, S6, S7, S9, S11, S13, K1, K2, K3, and K4), domestic wastewater (P1), poultry farm (P2), fish farm discharge (P3), and agricultural wastewater (P4).

The diversity of the phylogenetic groups of *E. coli* indicated that there were several groups in each of the water sample types or each water sampling point. The *E. coli* strains belonging to phylogenetic group B2 were only found in the water samples from the dry season, and all isolates harboured ARGs. The B2 phylogenetic group samples harbouring the ARGs isolates had the *mcr-8* and *mcr-9* genes at S4 (the sampling point of the surface water of the Namsuay River near the untreated domestic wastewater), the *mcr-8*, *mcr-9*, and $bla_{oxa-48-like}$ genes at S13 (the sampling point at the river mouth of the Namsuay River), the *mcr-8* and *mcr-9* genes at K3 (the sampling point at the surface of the Mekong River), and the $bla_{oxa-48-like}$ and *aac(6')-bl-cr* genes at P5 (the sampling point for the hospital discharge water).

2.6. Associations of Phenotypic and Genotypic Antibiotic Resistance in E. coli with the Phylogenetic Groups and Seasons

As shown in Table 5, Fisher's exact test showed a significant association between the antibiotic resistance phenotype of *E. coli* and phylogroup non-B1 ($p < 0.001$). In contrast, there was no association between the resistance genes and phylogroups.

Table 5. Associations between the antibiotic susceptibility and antibiotic resistance genes of *E. coli* and Phylogenetic Group (B1 and Non-B1).

Phenotypic and Genotypic Antibiotic Resistance in *E. coli*	B1 (*n* = 48)	Non-B1 (*n* = 65)	*p*-Values
Antibiotic resistance	8	33	<0.001
Antibiotic susceptibility	40	32	
Antibiotic resistance genes	18	34	0.131
Non-antibiotic resistance genes	30	31	

In the case of the season, the antibiotic resistance and the resistance genes of *E. coli* were significantly different between seasons ($p < 0.001$; Table 6).

Table 6. Association between antibiotic susceptibility and antibiotic resistance genes of *E. coli* and season (dry and wet).

Phenotypic and Genotypic Antibiotic Resistance in *E. coli*	Dry (*n* = 21)	Wet (*n* = 92)	*p*-Values
Antibiotic resistance	15	26	<0.001
Antibiotic susceptibility	6	66	
Antibiotic resistance genes	17	35	<0.001
Non-antibiotic resistance genes	4	57	

3. Discussion

This study investigated the numerous ARG- and AR-*E. coli* isolates found in the Namsuay watershed sources. Several reports have indicated that bacterial isolates carry many ARGs in aquatic environments in Thailand [15–17]. One study revealed that the AR bacteria and ARGs in aquatic settings could be harmful to human health [18].

According to the current results, most of the *E. coli* isolates were resistant to ciprofloxacin, which belongs to the fluoroquinolone class and was found in all settings. The global antimicrobial resistance surveillance system (GLASS) reported the prevalence of resistance of *E. coli* from patients in Thailand to fluoroquinolone (54%), third-generation cephalosporin (38%), polymyxin (13%), and carbapenems (2%) [19]. The current study identified high fluoroquinolone-nonsusceptible *E. coli*, perhaps due to the higher levels of quinolone used in agriculture or communities that may transmit to humans via the food-chain system [20].

The prevalence levels of the ARGs in *E. coli* from the discharge water and wastewater were higher than for the surface water because the discharge water (a hospital and a fish farm) and the wastewater are anthropogenic sources that have a well-known origin of contributing to the spread of antibiotic resistance in the environment [21–23]. The most prevalent PMQR gene was *oqxAB*, which was consistent with the results of a study from China [24] and Thailand [25]. The *oqxAB* was more prevalent in the wet season than in the dry season. We carried the assumption that the dry season had less rainfall than the wet season because the runoff associated with rainfall was a driver of AR gene dissemination and contamination in water [26]. The most prevalent *mcr* gene was *mcr-9*. Other studies reported *mcr-9* in *E. coli* from animals in China and the environment in Germany [9]. In Thailand, *mcr-9* was detected in *Enterobacter cloacae* from patients with community-acquired urinary tract infections [27] and in *E. coli* from slaughtered pigs [28], indicating that *mcr-9* had spread in the environment and was circulating in the human-animal-environment.

The levels of diversity of the ARGs and antibiotic resistance in the dry and wet seasons were significantly different. Similarly, another study reported that the ARGs of E. coli in summer were more diverse than in spring, fall, and winter because of environmental factors, such as temperature, suited to the survival of bacteria [29]. A study in Bangladesh showed that the carbapenem-resistant E. coli from river water samples only had a higher prevalence level in summer compared to winter and that seasonal factors were not positively correlated in any other water systems [30]. The possible reasons for the seasonal variation were the differences in the temperature, pH, and electrical conductivity of the water. The dry season has less rainfall than the wet season, thus reducing the flow of water in rivers and causing a greater accumulation of bacteria in the water sources than in the wet season [26]. The runoff and leaching of rainwater could dissolve environmental contaminants as a part of natural recovery. In addition, the temperatures in the dry season are higher than in the wet season, allowing bacteria to develop better and resulting in a greater likelihood of finding bacteria resistant to antibiotics in the dry season.

Our study demonstrated that the phylogroup B1 was predominant, and its occurrence was generally commensal with faecal flora *E. coli* strains [31,32]. In Kuwait, most *E. coli* from sewage belonged to groups A and B1 [33]. Another study showed that pathogenic *E. coli* isolates were mostly in phylogroup B2, while the isolates from faecal flora were mostly in phylogroup B1 [32]. Although phylogenetic group B1 was related to commensal strains, it carried more ARGs and AR than the other groups. This might provide a reservoir for the spread or transmission of ARGs to other bacteria, as well as provide a human-animal-environmental interface.

4. Materials and Methods

4.1. Study Area and Sampling Sites

The study area for sampling was the Namsuay watershed (1321.91 km^2) within the northeast Mekong watershed. The Namsuay River originates in the Udonthani province, from where it flows into the Mekong River in the Nongkhai province (Figure 1). The sample sites were selected to represent the different land uses and critical sites, such as agricultural, residential, cattle, and recreational sites.

In total, 44 water samples from 22 sites in the Nongkhai province (Figure 1) were collected from the Namsuay River surface water ($n = 26$), Mekong river surface water ($n = 8$), wastewater ($n = 6$), and discharge water ($n = 4$). At each sampling point, approximately 400 mL of water was collected in a sterile 500 mL glass bottle. Na$_2$S$_2$O$_3$ was added for de-chlorination, and all samples were transported to the laboratory in a cold box within 24 h. The water samples from each site were collected seasonally in January 2021 during the dry season and in May 2021 during the wet season.

4.2. Microbiological Quality Assessment

The MPN analysis was performed to determine the total coliform bacteria and faecal coliform bacteria in the water samples using the American public health association method [4]. Metallic green sheen colonies from the completed phase of the MPN test in eosin methylene blue agar were selected to culture on trypticase soy agar to confirm the *E. coli* isolates using a polymerase chain reaction (PCR) as described elsewhere [34].

4.3. Detection of the Antibioic Resistance Genes in the E. coli Isolates

Mobile-colistin-resistant genes, *mcr-1* to *mcr-9*, were detected based on the PCR as described previously [28], and all *mcr* PCR products were subjected to Sanger sequencing for confirmation by Apical Scientific Sdn Bhd (Selangor, Malaysia). The CEGs (bla_{IMP}, bla_{KPC}, bla_{NDM}, and $bla_{OXA-48-like}$) were identified using multiplex PCR described elsewhere [35]. The PMQR genes (*qnrA*, *qnrB*, *qnrC*, *qnrS*, *aac(6′)-Ib* and *qepA*) were identified using multiplex PCR as described by [36].

4.4. Antibiotic Susceptibility Profiles of the E. coli Isolates

The antibiotic susceptibility testing was performed using disk diffusion and broth microdilution (colistin only). Both methods were carried out in accordance with the 2020 Clinical and Laboratory Standards Institute (CLSI) guidelines [37]. *E. coli* strain ATCC 25922^{TM} was used as the control. The four antibiotic classes selected for the disk diffusion assay were fluoroquinolones: ciprofloxacin (CIP, 5 μg), third-generation cephalosporins: cefotaxime (CTX, 30 μg) and ceftazidime (CTZ, 30 μg), and the carbapenem: imipenem (IMI, 10 μg). The minimum inhibitory concentration (MIC) for colistin in the polymyxins class of antibiotics was performed using the broth microdilution method at concentrations of 1, 2, 4, 8, 16, and 32 μg/mL. The results were interpreted according to the CLSI [37], with a colistin MIC of >4 μg/mL against *E. coli*, corresponding to resistance.

4.5. E. coli Phylogenetic Group

Clermont PCR typing was applied to classily all *E. coli* isolates into phylogroups A, B1, B2, C, D, E, F, clade I, or clade II, as described elsewhere [38].

4.6. Statistical Analysis

Fisher's exact test (two-tailed) [39] was applied to find the associations between the antibiotic resistance phenotypes and antibiotic-resistant genes of the E. coli isolates and the phylogenetic groups (B1 and non-B1) and the seasons (dry and wet).

5. Conclusions

This study described the antibiotic resistance phenotypes and genotypes of *E. coli* in the Namsuay watershed, northeast rural Thailand. The results indicated that *E. coli* was resistant to the following classes of antibiotics: fluoroquinolone, third-generation cephalosporin, polymyxin, and carbapenem. The *E. coli* isolates carried the antibiotic resistance genes *mcr-1*, *mcr-8*, *mcr-9*, $bla_{OXA-48-like}$, *aac(6′)-bl-cr*, *qepA*, and *oqxAB*. Furthermore, this study showed that there was a significant association between antibiotic resistance and the antibiotic-resistance genes of *E. coli* isolates and seasons. The *E. coli* isolates from discharge water (from a hospital and a fish farm) showed a prevalence of resistance to antibiotics and harboured ARGs at higher levels than the other water sample sources. The presence of antibiotic-resistant *E. coli* in surface water, wastewater, and discharge water provided evidence that there is a public health risk associated with human exposure to water such as the Namsuay watershed.

Author Contributions: Conceptualization, P.T., R.Y. and A.K.; methodology; P.T., R.Y. and A.K.; formal analysis, P.T., R.Y., A.K. and R.U.; resources, P.T. and A.K.; data curation P.T. and A.K.; writing—original draft prep-aration, P.T. and R.Y.; writing—review and editing P.T., R.Y. and A.K. All authors have read and agreed to the published version of the manuscript.

Funding: This research received no external funding.

Institutional Review Board Statement: Not applicable.

Informed Consent Statement: Not applicable.

Data Availability Statement: Not applicable.

Acknowledgments: The authors are pleased to acknowledgments the Faculty of Public Health, Kasetsart University Chalermphrakiat Sakon Nakhon campus for their support during the laboratory analysis.

Conflicts of Interest: The authors declare no conflict of interest.

References

1. World Health Organization. *Global Antimicrobial Resistance Surveillance System (GLASS) Report: Early Implementation 2020*; World Health Organization: Geneva, Switzerland, 2020; pp. 109–115.
2. Sapkota, A.R. Other Water Pollutants: Antibiotic-Resistant Bacteria. In *Water and Sanitation-Related Diseases and the Environment*; John Wiley & Sons, Ltd.: Hoboken, NJ, USA, 2011; pp. 329–335.
3. Anthony, A.A.; Adekunle, C.F.; Thor, A.S. Residual antibiotics, antibiotic resistant superbugs and antibiotic resistance genes in surface water catchments: Public health impact. *Phys. Chem. Earth* **2018**, *105*, 177–183. [CrossRef]
4. Association, A.P.H. Microbiological examination. In *Standard Methods for the Examination of Water and Wastewater*, 23rd ed.; Baird, R.B., Eaton, A.D., Rice, E.W., Eds.; American Public Health Association: Washington, DC, USA, 2017; pp. 1–99.
5. Croxen, M.A.; Law, R.J.; Scholz, R.; Keeney, K.M.; Wlodarska, M.; Finlay, B.B. Recent advances in understanding enteric pathogenic *Escherichia coli*. *Clin. Microbiol. Rev.* **2013**, *26*, 822–880. [CrossRef] [PubMed]
6. Bungau, S.; Tit, D.M.; Behl, T.; Aleya, L.; Zaha, D.C. Aspects of excessive antibiotic consumption and environmental influences correlated with the occurrence of resistance to antimicrobial agents. *Curr. Opin. Environ. Sci.* **2021**, *19*, 100224. [CrossRef]
7. Zarei-Baygi, A.; Smith, A.L. Intracellular versus extracellular antibiotic resistance genes in the environment: Prevalence, horizontal transfer, and mitigation strategies. *Bioresour. Technol.* **2021**, *319*, 124181. [CrossRef]
8. Elbediwi, M.; Li, Y.; Paudyal, N.; Pan, H.; Li, X.; Xie, S.; Rajkovic, A.; Feng, Y.; Fang, W.; Rankin, S.C.; et al. Global burden of colistin-resistant bacteria: Mobilized colistin resistance genes study (1980–2018). *Microorganisms* **2019**, *7*, 461. [CrossRef]
9. Li, Y.; Dai, X.; Zeng, J.; Gao, Y.; Zhang, Z.; Zhang, L. Characterization of the global distribution and diversified plasmid reservoirs of the colistin resistance gene *mcr-9*. *Sci. Rep.* **2020**, *10*, 8113. [CrossRef] [PubMed]
10. Hooban, B.; Joyce, A.; Fitzhenry, K.; Chique, C.; Morris, D. The role of the natural aquatic environment in the dissemination of extended spectrum beta-lactamase and carbapenemase encoding genes: A scoping review. *Water Res.* **2020**, *180*, 115880. [CrossRef]
11. Yassine, I.; Rafei, R.; Osman, M.; Mallat, H.; Dabboussi, F.; Hamze, M. Plasmid-mediated quinolone resistance: Mechanisms, detection, and epidemiology in the Arab countries. *Infect. Genet. Evol.* **2019**, *76*, 104020. [CrossRef]
12. Varela, A.R.; Macedo, G.N.; Nunes, O.C.; Manaia, C.M. Genetic characterization of fluoroquinolone resistant *Escherichia coli* from urban streams and municipal and hospital effluents. *FEMS Microbiol. Ecol.* **2015**, *91*, fiv015. [CrossRef] [PubMed]
13. Graham, D.W.; Bergeron, G.; Bourassa, M.W.; Dickson, J.; Gomes, F.; Howe, A.; Kahn, L.H.; Morley, P.S.; Scott, H.M.; Simjee, S.; et al. Complexities in understanding antimicrobial resistance across domesticated animal, human, and environmental systems. *Ann. N. Y. Acad. Sci.* **2019**, *1441*, 17–30. [CrossRef] [PubMed]
14. Zhou, Z.C.; Feng, W.Q.; Han, Y.; Zheng, J.; Chen, T.; Wei, Y.Y.; Gillings, M.; Zhu, Y.G.; Chen, H. Prevalence and transmission of antibiotic resistance and microbiota between humans and water environments. *Environ. Int.* **2018**, *121*, 1155–1161. [CrossRef]
15. Dawangpa, A.; Lertwatcharasarakul, P.; Ramasoota, P.; Boonsoongnern, A.; Ratanavanichrojn, N.; Sanguankiat, A.; Phatthanakunanan, S.; Tulayakul, P. Genotypic and phenotypic situation of antimicrobial drug resistance of *Escherichia coli* in water and manure between biogas and non-biogas swine farms in central Thailand. *J. Environ. Manag.* **2021**, *279*, 111659. [CrossRef]
16. Tansawai, U.; Walsh, T.R.; Niumsup, P.R. Extended spectrum ß-lactamase-producing *Escherichia coli* among backyard poultry farms, farmers, and environments in Thailand. *Poult. Sci.* **2019**, *98*, 2622–2631. [CrossRef]
17. Thamlikitkul, V.; Tiengrim, S.; Thamthaweechok, N.; Buranapakdee, P.; Chiemchaisri, W. Contamination by Antibiotic-Resistant Bacteria in Selected Environments in Thailand. *Int. J. Environ. Res. Public Health* **2019**, *16*, 3753. [CrossRef]
18. Amarasiri, M.; Sano, D.; Suzuki, S. Understanding human health risks caused by antibiotic resistant bacteria (ARB) and antibiotic resistance genes (ARG) in water environments: Current knowledge and questions to be answered. *Crit. Rev. Environ. Sci. Technol.* **2020**, *50*, 2016–2059. [CrossRef]
19. ResistanceMap: Antibiotic Resistance. Available online: https://resistancemap.cddep.org/AntibioticResistance.php (accessed on 12 September 2022).

20. Kenyon, C. Positive Association between the Use of Quinolones in Food Animals and the Prevalence of Fluoroquinolone Resistance in *E. coli* and *K. pneumoniae*, *A. baumannii* and *P. aeruginosa*: A Global Ecological Analysis. *Antibiotics* **2021**, *10*, 1193. [CrossRef]

21. Hooban, B.; Fitzhenry, K.; Cahill, N.; Joyce, A.; O' Connor, L.; Bray, J.E.; Brisse, S.; Passet, V.; Abbas Syed, R.; Cormican, M.; et al. A Point Prevalence Survey of Antibiotic Resistance in the Irish Environment, 2018–2019. *Environ. Int.* **2021**, *152*, 106466. [CrossRef]

22. Huijbers, P.M.C.; Larsson, D.G.J.; Flach, C.-F. Surveillance of antibiotic resistant *Escherichia coli* in human populations through urban wastewater in ten European countries. *Environ. Pollut.* **2020**, *261*, 114200. [CrossRef]

23. Kunhikannan, S.; Thomas, C.J.; Franks, A.E.; Mahadevaiah, S.; Kumar, S.; Petrovski, S. Environmental hotspots for antibiotic resistance genes. *Microbiologyopen* **2021**, *10*, e1197. [CrossRef]

24. Cheng, P.; Yang, Y.; Li, F.; Li, X.; Liu, H.; Fazilani, S.A.; Guo, W.; Xu, G.; Zhang, X. The prevalence and mechanism of fluoroquinolone resistance in *Escherichia coli* isolated from swine farms in China. *BMC Vet. Res.* **2020**, *16*, 258. [CrossRef]

25. Lekagul, A.; Tangcharoensathien, V.; Liverani, M.; Mills, A.; Rushton, J.; Yeung, S. Understanding antibiotic use for pig farming in Thailand: A qualitative study. *Antimicrob. Resist. Infect. Control* **2021**, *10*, 3. [CrossRef]

26. Zhang, X.; Zhi, X.; Chen, L.; Shen, Z. Spatiotemporal variability and key influencing factors of river fecal coliform within a typical complex watershed. *Water Res.* **2020**, *178*, 115835. [CrossRef]

27. Assawatheptawee, K.; Treebupachatsakul, P.; Luangtongkum, T.; Niumsup, P.R. Risk Factors for Community-Acquired Urinary Tract Infections Caused by Multidrug-Resistant Enterobacterales in Thailand. *Antibiotics* **2022**, *11*, 1039. [CrossRef]

28. Khanawapee, A.; Kerdsin, A.; Chopjitt, P.; Boueroy, P.; Hatrongjit, R.; Akeda, Y.; Tomono, K.; Nuanualsuwan, S.; Hamada, S. Distribution and Molecular Characterization of *Escherichia coli* Harboring *mcr* Genes Isolated from Slaughtered Pigs in Thailand. *Microb. Drug Resist.* **2021**, *27*, 971–979. [CrossRef]

29. Yasmin, S.; Karim, A.M.; Lee, S.H.; Zahra, R. Temporal Variation of Meropenem Resistance in *E. coli* Isolated from Sewage Water in Islamabad, Pakistan. *Antibiotics* **2022**, *11*, 635. [CrossRef]

30. Asaduzzaman, M.; Rousham, E.; Unicomb, L.; Islam, M.R.; Amin, M.B.; Rahman, M.; Hossain, M.I.; Mahmud, Z.H.; Szegner, M.; Wood, P.; et al. Spatiotemporal distribution of antimicrobial resistant organisms in different water environments in urban and rural settings of Bangladesh. *Sci. Total Environ.* **2022**, *831*, 154890. [CrossRef]

31. Duriez, P.; Clermont, O.; Bonacorsi, S.; Bingen, E.; Chaventré, A.; Elion, J.; Picard, B.; Denamur, E. Commensal *Escherichia coli* isolates are phylogenetically distributed among geographically distinct human populations. *Microbiology* **2001**, *147*, 1671–1676. [CrossRef]

32. Mojaz-Dalfardi, N.; Kalantar-Neyestanaki, D.; Hashemizadeh, Z.; Mansouri, S. Comparison of virulence genes and phylogenetic groups of *Escherichia coli* isolates from urinary tract infections and normal fecal flora. *Gene Rep.* **2020**, *20*, 100709. [CrossRef]

33. Redha, M.A.; Al Sweih, N.; Albert, M.J. Virulence and phylogenetic groups of *Escherichia coli* cultured from raw sewage in Kuwait. *Gut Pathog.* **2022**, *14*, 18. [CrossRef]

34. Molina, F.; López-Acedo, E.; Tabla, R.; Roa, I.; Gómez, A.; Rebollo, J.E. Improved detection of *Escherichia coli* and coliform bacteria by multiplex PCR. *BMC Biotechnol.* **2015**, *15*, 48. [CrossRef]

35. Hatrongjit, R.; Kerdsin, A.; Akeda, Y.; Hamada, S. Detection of plasmid-mediated colistin-resistant and carbapenem-resistant genes by multiplex PCR. *MethodsX* **2018**, *5*, 532–536. [CrossRef]

36. Ciesielczuk, H.; Hornsey, M.; Choi, V.; Woodford, N.; Wareham, D.W. Development and evaluation of a multiplex PCR for eight plasmid-mediated quinolone-resistance determinants. *J. Med. Microbiol.* **2013**, *62*, 1823–1827. [CrossRef]

37. CLSI. *Performance Standards for Antimicrobial Susceptibility Testing*, 30th ed.; Clinical Laboratory Standard Institute: Wayne, PA, USA, 2020; pp. 1–41.

38. Clermont, O.; Christenson, J.K.; Denamur, E.; Gordon, D.M. The Clermont *Escherichia coli* phylo-typing method revisited: Improvement of specificity and detection of new phylo-groups. *Environ. Microbiol. Rep.* **2013**, *5*, 58–65. [CrossRef]

39. Yates, F. Tests of Significance for 2 × 2 Contingency Tables. *J. R. Stat. Soc. Ser. A Gen.* **1984**, *147*, 426–449. [CrossRef]

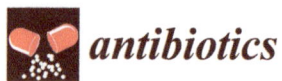

MDPI

Article

Irrigation Ponds as Sources of Antimicrobial-Resistant Bacteria in Agricultural Areas with Intensive Use of Poultry Litter

Eliene S. Lopes [1], Cláudio E. T. Parente [2], Renata C. Picão [3] and Lucy Seldin [1,*]

[1] Laboratório de Genética Microbiana, Instituto de Microbiologia Paulo de Góes, Universidade Federal do Rio de Janeiro (UFRJ), Rio de Janeiro 21941-902, Brazil
[2] Laboratório de Radioisótopos Eduardo Penna Franca, Instituto de Biofísica Carlos Chagas Filho, Universidade Federal do Rio de Janeiro (UFRJ), Rio de Janeiro 21941-902, Brazil
[3] Laboratório de Investigação em Microbiologia Médica, Instituto de Microbiologia Paulo de Góes, Universidade Federal do Rio de Janeiro (UFRJ), Rio de Janeiro 21941-902, Brazil
* Correspondence: lseldin@micro.ufrj.br; Tel.: +55-21-3938-6741; Fax: +55-21-2560-8344

Abstract: Poultry litter is widely used worldwide as an organic fertilizer in agriculture. However, poultry litter may contain high concentrations of antibiotics and/or antimicrobial-resistant bacteria (ARB), which can be mobilized through soil erosion to water bodies, contributing to the spread of antimicrobial resistance genes (ARGs) in the environment. To better comprehend this kind of mobilization, the bacterial communities of four ponds used for irrigation in agricultural and poultry production areas were determined in two periods of the year: at the beginning (low volume of rainfall) and at the end of the rainy season (high volume of rainfall). 16S rRNA gene sequencing revealed not only significantly different bacterial community structures and compositions among the four ponds but also between the samplings. When the DNA obtained from the water samples was PCR amplified using primers for ARGs, those encoding integrases (*intI1*) and resistance to sulfonamides (*sul1* and *sul2*) and β-lactams (*bla*$_{GES}$, *bla*$_{TEM}$ and *bla*$_{SHV}$) were detected in three ponds. Moreover, bacterial strains were isolated from CHROMagar plates supplemented with sulfamethoxazole, ceftriaxone or ciprofloxacin and identified as belonging to clinically important Enterobacteriaceae. The results presented here indicate a potential risk of spreading ARB through water resources in agricultural areas with extensive fertilization with poultry litter.

Keywords: poultry litter; antimicrobial resistance genes; bacterial community; irrigation ponds; fluoroquinolones; β-lactams; sulfonamides

Citation: Lopes, E.S.; Parente, C.E.T.; Picão, R.C.; Seldin, L. Irrigation Ponds as Sources of Antimicrobial-Resistant Bacteria in Agricultural Areas with Intensive Use of Poultry Litter. *Antibiotics* **2022**, *11*, 1650. https://doi.org/10.3390/antibiotics11111650

Academic Editors: Jonathan Frye, Athanasios Tsakris, Anusak Kerdsin and Jinquan Li

Received: 11 October 2022
Accepted: 15 November 2022
Published: 18 November 2022

Publisher's Note: MDPI stays neutral with regard to jurisdictional claims in published maps and institutional affiliations.

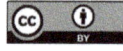
1. Introduction

Antimicrobial resistance (AMR) is a global public health problem that generates social and economic impacts [1,2]. Although AMR is a natural evolutionary phenomenon, its main driver is the widespread use of antimicrobials in human and veterinary medicine [3].

In animal husbandry, it is estimated that the use of antimicrobials will increase by 70% between 2010 and 2030 with the intensification of production to meet the growing demand for cheap animal protein [4–6]. The poultry industry draws attention to the wide use of antimicrobials, such as β-lactams, sulfonamides, and fluoroquinolones, which are widely used due to their broad spectrum against Gram-positive and Gram-negative pathogens [7–9]. The use of antimicrobial agents as growth promoters is controlled in animal husbandry in Brazil. However, many molecules may still be used for therapeutic, prophylactic and metaphylactic purposes [4,10]. This constant exposure to antimicrobials, especially in subtherapeutic doses, may result in selective pressure on the poultry microbiota. Therefore, increased expression and transfer of antimicrobial resistance genes (ARGs) from one organism to another, triggering a reduction in the sensitivity of microorganisms to these drugs, can be observed [11].

Additionally, most antimicrobials are not completely metabolized by the animal organism, and bioactive compounds are excreted without changes. These bioactive compounds are able to reach the environment mainly through the application of poultry litter in agricultural soils [12,13]. Poultry litter, mainly composed of chicken manure, spilled feed, feathers, and bedding materials, is the main waste of poultry farming, and millions of tons are generated annually worldwide, providing macronutrients and improving the physical, chemical and biological characteristics of soils [14]. However, considering the risks to public health, it is necessary to comprehensively verify the environmental fate of contaminants due to poultry litter fertilization in agricultural environments [15].

Previous studies have reported that antimicrobials can accumulate in soils and reach surface and groundwater through erosive processes, such as leaching and surface runoff, increasing selective pressure in these environments [12,16–19]. Contaminated water can be an important route of transmission of pathogens through animal watering, human supply, and irrigation of agricultural crops [20,21].

In this context, to better understand the influence of the use of poultry litter on the spread of antimicrobial-resistant bacteria (ARB) and antimicrobial resistance genes (ARGs) and to predict possible risks to human health, the bacterial communities found in the water of four irrigation ponds surrounded by agricultural areas with intensive use of poultry litter were characterized. Moreover, the presence of clinically important ARB and the occurrence of β-lactam, sulfonamide and fluoroquinolone resistance genes were also investigated. As the study area is situated in a highly weathered tropical region (average annual rainfall greater than 2500 mm [22,23], and considering that the wet season is the period of the greatest mobilization (soil–water) of contaminants (through soil leaching and surface water runoff), two periods of the year—high and low rainfall (end and beginning of rainy season, respectively)—were evaluated to understand seasonal influences on the evaluated bacterial communities.

2. Materials and Methods

2.1. Study Area and Sampling Design

The study area comprises agricultural areas in the municipality of São José do Vale do Rio Preto (SJVRP; 220 km^2 and 615 m.a.s.l. mean elevation), located in the upland region of Rio de Janeiro state, in southeastern Brazil (Figure S1, [24,25]). The climate of the region is classified as Altitude Tropical, with dry winters and humid summers [22,23].

The municipality stands out as the largest poultry producer in Rio de Janeiro state (RJ), housing approximately one hundred poultry farms surrounded by agricultural areas that supply fresh products to the RJ metropolitan region [24]. In SJVRP, agricultural soils are periodically fertilized with poultry litter contaminated with veterinary antimicrobials [24,25] and irrigated with water from surrounding ponds. The relief features with slopes and agricultural valleys can favor erosive processes, such as leaching and surface runoff along drainage basins, reaching irrigation ponds. The wet season is considered the critical period for the mobilization (soil–water) of contaminants. Therefore, two samplings (denoted S1 and S2) were carried out in the wet season to assess periods with high (S1; on 14 March 2019) and low monthly rainfall (S2; on 25 November 2019). The amount of rain was significantly different between samplings: S1 (187 mm) and S2 (107 mm) [26].

Water samples were collected in four artificial ponds used for crop irrigation: LA (22°11′35.4″ S, 42°55′11.0″ W) with 245 m^2; LB (22°11′31.8″ S, 42°55′06.3″ W) with 147 m^2; LC (22°06′52.7″ S, 42°57′04.2″ W) with 665 m^2 and LD (22°08′57.4″ S, 42°52′54.4″ W) with 294 m^2 (Figure S2). The main crops in the surroundings were chayote, tomato, zucchini, bell pepper, among others.

The water samples (1 L) were collected (up to 30 cm deep) in triplicate with distances ranging from 1 to 10 m between each replicate in sterile glass bottles. They were identified by capital letters followed by the number of replicates: LA (LA1, LA2 and LA3), LB (LB1, LB2 and LB3), LC (LC1, LC2 and LC3) and LD (LD1, LD2 and LD3).

The physicochemical parameters of the pond waters—pH, salinity, and temperature—were measured using a portable meter (Mettler Toledo, Inc., Schwerzenbach, Switzerland). These data are shown in Table S1.

2.2. DNA Extraction from Water Samples

For the extraction of total DNA, 250 mL of each water sample was filtered through Millipore filters with 0.45 μm pore size membranes using a Kitassato connected to a vacuum pump. DNA extraction from water samples was performed from the membranes using the FastDNA Spin kit (MP Biomedicals, Santa Ana, CA, USA) according to the protocol provided by the manufacturer. After extraction, the concentration of the obtained DNA samples was evaluated using a Qubit 4 fluorometer (Thermo Fisher Scientific, Waltham, MA, USA).

2.3. Detection of β-Lactam, Sulfonamide and Fluoroquinolone Resistance Genes

Simplex and multiplex PCRs were performed using the DNA extracted from the four ponds to detect genes encoding class 1 and 2 integrases (*intI1* and *intI2*) and genes encoding resistance to β-lactams (bla_{CTX-M}, bla_{TEM}, bla_{SHV}, bla_{GES}, $bla_{FOX-like}$, $bla_{MOX-like}$, $bla_{CIT-like}$, $bla_{EBC-like}$, $bla_{DHA-like}$, $bla_{ACC-like}$, bla_{MIR} and bla_{ACT}), sulfonamides (*sul1* and *sul2*) and fluoroquinolones (*qnrA*, *qnrS*, *qnrC*, *qnrD*, *qnrB*, *qnrVC* and *qepA*). The primer sequences used and the amplification conditions are presented in Table S2 [27–34]. The PCR products were visualized after electrophoresis in a 1.4% agarose gel in 1X TBE buffer [35]. The presence or absence of common bands among the different ponds was compared and presented in a Venn diagram.

2.4. Amplicon Sequencing of 16S rRNA Genes from Water Samples

Total DNA extracted (approximately 10–20 ng/μL) from the 24 samples (four ponds in triplicate and two samplings) was sequenced using the MiSeq system (Illumina, USA) paired-end by Novogene Corporation (Beijing, China). The primers used for PCR amplification of the V4 region of the *rrs* gene (encoding 16S rRNA) were 515F (GTGCCAGCMGC-CGCGGTAA) and 806R (GGACTACHVGGGTWTCTAAT) [36,37], which generated fragments of approximately 250 bp.

2.5. Bioinformatics Analysis

The sequences obtained from sequencing were analyzed using Mothur v.1.44.3 software [38]. The forward and reverse sequences were paired in contigs, and sequences with sizes incompatible with these fragments, ambiguities and homopolymers (>8) were removed from the analysis, while similar sequences were grouped to eliminate redundancies. Virtual PCR was performed using primers 515F and 806R [36,37] to align the consensus sequences based on the Silva v138 database [39]. Sequences with insufficient alignments and columns without nucleotides were removed. A precluster was performed for error correction in rare sequences. The sequences were classified using the Ribosomal Database Project (RDP) [40] to remove contaminants such as mitochondrial DNA, chloroplasts, Archaea, Eukarya, chimeric sequences and nontaxon organisms. The Bayesian method was used for the classification of sequences based on the RDP dataset [40]. Using a cutoff of 97% similarity, the sequences were grouped into operational taxonomic units (OTUs), and singletons were removed. Finally, the data related to α-diversity and β-diversity indexes, rarefaction curves, and taxonomic relative abundance were used in further statistical analyses.

Raw sequence data were deposited in the NCBI Sequence Read Archive (SRA) and are available under Bioproject accession number (PRJNA895046).

2.6. Statistical Analyses

The statistical analyses of sequencing data were performed in Past v4.03 software [41] based on two independent variables: the sampling period (March and November 2019, corresponding to the first (S1)—high rainfalls—and second (S2)—low rainfalls—samplings, respectively) and the area (the four studied ponds). The richness and diversity indexes, as well as the relative abundance of the taxa (phylum, class and genus), were checked for distribution normality by the Shapiro–Wilk test or homoscedasticity among samples by the Levene test. The resulting data were submitted to normalization by Box Cox [42] when necessary. Student's *t* test was applied to parametric data, while the Mann–Whitney test was applied to nonparametric data to compare the bacterial communities between the two samplings from each pond. Parametric data were submitted to one-way analysis of variance (ANOVA), and the nonparametric data were submitted to the Kruskal–Wallis test to compare the bacterial communities of the four ponds at each sampling. In addition, richness and diversity indexes were also submitted to ANOVA.

Finally, nonmetric multidimensional scaling (nMDS) was performed with the Bray–Curtis dissimilarity index using the OTU distribution matrix followed by two-way PERMANOVA to test the distribution of OTUs considering the sampling periods and the ponds studied. The physical–chemical variables (pH, salinity and temperature) were integrated into nMDS as metadata.

2.7. Isolation of ARB from Water Samples

Bacterial strains resistant to different antimicrobials were isolated from water samples in the second sampling campaign (S2, low rainfall sampling). The triplicates were mixed (750 mL of water from each replicate), and 1000 mL of water from each pond was filtered through 0.45 μm pore size Millipore® (Barueri, SP, Brazil) membranes using a Kitassato connected to a vacuum pump. The four membranes were washed individually in 20 mL of saline (NaCl 0.85%).

Aliquots of 100 μL of each sample and their respective dilutions (10^{-1} and 10^{-2}) were plated in Petri dishes containing CHROMagar Orientation culture medium (BD Diagnostics) supplemented with 50 μg/mL ciprofloxacin (Sigma®, Saint Louis, MI, USA), 60 μg/mL sulfamethoxazole (Sigma®, Buchs, Switzerland) or 8 μg/mL ceftriaxone (Sigma® Saint Louis, MI, USA) [43,44]. The plates were incubated at 37 °C for 24 h. After determination of colony forming units per milliliter (CFU/mL), three colonies of each morphology were reinoculated on CHROMagar and further identified at the genus level by MALDI-TOF (Bruker Daltonics Bremen, Germany). All isolated strains were maintained at −80 °C in tryptic soy broth medium (TSB) supplemented with the antibiotic used for their isolation, and 20% glycerol.

3. Results

3.1. PCR Amplification of Antimicrobial Resistance Genes in Water Samples

After DNA extraction from the water samples of the four ponds studied here in two periods of the year corresponding to high (S1) and low (S2) rainfall samplings, β-lactams resistance genes were detected in two ponds (LB and LC). The genes bla_{GES} and bla_{TEM} were detected in LB in S1 and S2, respectively, while both genes and the bla_{SHV} gene were also observed in LC, but only in S2 (Figures 1 and S3A–C).

Sulfonamide resistance genes were detected in three ponds (LB, LC and LD). Bands corresponding to *sul1* were observed in LB and LD (S1) and in LC and LD (S2), while bands corresponding to *sul2* were observed in LC (S1) and in LB, LC and LD (S2) (Figures 1 and S4A,B).

Genes encoding integrases were also detected in three of the four ponds (LB, LC and LD). Bands corresponding to the *intI1* gene were observed in the LB, LC and LD (S1) and in the LC and LD (S2) (Figures 1 and S5A).

Only in one pond (LA) was the presence of the abovementioned genes not observed. Furthermore, amplification of genes encoding resistance to fluoroquinolones (*qnrA*, *qnrS*, *qnrC*, *qnrD*, *qnrB*, *qnrVC* and *qepA*) was not detected in any of the studied ponds.

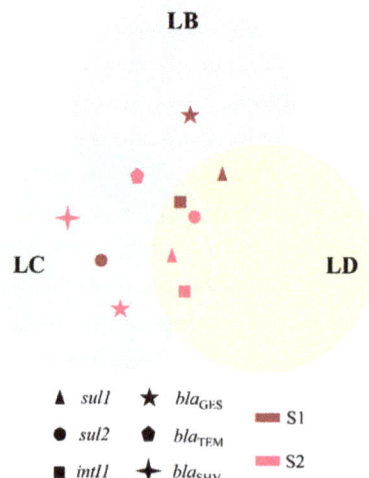

Figure 1. Presence of resistance genes in the studied ponds. Resistance genes are represented by geometric figures—dark pink in S1 and light pink in S2—in a Venn diagram. S1 and S2 correspond to the sampling period: high (S1; on 14 March 2019) and low monthly rainfall (S2; on 25 November 2019).

3.2. Structure and Composition of the Bacterial Communities of Water Samples

After sequencing the V4 region of the gene encoding 16S rRNA of the 24 DNA samples obtained from the four ponds, the sequences were analyzed and normalized to 47,990 sequences per sample. The number of sequences represented a sufficient coverage of the OTUs present in the bacterial communities, which can be observed by the tendency of the rarefaction curves to reach a plateau (Figure S6).

A significant difference was observed for richness (number of OTUs) between S1 and S2 for ponds LA (p = 0.0058288) and LD (p = 0.021009) (Figure 2A). Statistical differences were also observed in either S1 (p = 0.00584) or S2 (p = 0.003146) among the four ponds (Figure 2A). Considering the Shannon diversity index (Figure 2B), significant differences between S1 and S2 for LC (p = 0.011584) and for LD (p = 0.018024) were observed among the four ponds in S1 (p = 0.004127) and S2 (p = 0.004021). Moreover, an interaction between sampling periods (S1 and S2) and ponds (four water samples), related to both richness (p = 0.001341) (Figure 2A) and diversity (p = 0.01374) (Figure 2B), was observed using a two-way ANOVA.

Beta diversity was evaluated by nonmetric multidimensional scaling (nMDS) of OTUs based on the Bray–Curtis dissimilarity index (Figure 3). From a two-way PERMANOVA, it was observed that the structure of the bacterial communities of each pond was different between samplings (S1 and S2) (p = 0.0001). Additionally, a clear dispersion among the four ponds (p = 0.0001) was observed (Figure 3). With the integration of the physicochemical data to the NMDs, the temperature positively influenced the first sampling (S1) of LC, while pH and salinity positively influenced the second sampling (S2) of this pond (Figure 3).

The relative abundance of bacterial taxa in the four water samples was determined in S1 and S2. All phyla with at least 1% of the total relative abundance are shown in Figure 4. A significant difference was observed among the ponds in the relative abundance of Proteobacteria, Verrucomicrobia and Planctomycetes in S1 and S2. For Firmicutes, a significant difference among the ponds was observed only in S1, while for Actinobacteria and Bacteroidetes, a significant difference was observed only in S2. In addition, the following can be observed in Figure 4: (i) a significant difference in the relative abundance of Proteobacteria between S1 and S2 in LC and LD; (ii) a significant difference in the abundances of Actinobacteria and Verrucomicrobia between S1 and S2 in all water samples except in LB; (iii) the predominance of Actinobacteria and Verrucomicrobia in LC and LD (in S1) and in LA (in S2); and (iv) the predominance of Firmicutes in the four ponds in S1 and Bacteroidetes in LA (S1).

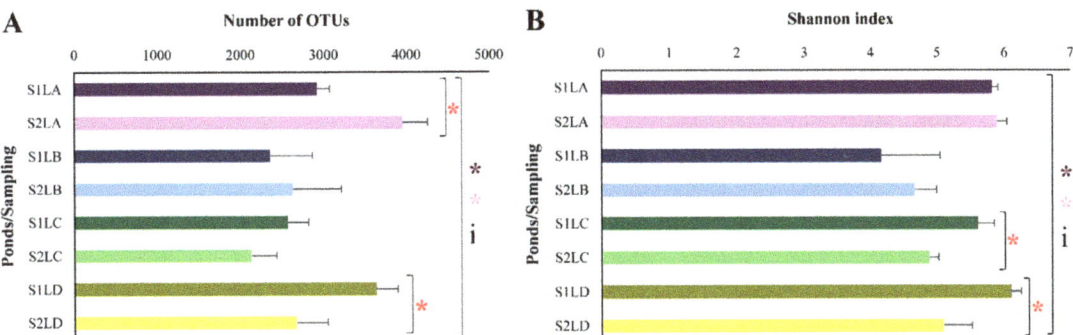

Figure 2. Alpha diversity evaluated by massive sequencing of the gene encoding 16S rRNA in water samples collected in LA (purple), LB (blue), LC (green) and LD (yellow) in S1 (high rainfall period—dark tones) and in S2 (low rainfall period—light tones). The bars represent the standard deviation. Species richness and alpha diversity showed significant differences between the ponds in the two samplings (parametric data submitted to a one-way ANOVA) represented by asterisks (dark pink for S1 and light pink for S2). A red asterisk represents the significant difference among the ponds at each sampling (parametric data submitted to the t test). The data were also submitted to a two-way ANOVA, and the interaction between the factors is represented by the letter i. (**A**) Richness evaluated by the number of OTUs; (**B**) Shannon diversity index.

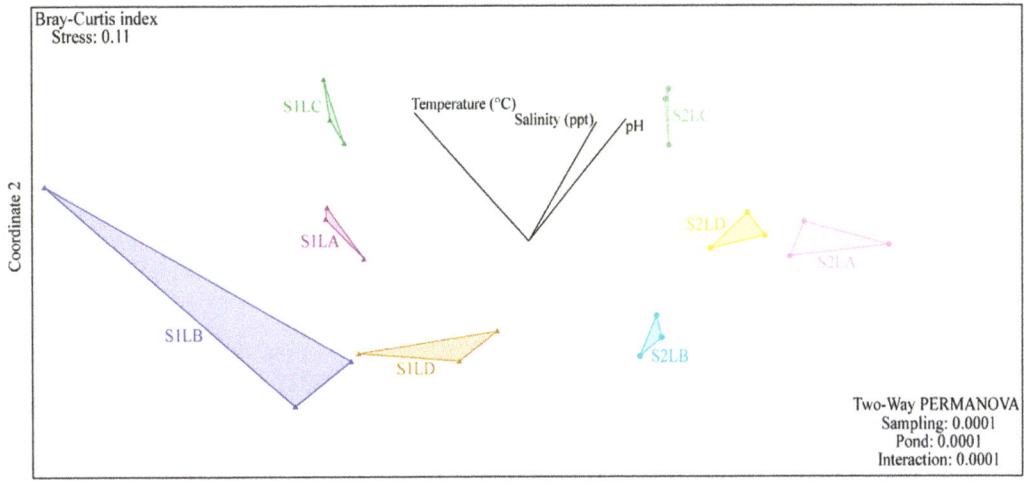

Figure 3. Nonmetric multidimensional scaling (nMDS) with the Bray–Curtis dissimilarity index. Representation of LA (purple), LB (blue), LC (green) and LD (yellow). The replicates are represented by triangles in dark tones (S1) and circles in light tones (S2). The physical–chemical data evaluated from the water samples from the ponds were integrated as metadata.

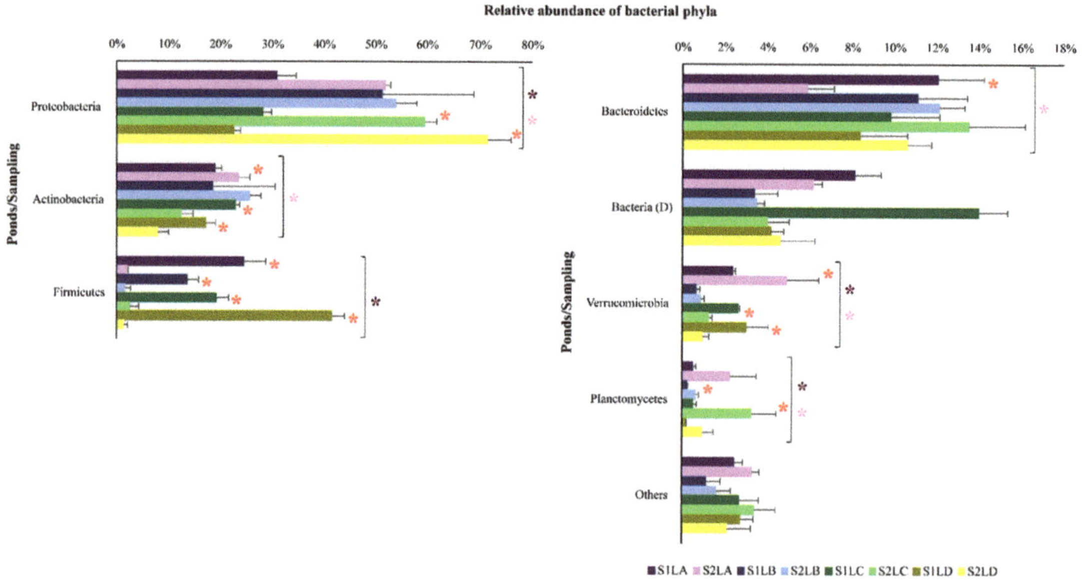

Figure 4. Relative abundance of bacterial phyla in water samples collected in LA (purple), LB (blue), LC (green) and LD (yellow) in S1 (high rainfall period—dark tones) and in S2 (low rainfall period—light tones). The bars represent the standard deviation. Asterisks (dark pink for S1 and light pink for S2) represent the significant differences among the ponds in the two samplings (parametric data submitted to a one-way ANOVA and nonparametric data submitted to Kruskal–Wallis). A red asterisk corresponds to the significant difference between the samples of each pond (parametric data submitted to the t test and nonparametric data submitted to Mann–Whitney). (D) next to the bacterial taxon means that the classification was at the domain level, and no statistical analysis was applied. The data represented by "others" were also not statistically analyzed because they are formed by more than one taxon.

At the class level, the relative abundance of the taxa also varied among the four ponds and between the two samplings (Figure S7). Significant differences were observed in S1 and S2 in the relative abundance of classes Betaproteobacteria, Alphaproteobacteria, Clostridia, Sphingobacteria, Gammaproteobacteria, Cytophaga, Deltaproteobacteria and Planctomycetia. The predominance of Actinobacteria and Bacilli varied among the ponds in S2 and S1, respectively. In addition, between the two samplings of the four ponds, Clostridia was the only class that predominated in S1. Ten classes showing relative abundances of at least 1% are represented in Figure S7.

More than 40% of the sequences were taxonomically classified at the genus level. A significant difference was observed among the four ponds in the relative abundance of the genera *Clostridium*, *Sediminibacterium*, *Pseudarcicella* and *Polynucleobacter* in both samplings. *Clostridium* was predominant in the four ponds in S1. The genera *Paenibacillus* and *Methylocystis* showed significant differences only in S1. The genus *Paenibacillus* was more prevalent in LC and LD (in S1). In S2, *Rhodobacter* was more abundant in LC, and the relative abundance of *Acidovorax*, *Novosphingobium* and *Rhodobacter* varied in the four ponds (Figure S8).

3.3. Strains of ARB Identified by MALDI-TOF

A total of 135 bacterial strains isolated from CHROMagar plates supplemented with the different antimicrobials were submitted to MALDI-TOF identification. From this total, 102 strains showed score values between 1700 and 2448.

No growth was observed from LC in cultures supplemented with ciprofloxacin. The highest number of colonies was observed in LA (8×10^2 CFU/mL). Three colonies of each morphology observed in the different plates (from LA, LB and LD) were reinoculated in ciprofloxacin-supplemented plates, but only three of these strains (isolated from LD) could be identified as belonging to the genus *Escherichia*, with score values between 1961 and 2238 (Table S3).

Fifty-four bacterial strains recovered from cultures supplemented with ceftriaxone were identified with score values between 1700 and 2402: 10 strains of LA; 11 strains of LB; 23 strains of LC and 10 strains of LD. Strains belonging to the genus *Chryseobacterium* were identified from samples from all four ponds. On the other hand, strains belonging to the genus *Elizabethkingia* were observed only in LB, *Acinetobacter* sp. and *Stenotrophomonas* sp. only in LC, while *Enterobacter* sp. and *Proteus* sp. only in LD (Table S4).

Forty-five strains recovered from sulfamethoxazole-supplemented cultures were identified with score values between 1700 and 2438: 14 of LA; 8 of LB; 14 of LC and 9 of LD. Strains belonging to the genera *Escherichia* and *Klebsiella* were isolated from all ponds, while strains of *Aeromonas* and *Cronobacter* were identified only in LA, and those belonging to the genus *Serratia* were identified only in LB. Strains belonging to the genera *Enterobacter* and *Proteus* were found in LA, LC and LD (Table S5).

3.4. Comparison of Bacterial Community Composition with the Prevalence of ARB

By sequencing the gene encoding 16S rRNA, different OTUs could be related to genera attributed to bacterial strains resistant to the different antimicrobials tested and identified by MALDI-TOF (Figure S9).

In general, isolated strains identified as belonging to the genera *Pseudomonas*, *Bacillus*, *Acinetobacter*, *Stenotrophomonas*, *Chryseobacterium*, *Aeromonas*, *Pantoea*, *Escherichia* and *Citrobacter* were also found in the taxonomic classification of the different OTUs in all ponds. Bacterial strains from other genera belonging to the Enterobacteriaceae family were also identified, such as *Cronobacter*, *Enterobacter*, *Proteus* and *Klebsiella*.

A significant difference was observed among the ponds (one-way ANOVA/Kruskal–Wallis) in the relative abundance of OTUs associated with the genera *Pseudomonas* and *Bacillus* in S1 and with *Aeromonas* and Enterobacteriaceae in S2. Statistical differences were also observed between S1 and S2 in the relative abundance of *Bacillus* and *Pantoea* in LC and of Enterobacteriaceae and *Bacillus* in LD (Student's *t* test/Mann–Whitney).

3.5. ARGs in Isolated Strains

Forty-four isolated strains were PCR amplified for the presence of ARGs using specific primers. Table 1 shows all strains where a PCR product was detected. Among the strains grown on ceftriaxone plates, *Escherichia* strains (isolated from LA) were positive for the bla_{TEM} gene. Strains of *Klebsiella* (isolated from LA) were positive for bla_{TEM} and bla_{SHV} (Table 1, Figure S3B). Among the strains previously isolated on sulfamethoxazole-containing plates, the *sul1* gene was detected in an *Enterobacter* strain (isolated from LA) (Table 1, Figure S4A) and the *sul2* gene was detected in strains belonging to the genera *Escherichia*, *Proteus* and *Aeromonas* (isolated from LA and LD) (Table 1, Figure S4B). The *intI1* gene was observed in *Escherichia* and *Enterobacter* strains (isolated from LA and LD) (Table 1, Figure S5), and the *intI2* gene was observed in *Enterobacter* and *Pantoea* strains (isolated from LA and LB) (Table 1, Figure S3).

Table 1. Presence of antimicrobial resistance genes in the isolated strains.

Ceftriaxone Resistant Strains	Antimicrobial Resistance Genes			
	bla_{TEM}		bla_{SHV}	
Escherichia sp. (CCA 1.2) *	1		0	
Escherichia sp. (CCA 1.3)	1		0	
Klebsiella sp. (CCA 2.1)	1		1	
Klebsiella sp. (CCA 2.2)	1		1	
Klebsiella sp. (CCA 2.3)	1		1	
Sulfamethoxazole resistant strains	*sul1*	*sul2*	*intI1*	*intI2*
Escherichia sp. (CSA 1.1) *	0	1	1	0
Proteus sp. (CSA 2.1A)	0	1	0	0
Aeromonas sp. (CSA 2.2)	0	1	0	0
Enterobacter sp. (CSA 2.3)	1	0	1	0
Enterobacter sp. (CSA 5.1)	0	0	0	1
Enterobacter sp. (CSA 5.2)	0	0	0	1
Pantoea sp. (CSB 1.1)	0	0	0	1
Escherichia sp. (CSD 1.2)	0	1	0	0
Escherichia sp. (CSD 1.3)	0	1	1	0

* The name of the strains corresponds to the origin of their isolation: CCA (CHROMagar containing ceftriaxone and LA), CSA, CSB and CSD (CHROMagar containing sulfamethoxazole and LA, LB and LD, respectively).

4. Discussion

It is well known that surface waters act as a sink for pollutants from terrestrial environments. Therefore, there is a great concern regarding the fate of antimicrobials and the role of bacterial communities in the dissemination of antimicrobial resistance genes in water sources. Several studies have demonstrated the presence of antibiotics, families of ARGs and ARB in aquatic ecosystems, including wastewaters, sea water, surface water (rivers, ponds, and lakes), recreational or drinking water [45–51]. This confirms the widespread dissemination of resistance in aquatic systems and the importance of the problem worldwide [49]. However, studies with this approach are still incipient not only in Brazil but also in other countries, especially when surface water in agricultural producing areas with the use of poultry litter is considered [52,53].

In this study, β-lactams resistance genes (bla_{GES}, bla_{TEM} and bla_{SHV}) were detected in two ponds (LB and LC). Furlan and Stehling (2018) [54] also detected the bla_{SHV} gene in water, feces, and soil from a pig farm in Brazil. However, the bla_{GES} gene could not be detected in the water samples analyzed. Indeed, GES β-lactamases (encoded by bla_{GES}) are less frequently found than other ESBLs (Extended Spectrum β-lactamases) and carbapenemases, except for bacterial strains isolated from clinical settings [54,55]. Therefore, the presence of the bla_{GES} gene in the ponds studied here corroborates the data obtained by Jurelevicius et al. (2021) [51], where this gene and the bla_{TEM} gene were observed in marine waters.

Sulfonamide resistance genes and genes encoding integrases were simultaneously detected in the three ponds. The detection of *sul1* and *intI1* genes in the same sample is not a surprise, as the *sul1* gene is often found in the conserved regions of class 1 integrons. Therefore, in addition to the potential risk of accumulation of *sul1* genes, this result may indicate the risk of dissemination of the *sul* genes by the frequent association of integrons with transposons and plasmids [56,57]. Lai et al. (2021) [50] also observed similar results in surface water sources in Sweden and highlighted the importance of the *intI1* and *sul1* genes as genetic markers of anthropogenic pollution. The *sul1* and *sul2* genes were also the most prevalent genes detected by PCR in river water samples from Germany and Australia, showing the environmental spread of these genes worldwide [45].

Although fluoroquinolone resistance genes were not detected on the water surface of the ponds in this study, we cannot exclude the possibility of their presence in a small amount, below the detection limit of the PCR technique. The occurrence of the *qnrS* gene and high concentrations of ciprofloxacin and enrofloxacin (fluoroquinolones) have already been reported in agricultural soils from the same region [24]. Moreover, fluoroquinolones have a low leaching potential and are usually detected in water at low concentrations, as they are strongly adsorbed to soils and sediments [58,59]. In contrast, sulfonamides have a high leaching potential and have been detected in high concentrations on water surfaces [60,61]. Vollú et al. (2018) [14] did not detect the *qnrA*, *qnrB* and *qnrS* genes in poultry litter samples in the presence of enrofloxacin and ciprofloxacin (fluoroquinolones) residues. The authors suggested that either these genes were not present or were present in low copy numbers, below the detection limit of the PCR technique.

The differences observed in the structure and composition of the bacterial communities in the four ponds may be related to soil fertilization and the amount of precipitation (which was significantly different between samplings), in addition to the physicochemical characteristics of the water samples. The phyla Firmicutes, Clostridia (class) and *Clostridium* (genus) were significantly more abundant in S1. Likewise, Clostridia has been described as an abundant class in the microbiota of poultries that are treated with penicillins [62,63]. Considering that S1 occurred in the wet season in a period of high rainfall volume, it is possible that bacteria of these taxa were mobilized from the soil fertilized with the poultry litter to the ponds by the surface runoff of water and leaching. Brooks et al. (2009) [62] reported that the species *Clostridium perfringens* can be an indicator of fecal contamination and of mobilization of poultry litter by surface runoff.

When ARB were isolated from the different ponds and further characterized, strains identified as enterobacteria (*Escherichia* sp., *Enterobacter* sp., *Aeromonas* sp., *Proteus* sp. and *Pantoea* sp.) were isolated from all sulfamethoxazole-containing plates. One of the most common mechanisms of sulfonamide resistance in enterobacteria is the acquisition of *sul* genes, which encode resistant variants of the dihydropteroate synthase (DHPS) enzyme. Usually, *sul1* and *sul2* genes are found among sulfonamide-resistant Enterobacteriaceae with the same frequency [64,65]. Considering the results obtained here using primers for *sul1*, *sul2*, *intI1* and *intI2* genes, there is a potential risk of dissemination of sulfonamide resistance among clinically important bacteria in the studied ponds.

In the same way, as genes encoding ESBLs were detected in water samples (bla_{GES}, bla_{SHV} and bla_{TEM}) and in *Klebsiella* and *Escherichia* strains, there is a potential risk of dissemination of β-lactam resistance in these environments, especially considering that the genes bla_{SHV} and bla_{TEM} are plasmid-mediated and often reported in these genera. These genes encode narrow-spectrum β-lactamases or ESBLs that hydrolyze broad spectrum cephalosporins and monobactams [66]. The production of these enzymes by pathogenic strains of *E. coli* and *K. pneumoniae* has been reported by researchers worldwide, and their prevalence has been increasing from 6% to 88% in healthcare settings [66–68]. The presence of these ARGs in surface water sources indicates the dissemination of AMR in the environment. Elshafiee et al. (2022) [69] also detected the presence of bla_{SHV} and bla_{TEM} genes in *K. pneumoniae* isolates in irrigation waters from fresh produce farms in Egypt. Likewise, Amato et al. (2021) [49] also detected a high prevalence of bla_{TEM} in *E. coli* strains isolated from irrigation water surface sources in Spain. These studies indicate the risk of transmission of resistant β-lactams for farmers and through the consumption of commercialized products. Bacteria of the Enterobacteriaceae family are often associated with intra-abdominal infections and can be transmitted by contaminated food and water, such as pathogenic strains of *E. coli* and *K. pneumoniae* that can cause gastrointestinal and urinary tract infections (UTIs) [69,70].

Finally, some bacterial genera isolated here, such as those of the CESP group (*Citrobacter*, *Enterobacter*, *Serratia* and *Providencia*), are producers of inducible AmpC-type β-lactamases, which mediate intrinsic resistance to most third-generation cephalosporins [71]. Intrinsic resistance is increasingly considered relevant mainly when it is detected in opportunistic pathogens. *Stenotrophomonas* sp. has been described as a reservoir and as a vector of acquired ARGs that encode carbapenemases, such as the bla_{KPC} gene, especially in aquatic environments [72].

Indeed, ESBL- and carbapenemase-producing Gram-negative bacteria of the Enterobacteriaceae family represent a global threat to human and animal health. These bacteria are the main propagators of the AMR pandemic and are on the World Health Organization priority pathogens list to guide research, discovery, and development of new antimicrobials [73,74].

According to Lapidot and Yaron (2009) [75], contaminated water can increase the ability of pathogens to colonize agricultural crops, favoring resistant bacteria dissemination in the environment and resistant pathogen transmission to humans and animals [76]. Water used in irrigation has already been identified as the likely source of several outbreaks of diseases transmitted by fresh and raw foods, such as fruits and vegetables, which are the most common agricultural crops associated with outbreaks [77].

5. Conclusions

This study demonstrates that surface water sources can be considered reservoirs of resistant bacteria and resistance genes in agricultural areas with extensive use of poultry litter as an organic fertilizer. The presence of *sul1*, *sul2*, *intI1* and *intI2* genes and in strains isolated from the studied ponds may indicate the accumulation of resistance to sulfonamides in the environment. The detection of genes encoding ESBLs, mainly bla_{GES}, which are found less frequently in the environment, also suggests the spread of resistance to β-lactams in the environment. In addition, seasonal influences on the evaluated bacterial communities (mainly periods of high rainfall) are an additional aggravating factor for antimicrobial-resistant bacteria mobilization (soil–water). Considering the extensive use of surface water sources, this study suggests the potential risk of dissemination and transmission of AMR, through different forms of water use, mainly in the irrigation of agricultural crops, which favors the entry of pathogens into the food chain. Therefore, monitoring and understanding of aquatic resistomes under anthropic influence is of great importance to control the environmental spread of AMR. It is still necessary to contain the irrational use of antimicrobials in human medicine, veterinary medicine, and especially in livestock and agriculture.

Supplementary Materials: The following supporting information can be downloaded at: https://www.mdpi.com/article/10.3390/antibiotics11111650/s1.

Author Contributions: L.S., E.S.L., C.E.T.P. and R.C.P. conceived the study. L.S. was responsible for project administration and funding acquisition. E.S.L. and C.E.T.P. collected the water samples. E.S.L. analyzed data from 16S rRNA amplicon metagenomic sequencing, isolated, identified and characterized the AMR bacteria. L.S., E.S.L. and C.E.T.P. drafted the manuscript. All authors have read and agreed to the published version of the manuscript.

Funding: This study was supported by grants from Conselho Nacional de Desenvolvimento Científico e Tecnológico (CNPq), Coordenação de Aperfeiçoamento de Pessoal de Nível Superior (CAPES, financial code 001) and Fundação de Amparo à Pesquisa do Estado do Rio de Janeiro (FAPERJ).

Institutional Review Board Statement: Not applicable.

Informed Consent Statement: Not applicable.

Data Availability Statement: The datasets used and/or analyzed under the current study are available from the corresponding author upon reasonable request.

Conflicts of Interest: The authors declare no conflict of interest.

References

1. World Health Organization. *Antimicrobial Resistance-Global Report on Surveillance*; World Health Organization: Geneva, Switzerland, 2014; Volume 61, pp. 383–394.
2. Chow, L.K.M.; Ghaly, T.M.; Gillings, M.R. A Survey of Sub-Inhibitory Concentrations of Antibiotics in the Environment. *J. Environ. Sci.* **2021**, *99*, 21–27. [CrossRef] [PubMed]
3. Maillard, J.Y.; Bloomfield, S.F.; Courvalin, P.; Essack, S.Y.; Gandra, S.; Gerba, C.P.; Rubino, J.R.; Scott, E.A. Reducing Antibiotic Prescribing and Addressing the Global Problem of Antibiotic Resistance by Targeted Hygiene in the Home and Everyday Life Settings: A Position Paper. *Am. J. Infect. Control* **2020**, *48*, 1090–1099. [CrossRef] [PubMed]

4.	Rabello, R.F.; Bonelli, R.R.; Penna, B.A.; Albuquerque, J.P.; Souza, R.M.; Cerqueira, A.M.F. Antimicrobial Resistance in Farm Animals in Brazil: An Update Overview. *Animals* **2020**, *10*, 552. [CrossRef] [PubMed]
5.	van Boeckel, T.P.; Brower, C.; Gilbert, M.; Grenfell, B.T.; Levin, S.A.; Robinson, T.P.; Teillant, A.; Laxminarayan, R. Global Trends in Antimicrobial Use in Food Animals. *Proc. Natl. Acad. Sci. USA* **2015**, *112*, 5649–5654. [CrossRef] [PubMed]
6.	Gouvêa, R.; Dos Santos, F.F.; De Aquino, M.H.C. Fluoroquinolones in Industrial Poultry Production, Bacterial Resistance and Food Residues: A Review. *Braz. J. Poult. Sci.* **2015**, *17*, 1–10. [CrossRef]
7.	Meletis, G. Carbapenem Resistance: Overview of the Problem and Future Perspectives. *Ther. Adv. Infect. Dis.* **2016**, *3*, 15–21. [CrossRef]
8.	Morales-Gutiérrez, F.J.; Barbosa, J.; Barrón, D. Metabolic Study of Enrofloxacin and Metabolic Profile Modifications in Broiler Chicken Tissues after Drug Administration. *Food Chem.* **2015**, *172*, 30–39. [CrossRef]
9.	van Duijkeren, E.; Schink, A.-K.; Roberts, M.C.; Wang, Y.; Schwarz, S. Mechanisms of Bacterial Resistance to Antimicrobial Agents. *Microbiol. Spectr.* **2018**, *6*, 52–82. [CrossRef]
10.	Cardoso, M. Antimicrobial Use, Resistance and Economic Benefits and Costs to Livestock Producers in Brazil. *OECD Food Agric. Fish. Pap.* **2019**, *135*, 1–44.
11.	Palma, E.; Tilocca, B.; Roncada, P. Antimicrobial Resistance in Veterinary Medicine: An Overview. *Int. J. Mol. Sci.* **2020**, *21*, 1914. [CrossRef]
12.	Sarmah, A.K.; Meyer, M.T.; Boxall, A.B.A. A Global Perspective on the Use, Sales, Exposure Pathways, Occurrence, Fate and Effects of Veterinary Antibiotics (VAs) in the Environment. *Chemosphere* **2006**, *65*, 725–759. [CrossRef] [PubMed]
13.	Kemper, N. Veterinary Antibiotics in the Aquatic and Terrestrial Environment. *Ecol. Indic.* **2008**, *8*, 1–13. [CrossRef]
14.	Vollú, R.E.; Cotta, S.R.; Jurelevicius, D.; Leite, D.C.D.A.; Parente, C.E.T.; Malm, O.; Martins, D.C.; Resende, Á.V.; Marriel, I.E.; Seldin, L. Response of the Bacterial Communities Associated with Maize Rhizosphere to Poultry Litter as an Organomineral Fertilizer. *Front. Environ. Sci.* **2018**, *6*, 118. [CrossRef]
15.	Ljubojevic, D.; Puvača, N.; Pelic, M.; Todorovic, D.; Pajic, M.; Milanov, D.; Velhner, M. Epidemiological Significance of Poultry Litter for Spreading the Antibiotic-Resistant Strains of *Escherichia coli*. *Worlds Poult. Sci. J.* **2016**, *72*, 485–494. [CrossRef]
16.	Lamshöft, M.; Sukul, P.; Zühlke, S.; Spiteller, M. Behaviour of 14C-Sulfadiazine and 14C-Difloxacin during Manure Storage. *Sci. Total Environ.* **2010**, *408*, 1563–1568. [CrossRef]
17.	Jechalke, S.; Heuer, H.; Siemens, J.; Amelung, W.; Smalla, K. Fate and Effects of Veterinary Antibiotics in Soil. *Trends Microbiol.* **2014**, *22*, 536–545. [CrossRef]
18.	Xie, W.Y.; Shen, Q.; Zhao, F.J. Antibiotics and Antibiotic Resistance from Animal Manures to Soil: A Review. *Eur. J. Soil Sci.* **2018**, *69*, 181–195. [CrossRef]
19.	Muhammad, J.; Khan, S.; Su, J.Q.; Hesham, A.E.L.; Ditta, A.; Nawab, J.; Ali, A. Antibiotics in Poultry Manure and Their Associated Health Issues: A Systematic Review. *J. Soils Sediments* **2020**, *20*, 486–497. [CrossRef]
20.	Wright, G.D. Antibiotic Resistance in the Environment: A Link to the Clinic? *Curr. Opin. Microbiol.* **2010**, *13*, 589–594. [CrossRef]
21.	Jones, L.A.; Worobo, R.W.; Smart, C.D. Plant-Pathogenic Oomycetes, *Escherichia coli* Strains, and *Salmonella* spp. Frequently Found in Surface Water Used for Irrigation of Fruit and Vegetable Crops in New York State. *Appl. Environ. Microbiol.* **2014**, *80*, 4814–4820. [CrossRef]
22.	Dourado, F.; Arraes, T.C.; Silva, M.F. The "Megadesastre" in the Mountain Region of Rio de Janeiro State-Causes, Mechanisms of Mass Movements and Spatial Allocation of Investments for Reconstruction Post Disaster. *Anuário Inst. Geociências-UFRJ* **2012**, *35*, 43–54. [CrossRef]
23.	Rosi, A.; Canavesi, V.; Segoni, S.; Dias Nery, T.; Catani, F.; Casagli, N. Landslides in the Mountain Region of Rio de Janeiro: A Proposal for the Semi-Automated Definition of Multiple Rainfall Thresholds. *Geosciences* **2019**, *9*, 203. [CrossRef]
24.	Parente, C.E.T.; Azeredo, A.; Vollú, R.E.; Zonta, E.; Azevedo-Silva, C.E.; Brito, E.M.S.; Seldin, L.; Torres, J.P.M.; Meire, R.O.; Malm, O. Fluoroquinolones in Agricultural Soils: Multi-Temporal Variation and Risks in Rio de Janeiro Upland Region. *Chemosphere* **2019**, *219*, 409–417. [CrossRef] [PubMed]
25.	Parente, C.E.T.; Brusdzenski, G.S.; Zonta, E.; Lino, A.S.; Azevedo-Silva, C.E.; Dorneles, P.R.; Azeredo, A.; Torres, J.P.M.; Meire, R.O.; Malm, O. Fluoroquinolones and Trace Elements in Poultry Litter: Estimation of Environmental Load Based on Nitrogen Requirement for Crops. *J. Environ. Sci. Health B* **2020**, *55*, 1087–1098. [CrossRef] [PubMed]
26.	Instituto Nacional de Meteorologia Histórico de Dados Meteorológicos. Available online: https://portal.inmet.gov.br/ (accessed on 5 March 2021).
27.	Xu, X.; Kong, F.; Cheng, X.; Yan, B.; Du, X.; Gai, J.; Ai, H.; Shi, L.; Iredell, J. Integron Gene Cassettes in *Acinetobacter* spp. Strains from South China. *Int. J. Antimicrob. Agents* **2008**, *32*, 441–445. [CrossRef] [PubMed]
28.	Campana, E.H.; Xavier, D.E.; Petrolini, F.V.B.; Cordeiro-Moura, J.R.; de Araujo, M.R.E.; Gales, A.C. Carbapenem-Resistant and Cephalosporin-Susceptible: A Worrisome Phenotype among *Pseudomonas aeruginosa* Clinical Isolates in Brazil. *Braz. J. Infect. Dis.* **2017**, *21*, 57–62. [CrossRef]
29.	Picão, R.C.; Poirel, L.; Gales, A.C.; Nordmann, P. Diversity of β-Lactamases Produced by Ceftazidime-Resistant *Pseudomonas aeruginosa* Isolates Causing Bloodstream Infections in Brazil. *Antimicrob. Agents Chemother.* **2009**, *53*, 3908–3913. [CrossRef]
30.	Pérez-Pérez, F.J.; Hanson, N.D. Detection of Plasmid-Mediated AmpC β-Lactamase Genes in Clinical Isolates by Using Multiplex PCR. *J. Clin. Microbiol.* **2002**, *40*, 2153–2162. [CrossRef]
31.	Toleman, M.A.; Bennett, P.M.; Bennett, D.M.C.; Jones, R.N.; Walsh, T.R. Global Emergence of Trimethoprim/Sulfamethoxazole Resistance in *Stenotrophomonas maltophilia* Mediated by Acquisition of *sul* Genes. *Emerg. Infect. Dis.* **2007**, *13*, 559–565. [CrossRef]

32. Cattoir, V.; Poirel, L.; Rotimi, V.; Soussy, C.J.; Nordmann, P. Multiplex PCR for Detection of Plasmid-Mediated Quinolone Resistance Qnr Genes in ESBL-Producing Enterobacterial Isolates. *J. Antimicrob. Chemother.* **2007**, *60*, 394–397. [CrossRef]
33. Kraychete, G.B.; Botelho, L.A.B.; Campana, E.H.; Picão, R.C.; Bonelli, R.R. Updated Multiplex PCR for Detection of All Six Plasmid-Mediated Qnr Gene Families. *Antimicrob. Agents Chemother.* **2016**, *60*, 7524–7526. [CrossRef] [PubMed]
34. Yamane, K.; Wachino, J.I.; Suzuki, S.; Kimura, K.; Shibata, N.; Kato, H.; Shibayama, K.; Konda, T.; Arakawa, Y. New Plasmid-Mediated Fluoroquinolone Efflux Pump, QepA, Found in an *Escherichia coli* Clinical Isolate. *Antimicrob. Agents Chemother.* **2007**, *51*, 3354–3360. [CrossRef] [PubMed]
35. Sambrook, J.; Fritsch, E.F.; Maniatis, T. *Molecular Cloning: A Laboratory Manual*, 2nd ed.; Cold Spring Harbor Laboratory Press: New York, NY, USA, 1989.
36. Apprill, A.; Mcnally, S.; Parsons, R.; Weber, L. Minor Revision to V4 Region SSU rRNA 806R Gene Primer Greatly Increases Detection of SAR11 Bacterioplankton. *Aquatic. Microbial. Ecol.* **2015**, *75*, 129–137. [CrossRef]
37. Caporaso, J.G.; Lauber, C.L.; Walters, W.A.; Berg-Lyons, D.; Lozupone, C.A.; Turnbaugh, P.J.; Fierer, N.; Knight, R. Global Patterns of 16S rRNA Diversity at a Depth of Millions of Sequences per Sample. *Proc. Natl. Acad. Sci. USA* **2011**, *108*, 4516–4522. [CrossRef] [PubMed]
38. Schloss, P.D.; Westcott, S.L.; Ryabin, T.; Hall, J.R.; Hartmann, M.; Hollister, E.B.; Lesniewski, R.A.; Oakley, B.B.; Parks, D.H.; Robinson, C.J.; et al. Introducing Mothur: Open-Source, Platform-Independent, Community-Supported Software for Describing and Comparing Microbial Communities. *Appl. Environ. Microbiol.* **2009**, *75*, 7537–7541. [CrossRef]
39. Quast, C.; Pruesse, E.; Yilmaz, P.; Gerken, J.; Schweer, T.; Yarza, P.; Peplies, J.; Glöckner, F.O. The SILVA Ribosomal RNA Gene Database Project: Improved Data Processing and Web-Based Tools. *Nucleic Acids Res.* **2013**, *41*, 590–596. [CrossRef]
40. Cole, J.R.; Wang, Q.; Cardenas, E.; Fish, J.; Chai, B.; Farris, R.J.; Kulam-Syed-Mohideen, A.S.; McGarrell, D.M.; Marsh, T.; Garrity, G.M.; et al. The Ribosomal Database Project: Improved Alignments and New Tools for rRNA Analysis. *Nucleic Acids Res.* **2009**, *37*, 141–145. [CrossRef]
41. Hammer, R.; Harper, D.A.T.; Ryan, P.D. PAST: Paleontological Statistics Software Package for Education and Data Analysis. *Palaeontol. Electron.* **2001**, *4*, 9.
42. Box, G.E.P.; Cox, D.R. An Analysis of Transformations. *J. R. Stat. Soc. Ser. B* **1964**, *26*, 211–243. [CrossRef]
43. Suzuki, S.; Ogo, M.; Miller, T.W.; Shimizu, A.; Takada, H.; Siringan, M.A.T. Who Possesses Drug Resistance Genes in the Aquatic Environment?: Sulfamethoxazole (SMX) Resistance Genes among the Bacterial Community in Water Environment of Metro-Manila, Philippines. *Front. Microbiol.* **2013**, *4*, 102. [CrossRef]
44. Röderova, M.; Halova, D.; Papousek, I.; Dolejska, M.; Masarikova, M.; Hanulik, V.; Pudova, V.; Broz, P.; Htoutou-Sedlakova, M.; Sauer, P.; et al. Characteristics of Quinolone Resistance in *Escherichia coli* Isolates from Humans, Animals, and the Environment in the Czech Republic. *Front. Microbiol.* **2017**, *7*, 2147. [CrossRef] [PubMed]
45. Stoll, C.; Sidhu, J.P.S.; Tiehm, A.; Toze, S. Prevalence of Clinically Relevant Antibiotic Resistance Genes in Surface Water Samples Collected from Germany and Australia. *Environ. Sci. Technol.* **2012**, *46*, 9716–9726. [CrossRef] [PubMed]
46. Christou, A.; Agüera, A.; Bayona, J.M.; Cytryn, E.; Fotopoulos, V.; Lambropoulou, D.; Manaia, C.M.; Michael, C.; Revitt, M.; Schröder, P.; et al. The Potential Implications of Reclaimed Wastewater Reuse for Irrigation on the Agricultural Environment: The Knowns and Unknowns of the Fate of Antibiotics and Antibiotic Resistant Bacteria and Resistance Genes—A Review. *Water Res.* **2017**, *123*, 448–467. [CrossRef] [PubMed]
47. Niu, Z.G.; Zhang, K.; Zhang, Y. Occurrence and Distribution of Antibiotic Resistance Genes in the Coastal Area of the Bohai Bay, China. *Mar. Pollut. Bull.* **2016**, *107*, 245–250. [CrossRef]
48. Proia, L.; von Schiller, D.; Sànchez-Melsió, A.; Sabater, S.; Borrego, C.M.; Rodríguez-Mozaz, S.; Balcázar, J.L. Occurrence and Persistence of Antibiotic Resistance Genes in River Biofilms after Wastewater Inputs in Small Rivers. *Environ. Pollut.* **2016**, *210*, 121–128. [CrossRef]
49. Amato, M.; Dasí, D.; González, A.; Ferrús, M.A.; Castillo, M.Á. Occurrence of Antibiotic Resistant Bacteria and Resistance Genes in Agricultural Irrigation Waters from Valencia City (Spain). *Agric. Water Manag.* **2021**, *256*, 107097. [CrossRef]
50. Lai, F.Y.; Muziasari, W.; Virta, M.; Wiberg, K.; Ahrens, L. Profiles of Environmental Antibiotic Resistomes in the Urban Aquatic Recipients of Sweden Using High-Throughput Quantitative PCR Analysis. *Environ. Pollut.* **2021**, *287*, 117651. [CrossRef]
51. Jurelevicius, D.; Cotta, S.R.; Montezzi, L.F.; Dias, A.C.F.; Mason, O.U.; Picão, R.C.; Jansson, J.K.; Seldin, L. Enrichment of Potential Pathogens in Marine Microbiomes with Different Degrees of Anthropogenic Activity. *Environ. Pollut.* **2021**, *268*, 115757. [CrossRef]
52. Amarasiri, M.; Sano, D.; Suzuki, S. Understanding Human Health Risks Caused by Antibiotic Resistant Bacteria (ARB) and Antibiotic Resistance Genes (ARG) in Water Environments: Current Knowledge and Questions to Be Answered. *Crit. Rev. Environ. Sci. Technol.* **2020**, *50*, 2016–2059. [CrossRef]
53. Liu, X.; Wang, Z.; Zhang, L.; Fan, W.; Yang, C.; Li, E.; Du, Y.; Wang, X. Inconsistent Seasonal Variation of Antibiotics between Surface Water and Groundwater in the Jianghan Plain: Risks and Linkage to Land Uses. *J. Environ. Sci.* **2021**, *109*, 102–113. [CrossRef]
54. Furlan, J.P.R.; Stehling, E.G. Detection of β-Lactamase Encoding Genes in Feces, Soil and Water from a Brazilian Pig Farm. *Environ. Monit. Assess.* **2018**, *190*, 76. [CrossRef] [PubMed]
55. Queenan, A.M.; Bush, K. Carbapenemases: The Versatile β-Lactamases. *Clin. Microbiol. Rev.* **2007**, *20*, 440–458. [CrossRef]
56. Yang, Y.; Song, W.; Lin, H.; Wang, W.; Du, L.; Xing, W. Antibiotics and Antibiotic Resistance Genes in Global Lakes: A Review and Meta-Analysis. *Environ. Int.* **2018**, *116*, 60–73. [CrossRef]

57. Poirel, L.; Madec, J.-Y.; Lupo, A.; Schink, A.-K.; Kieffer, N.; Nordmann, P.; Schwarz, S. Antimicrobial Resistance in *Escherichia coli*. *Microbiol. Spectr.* **2018**, *6*, 289–316. [CrossRef] [PubMed]

58. Riaz, L.; Mahmood, T.; Khalid, A.; Rashid, A.; Ahmed Siddique, M.B.; Kamal, A.; Coyne, M.S. Fluoroquinolones (FQs) in the Environment: A Review on Their Abundance, Sorption and Toxicity in Soil. *Chemosphere* **2018**, *191*, 704–720. [CrossRef] [PubMed]

59. van Doorslaer, X.; Dewulf, J.; van Langenhove, H.; Demeestere, K. Fluoroquinolone Antibiotics: An Emerging Class of Environmental Micropollutants. *Sci. Total Environ.* **2014**, *500–501*, 250–269. [CrossRef] [PubMed]

60. Tang, J.; Wang, S.; Fan, J.; Long, S.; Wang, L.; Tang, C.; Tam, N.F.; Yang, Y. Predicting Distribution Coefficients for Antibiotics in a River Water–Sediment Using Quantitative Models Based on Their Spatiotemporal Variations. *Sci. Total Environ.* **2019**, *655*, 1301–1310. [CrossRef]

61. Leal, R.M.P.; Alleoni, L.R.F.; Tornisielo, V.L.; Regitano, J.B. Sorption of Fluoroquinolones and Sulfonamides in 13 Brazilian Soils. *Chemosphere* **2013**, *92*, 979–985. [CrossRef]

62. Brooks, J.P.; Adeli, A.; Read, J.J.; McLaughlin, M.R. Rainfall Simulation in Greenhouse Microcosms to Assess Bacterial-Associated Runoff from Land-Applied Poultry Litter. *J. Environ. Qual.* **2009**, *38*, 218–229. [CrossRef]

63. Singh, P.; Karimi, A.; Devendra, K.; Waldroup, P.W.; Cho, K.K.; Kwon, Y.M. Influence of Penicillin on Microbial Diversity of the Cecal Microbiota in Broiler Chickens. *Poult. Sci.* **2013**, *92*, 272–276. [CrossRef]

64. Shin, H.W.; Lim, J.; Kim, S.; Kim, J.; Kwon, G.C.; Koo, S.H. Characterization of Trimethoprim-Sulfamethoxazole Resistance Genes and Their Relatedness to Class 1 Integron and Insertion Sequence Common Region in Gram-Negative Bacilli. *J. Microbiol. Biotechnol.* **2015**, *25*, 137–142. [CrossRef] [PubMed]

65. Eliopoulos, G.M.; Huovinen, P. Resistance to Trimethoprim-Sulfamethoxazole. *Antimicrob. Resist.* **2001**, *32*, 1608–1614. [CrossRef] [PubMed]

66. Ugbo, E.N.; Anyamene, C.O.; Moses, I.B.; Iroha, I.R.; Babalola, O.O.; Ukpai, E.G.; Chukwunwejim, C.R.; Egbule, C.U.; Emioye, A.A.; Okata-Nwali, O.D.; et al. Prevalence of *bla*TEM, *bla*SHV, and *bla*CTX-M Genes among Extended Spectrum Beta-Lactamase-Producing *Escherichia coli* and *Klebsiella pneumoniae* of Clinical Origin. *Gene Rep.* **2020**, *21*, 100909. [CrossRef]

67. Fadil Saedii, A.A.; Abdelraheim, A.R.; Abdel Aziz, A.A.; Swelam, S.H. ESBL-Producing *E. coli* and *Klebsiella* among Patients Treated at Minia University Hospitals. *J. Infect. Dis. Prev. Med.* **2017**, *5*, 156. [CrossRef]

68. Zongo, K.J.; Dabire, A.M.; Compaore, L.G.; Sanou, I.; Sangare, L.; Simpore, J.; Zeba, B. First Detection of *bla* TEM, SHV and CTX-M among Gram Negative Bacilli Exhibiting Extended Spectrum -Lactamase Phenotype Isolated at University Hospital Center, Yalgado Ouedraogo, Ouagadougou, Burkina Faso. *Afr. J. Biotechnol.* **2015**, *14*, 1174–1180. [CrossRef]

69. Elshafiee, E.A.; Kadry, M.; Nader, S.M.; Ahmed, Z.S. Extended-Spectrum-Beta-Lactamases and Carbapenemase-Producing *Klebsiella pneumoniae* Isolated from Fresh Produce Farms in Different Governorates of Egypt. *Vet. World* **2022**, *15*, 1191–1196. [CrossRef]

70. Schuetz, A.N. Emerging Agents of Gastroenteritis: *Aeromonas, Plesiomonas*, and the Diarrheagenic Pathotypes of *Escherichia coli*. *Semin. Diagn Pathol.* **2019**, *36*, 187–192. [CrossRef]

71. Meurant, A.; Guérin, F.; le Hello, S.; Saint-Lorant, G.; de La Blanchardière, A. Cefepime Use: A Need for Antimicrobial Stewardship. *Infect. Dis. Now* **2021**, *51*, 445–450. [CrossRef]

72. Mançano, S.M.C.N.; Campana, E.H.; Felix, T.P.; Barrueto, L.R.L.; Pereira, P.S.; Picão, R.C. Frequency and Diversity of *Stenotrophomonas* Spp. Carrying *bla*KPC in Recreational Coastal Waters. *Water Res.* **2020**, *185*, 116210. [CrossRef]

73. Falgenhauer, L.; Schwengers, O.; Schmiedel, J.; Baars, C.; Lambrecht, O.; Heß, S.; Berendonk, T.U.; Falgenhauer, J.; Chakraborty, T.; Imirzalioglu, C. Multidrug-Resistant and Clinically Relevant Gram-Negative Bacteria Are Present in German Surface Waters. *Front. Microbiol.* **2019**, *10*, 2779. [CrossRef]

74. WHO. *Prioritization of Pathogens to Guide Discovery, Research and Development of New Antibiotics for Drug-Resistant Bacterial Infections, Including Tuberculosis*; WHO/EMP/IAU/2017.12; World Health Organization: Geneva, Switzerland, 2017.

75. Lapidot, A.; Yaron, S. Transfer of *Salmonella enterica* Serovar Typhimurium from Contaminated Irrigation Water to Parsley Is Dependent on Curli and Cellulose, the Biofilm Matrix Components. *J. Food Prot.* **2009**, *72*, 618–623. [CrossRef] [PubMed]

76. Marques, R.Z.; Wistuba, N.; Brito, J.C.M.; Bernardoni, V.; Rocha, D.C.; Gomes, M.P. Crop Irrigation (Soybean, Bean, and Corn) with Enrofloxacin-Contaminated Water Leads to Yield Reductions and Antibiotic Accumulation. *Ecotoxicol. Environ. Saf.* **2021**, *216*, 112193. [CrossRef] [PubMed]

77. Uyttendaele, M.; Jaykus, L.A.; Amoah, P.; Chiodini, A.; Cunliffe, D.; Jacxsens, L.; Holvoet, K.; Korsten, L.; Lau, M.; McClure, P.; et al. Microbial Hazards in Irrigation Water: Standards, Norms, and Testing to Manage Use of Water in Fresh Produce Primary Production. *Compr. Rev. Food Sci. Food Saf.* **2015**, *14*, 336–356. [CrossRef]

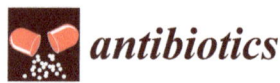

Article

Unveiling the Microbiome Landscape: A Metagenomic Study of Bacterial Diversity, Antibiotic Resistance, and Virulence Factors in the Sediments of the River Ganga, India

Ajaya Kumar Rout [1,2], Partha Sarathi Tripathy [3], Sangita Dixit [4], Dibyajyoti Uttameswar Behera [4], Bhaskar Behera [2], Basanta Kumar Das [1] and Bijay Kumar Behera [1,*]

[1] Aquatic Environmental Biotechnology and Nanotechnology Division, ICAR—Central Inland Fisheries Research Institute, Kolkata 700120, WB, India; ajayabi2012@gmail.com (A.K.R.); basantakumar@gmail.com (B.K.D.)

[2] Department of Biosciences and Biotechnology, Fakir Mohan University, Balasore 756089, OD, India; drbhaskarbehera@gmail.com

[3] Faculty of Biosciences and Aquaculture, Nord University, Universitetsalléen 11, 8026 Bodø, Norway; rabul92@gmail.com

[4] Center for Biotechnology, School of Pharmaceutical Sciences, Siksha 'O' Anusandhan (Deemed to Be University), Bhubaneswar 751030, OD, India; sangitadixit2011@gmail.com (S.D.); dibya01bioinfo@gmail.com (D.U.B.)

* Correspondence: beherabk18@yahoo.co.in; Tel.: +91-9163209580

Abstract: The global rise in antibiotic resistance, fueled by indiscriminate antibiotic usage in medicine, aquaculture, agriculture, and the food industry, presents a significant public health challenge. Urban wastewater and sewage treatment plants have become key sources of antibiotic resistance proliferation. The present study focuses on the river Ganges in India, which is heavily impacted by human activities and serves as a potential hotspot for the spread of antibiotic resistance. We conducted a metagenomic analysis of sediment samples from six distinct locations along the river to assess the prevalence and diversity of antibiotic resistance genes (ARGs) within the microbial ecosystem. The metagenomic analysis revealed the predominance of Proteobacteria across regions of the river Ganges. The antimicrobial resistance (AMR) genes and virulence factors were determined by various databases. In addition to this, KEGG and COG analysis revealed important pathways related to AMR. The outcomes highlight noticeable regional differences in the prevalence of AMR genes. The findings suggest that enhancing health and sanitation infrastructure could play a crucial role in mitigating the global impact of AMR. This research contributes vital insights into the environmental aspects of antibiotic resistance, highlighting the importance of targeted public health interventions in the fight against AMR.

Keywords: metagenomics; diversity; ganga; sediment; AMR; virulence factors

Citation: Rout, A.K.; Tripathy, P.S.; Dixit, S.; Behera, D.U.; Behera, B.; Das, B.K.; Behera, B.K. Unveiling the Microbiome Landscape: A Metagenomic Study of Bacterial Diversity, Antibiotic Resistance, and Virulence Factors in the Sediments of the River Ganga, India. *Antibiotics* **2023**, *12*, 1735. https://doi.org/10.3390/antibiotics12121735

Academic Editors: Jonathan Frye, Anusak Kerdsin and Jinquan Li

Received: 21 November 2023
Revised: 12 December 2023
Accepted: 13 December 2023
Published: 14 December 2023

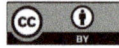

1. Introduction

The river Ganga, esteemed for its immense religious, cultural, spiritual, and ritual significance in India, is considered a sacred water body. It is exposed to considerable human impact as it serves nearly 400 million people, with a population density of around 520 individuals per square kilometer, as per recent estimates [1,2]. The river has increasingly become a focal point of pollution issues, notably the discovery of bacterial strains highly resistant to standard antibiotics [3,4]. Concurrently, research has identified bacterial and fungal strains within the Ganga's sediments capable of bioremediating potential and beneficial microbiomes [5,6]. Factors like rapid urbanization, industrial activities, population surges, and the release of agricultural waste have intensified pollution in the river. Additionally, the practice of mass religious bathing, drawing large crowds, including the elderly, consuming medicinal products, further impacts the river's condition. The Ganga's banks also attract tourists for spiritual pursuits, water sports, and hiking activities. Human settlements and industrial establishments within the river basin markedly affect the water quality, influencing the river's microbial composition [7–11]. Pollutants and toxic substances in the river significantly alter the dynamics of its microbial communities. A major concern is the rise of antibiotic resistance, a global health threat. Human activities have led to an increased prevalence of antibiotic resistance genes (ARGs) in the river [2]. Previous studies on Ganga's microorganisms have primarily relied on cultivation-based methods, offering a restricted view of its bacterial diversity [12,13]. However, recent research utilizing advanced metagenomic approaches has begun to unveil a bacterial population capable of bioremediating significant contaminants in the river's sediments [5,14–16]. A handful of studies have also employed metagenomic techniques to explore the presence of antibiotic resistance genes in the water and sediments of the Ganga [4,17,18].

The occurrence of microbial pollution presents additional risks, particularly due to the emergence of antibiotic-resistant bacteria (ARBs) and their associated ARGs [19]. The global public health community recognizes antibiotic resistance as a significant concern [20]. This issue is compounded by the likelihood of Horizontal Gene Transfer (HGT) events that facilitate the spread of ARGs among diverse microbial species [21]. In marine ecosystems, especially in coastal areas, antibiotic resistance is a prevalent phenomenon [19]. Human influences are major contributors to ARGs in environments impacted by anthropogenic activities [19]. Recent studies have linked the widespread occurrence of resistance genes primarily to fecal contamination [22]. Scientific investigations are increasingly focused on understanding the distribution, risks, and potential ecological consequences of antibiotics (ABs) and ARGs in various aquatic environments worldwide [20]. Additionally, there is an emerging hypothesis that resistance to heavy metals (HMs), evidenced through heavy metal resistance genes (HMRGs), may be linked to antibiotic (AB) resistance in environmental settings [23]. As a result, these resistance genes are crucial factors in assessing the ecological health of coastal waters.

Globally, various techniques have been established for assessing microbial pollution in aquatic environments, primarily focusing on detecting Fecal Indicator Bacteria (FIB) using cultivation-based methods. In contrast, high-throughput sequencing techniques, like shotgun metagenomics, offer a more advanced alternative to traditional microbial diversity studies. These innovative approaches facilitate a thorough investigation of environmental microbial communities. This includes examining the 16S rRNA genes to understand the breadth of microbial diversity and exploring genes related to pathogenicity, resistance to antibiotics and heavy metals, and virulence factors to evaluate their potential functions and impacts on ecosystems [24,25].

An analytical comparison of water and sediment provides a foundational understanding of the microbial interactions at the interface of these two environments. A recent study conducted a comparative analysis of the bacteriome and antibiotic resistance profile in the river Ganga, focusing on discerning the variations between samples taken from the river water and the sediment. This research undertakes a detailed comparison of both the bacteriome and ARGs within water and sediment samples collected across substantial stretches of the river Ganga.

2. Results

2.1. Sequencing Summary

The estimated sizes of the libraries varied between 8.4 Gb and 9.4 Gb (Table 1). The assembly statistics revealed that the average total contigs in the present study was 3,434,087. The average number of contigs $\geq$150 bp and $\leq$150 bp were found to be 3,307,063 and 127,024, respectively. The average total length of contigs was found to be 404,842,009 bp. A summary of all the statistics from all the samples is mentioned in Table 1.

Table 1. Summary of statistics from metagenome assembly.

Parameters	Bageswar	Bagwan	Koteswar	Rasulabad Ghat	Sahidabad	Triveni Sangam
Contigs (≤150 bp)	460,537	71,161	87,682	40,754	43,771	58,237
Contigs (≥150 bp)	1,008,926	1,766,259	5,172,327	3,263,830	3,839,878	4,791,158
Total contigs	1,469,463	1,837,420	5,260,009	3,304,584	3,883,649	4,849,395
Largest contig	887,047	897,272	1,192,971	343,376	789,499	645,470
Total length (in bp)	468,274,061	340,847,742	444,765,440	366,965,171	374,775,947	433,423,693
GC content (in %)	52	40	52	46	50	47
N50	1091	2615	1237	1517	1402	1471
N90	558	619	561	578	573	575
L50	91,382	21,741	66,190	41,780	48,856	55,263
L90	346,262	148,883	298,653	215,191	232,472	263,312
Ns per 100 kbp	0	0	0	0	0	0

2.2. Bacterial Diversity Analysis

Analysis of bacterial diversity conducted using Kraken2 and Pavian demonstrated that Proteobacteria were the most abundantly found across all surveyed locations in the river Ganga basin (Figures 1–6). In the specific sites of Bageswar, Koteswar, and Sahidabad, there was a notable abundance of *Flavobacterium* spp. (Figure 1, Figure 3, and Figure 5, respectively). Meanwhile, in the Rasulabad Ghat and Triveni Sangam locations, Pseudomonas spp. were observed to be prevalent (Figures 4 and 6, respectively). In Bagwan, *Sulfurospirillum* spp. ware dominant (Figure 2).

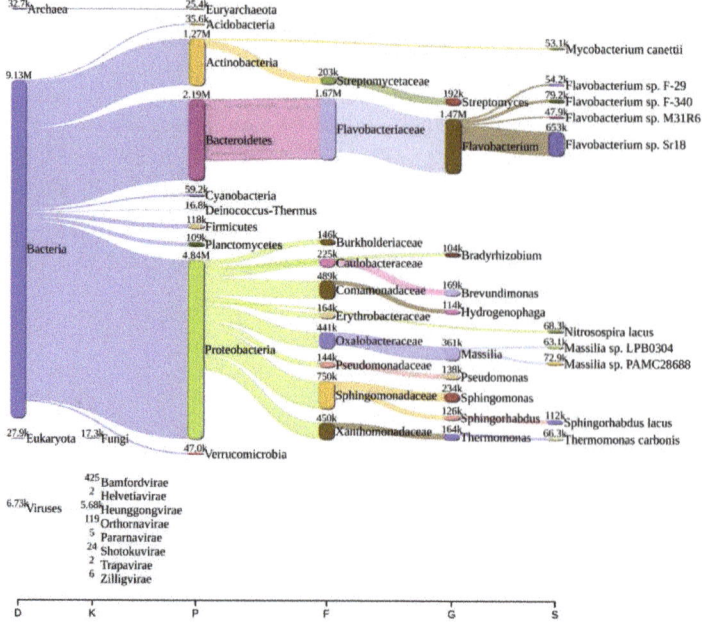

Figure 1. A sankey plot of comprehensive bacterial and viral community analysis in river Ganga sediment as analyzed from Pavian in Bageswar. This showcases the abundance and diversity of microbial taxa, including Proteobacteria, Flavobacterium, Sulfurospirillum, and various viral families. D: Domain, K: Kingdom, P: Phylum, F: Family, G: Genus, S: Species.

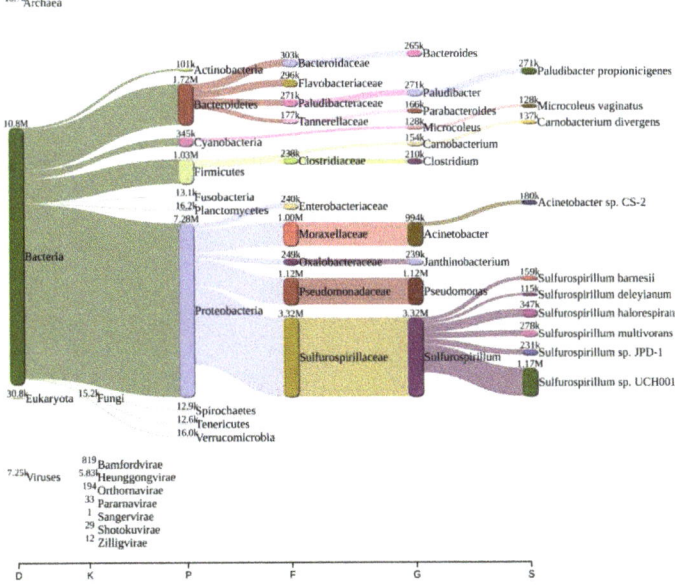

Figure 2. A sankey plot of comprehensive bacterial and viral community analysis in river Ganga sediment as analyzed from Pavian in Bagwan. This showcases the abundance and diversity of microbial taxa, including Proteobacteria, Flavobacterium, Sulfurospirillum, and various viral families. D: Domain, K: Kingdom, P: Phylum, F: Family, G: Genus, S: Species.

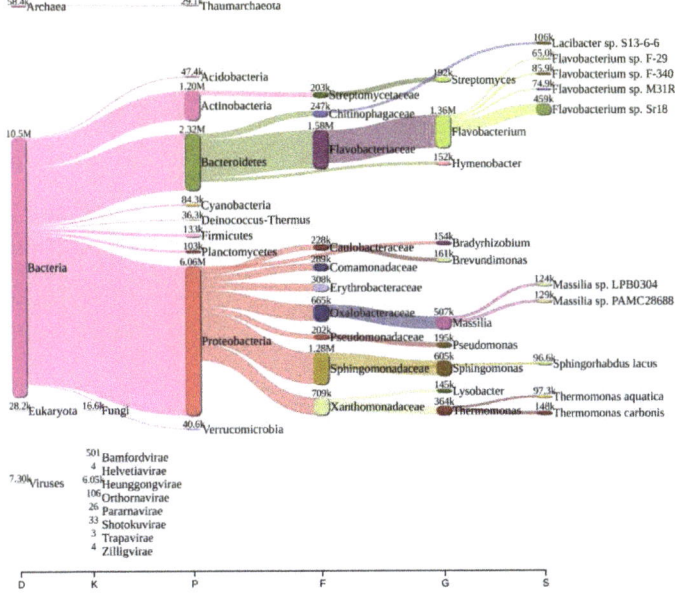

Figure 3. A sankey plot of comprehensive bacterial and viral community analysis in river Ganga sediment as analyzed from Pavian in Koteswar. This showcases the abundance and diversity of microbial taxa, including Proteobacteria, Flavobacterium, Sulfurospirillum, and various viral families. D: Domain, K: Kingdom, P: Phylum, F: Family, G: Genus, S: Species.

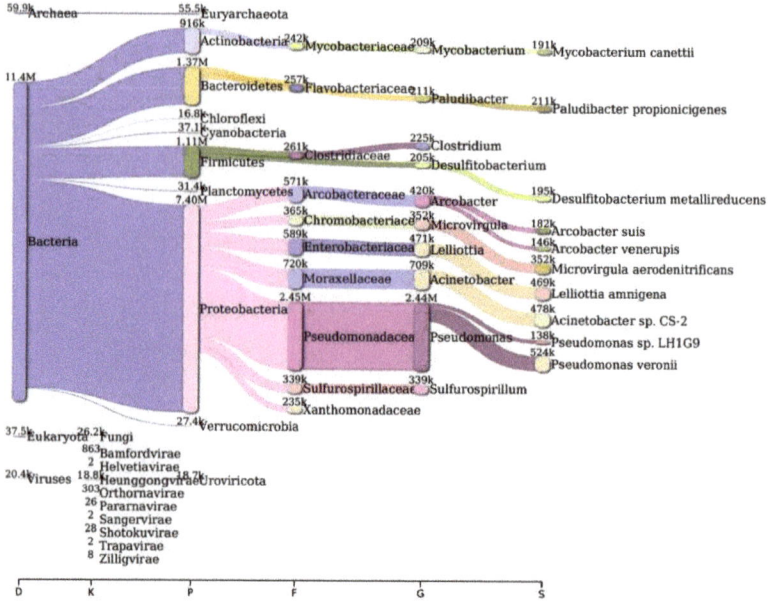

Figure 4. A sankey plot of comprehensive bacterial and viral community analysis in river Ganga sediment as analyzed from Pavian in Rasulabad Ghat. This showcases the abundance and diversity of microbial taxa, including Proteobacteria, Flavobacterium, Sulfurospirillum, and various viral families. D: Domain, K: Kingdom, P: Phylum, F: Family, G: Genus, S: Species.

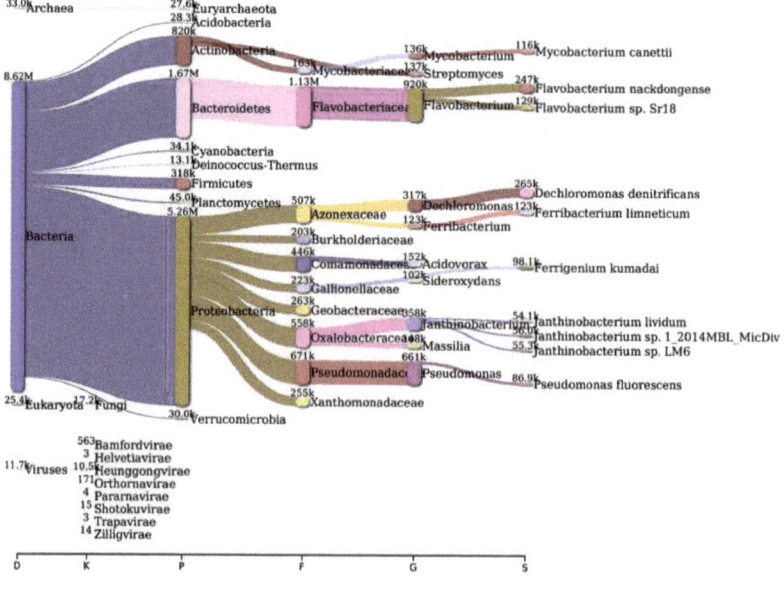

Figure 5. A sankey plot of comprehensive bacterial and viral community analysis in river Ganga sediment as analyzed from Pavian in Sahidabad. This showcases the abundance and diversity of microbial taxa, including Proteobacteria, Flavobacterium, Sulfurospirillum, and various viral families. D: Domain, K: Kingdom, P: Phylum, F: Family, G: Genus, S: Species.

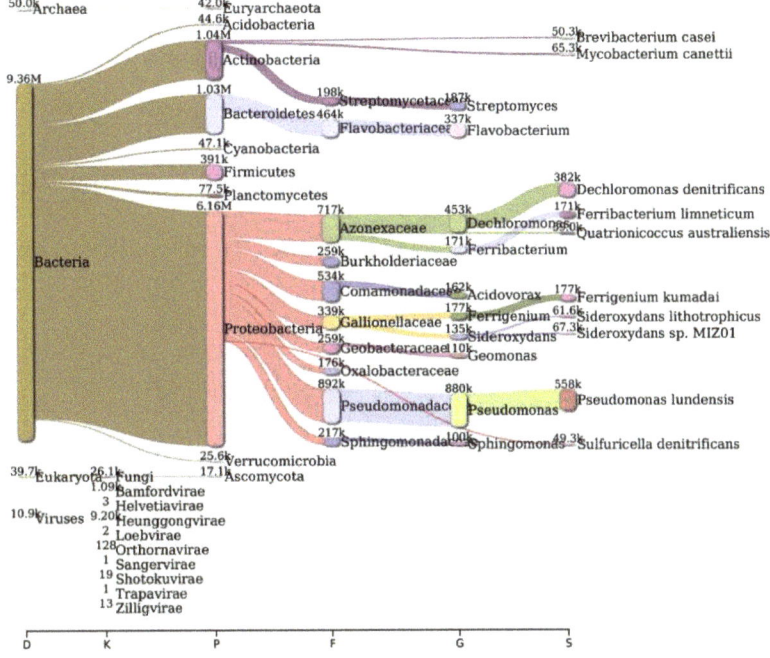

Figure 6. A sankey plot of comprehensive bacterial and viral community analysis in river Ganga sediment as analyzed from Pavian in Triveni Sangam. This showcases the abundance and diversity of microbial taxa, including Proteobacteria, Flavobacterium, Sulfurospirillum, and various viral families. D: Domain, K: Kingdom, P: Phylum, F: Family, G: Genus, S: Species.

2.3. AMR Genes Abundance

Geographical variability in ARG profiles was studied in the present study. This investigation delineated the geographical distribution patterns of antimicrobial resistance (AMR) genes across five discrete sites: Bageswar, Bagwan, Rasulabad Ghat, Sahidabad, and Triveni Sangam (Table 2). We did not find any AMR in the Koteswar sample. We found diverse categories of AMR, including but not limited to Aminoglycoside, Streptomycin, and Cephalosporin. The outcomes provide critical insights into the regional dissemination and the prevalence of AMR determinants. Aminoglycoside resistance determinants such as *aac(6′)-Ib*, *aadS*, *acrD*, and *ANT(2″)-Ia* were predominantly detected in Rasulabad Ghat, with *aadS* also present in Bagwan and Triveni Sangam. Rasulabad Ghat exclusively exhibited the presence of Streptomycin resistance genes (*aadA1*, *aadA5*, *aadA6*). Beta-lactam resistance markers, particularly *blaOXA-209*, were observed in Bagwan and Rasulabad Ghat, while *blaOXA-119* was exclusively found in Triveni Sangam. The *acrB* gene, associated with multi-drug resistance, was identified in Bagwan and Rasulabad Ghat.

This study highlighted distinct regional disparities in the distribution of AMR genes. Triveni Sangam displayed the unique presence of *blaOXA-119*, which was absent in other studied areas. Bagwan and Rasulabad Ghat were characterized by a higher incidence of genes, such as *acrB*, *blaOXA-209*, and *baeR*, indicative of a broader spectrum of drug resistance. Conversely, Bageswar showed a minimal presence of the surveyed AMR genes. The detection of *blaRm3* in Bagwan and Sahidabad, a gene conferring resistance to a wide array of antibiotics, signals the emergence of high-level resistance in these regions. The exclusive identification of *blaTHIN-B* in Sahidabad, linked to carbapenem resistance, highlights specific regional challenges in antibiotic resistance.

Table 2. List of AMRs found in the present study across the samples. "F" and "NF" represent whether the AMR was found or not found, respectively, across the samples.

Resistance	Gene Name	Number of Reads				
		Bageswar	Bagwan	Rasulabad Ghat	Sahidabad	Triveni Sangam
Aminoglycoside	*aac(6′)-Ib*	NF	NF	F	NF	NF
Streptomycin	*aadA1*	NF	NF	F	NF	NF
Streptomycin	*aadA5*	NF	NF	F	NF	NF
Streptomycin	*aadA6*	NF	NF	F	NF	NF
Aminoglycoside	*aadS*	NF	F	F	NF	F
Cephalosporin; Fluoroquinolone; Glycylcycline; Penam; Phenicol; Rifamycin; Tetracycline; Triclosan	*acrB*	NF	F	F	NF	NF
Aminoglycoside	*acrD*	NF	F	NF	NF	NF
Penam	*AER-1*	NF	NF	F	NF	NF
Aminoglycoside	*ANT(2″)-Ia*	NF	NF	F	NF	NF
Aminoglycoside	*ANT(3″)-Ia*	NF	NF	F	NF	NF
Aminoglycoside	*ANT(6)-Ia*	NF	NF	F	NF	NF
Aminoglycoside	*aph(3″)-Ib*	NF	NF	F	NF	F
Aminoglycoside	*aph(6)-Id*	NF	NF	F	NF	NF
Peptide	*arnA*	NF	F	NF	NF	NF
Rifamycin	*arr-2*	NF	NF	F	NF	NF
Peptide	*bacA*	NF	F	F	NF	NF
Aminocoumarin; Aminoglycoside	*baeR*	NF	F	F	NF	NF
BETA-LACTAM	*bla-A*	NF	NF	F	NF	NF
BETA-LACTAM	*blaAER-1*	NF	NF	F	NF	NF
Carbapenem	*blaGES-14*	NF	NF	F	NF	NF
Carbapenem	*blaGES-5*	NF	NF	F	NF	NF
BETA-LACTAM	*blaMCA*	NF	NF	F	NF	NF
BETA-LACTAM	*blaOXA-119*	NF	NF	NF	NF	F
BETA-LACTAM	*blaOXA-209*	F	NF	F	NF	NF
BETA-LACTAM	*blaOXA-296*	NF	F	NF	NF	NF
BETA-LACTAM	*blaOXA-347*	NF	NF	F	NF	NF
Carbapenem; Cephalosporin; Penam	*blaRm3*	NF	F	NF	F	NF
BETA-LACTAM	*blaRSD1-1*	NF	NF	NF	NF	F
Carbapenem	*blaTHIN-B*	NF	NF	NF	F	NF
Cephalosporin	*blaVEB-9*	NF	NF	F	NF	NF
Phenicol	*catQ*	NF	F	F	NF	NF
Aminoglycoside; Fluoroquinolone	*ceoB*	NF	NF	NF	F	F
Phenicol	*cmlA5*	NF	NF	F	NF	NF
Aminocoumarin; Aminoglycoside	*cpxA*	NF	NF	F	NF	NF
Fluoroquinolone; Macrolide; Penam	*CRP*	NF	F	F	NF	NF
Trimethoprim	*dfrA3*	NF	F	NF	NF	NF
Trimethoprim	*dfrG*	NF	NF	F	NF	NF

Table 2. *Cont.*

Resistance	Gene Name	Number of Reads				
		Bageswar	Bagwan	Rasulabad Ghat	Sahidabad	Triveni Sangam
Fluoroquinolone	*emrR*	NF	F	F	NF	NF
Cephalosporin; Fluoroquinolone; Glycylcycline; Penam; Phenicol; Rifamycin; Tetracycline; Triclosan	*Enterobacter cloacaeacrA*	NF	F	F	NF	NF
Macrolide	*ere(D)*	NF	NF	F	NF	NF
Chloramphenicol	*EstDL136*	F	NF	NF	NF	NF
Fosfomycin	*fos1*	NF	F	NF	NF	NF
Cephalosporin; Cephamycin; Fluoroquinolone; Macrolide; Penam; Tetracycline	*H-NS*	NF	F	F	NF	NF
Aminoglycoside; Carbapenem; Cephalosporin; Fluoroquinolone; Macrolide; Penam; Peptide	*Klebsiella pneumoniaeKpnH*	NF	F	F	NF	NF
Aminoglycoside; Carbapenem; Cephalosporin; Fluoroquinolone; Macrolide; Penem; Peptide	*KpnG*	NF	NF	F	NF	NF
Lincosamide	*lnu(D)*	NF	NF	F	NF	NF
Carbapenem; Cephalosporin; Cephamycin; Fluoroquinolone; Glycylcycline; Monobactam; Penem;phenicol; Rifamycin; Tetracycline; Triclosan	*marA*	NF	F	F	NF	NF
Aminocoumarin	*mdtB*	NF	F	F	NF	NF
Aminocoumarin	*mdtC*	NF	F	F	NF	NF
Macrolide	*mefA*	NF	NF	F	NF	NF
Macrolide	*mefB*	NF	NF	F	NF	NF
Macrolide	*mefC*	NF	NF	F	NF	NF
Lincosamide; Macrolide; Oxazolidinone; Phenicol; Pleuromutilin; Streptogramin; Tetracycline	*mel*	NF	NF	F	NF	NF
Aminocoumarin; Aminoglycoside; Cephalosporin; diaminopyrimidine; Fluoroquinolone; Macrolide; penam; Phenicol; Tetracycline	*MexD*	NF	NF	F	NF	NF
Diaminopyrimidine; Fluoroquinolone; Phenicol	*MexF*	NF	F	F	NF	F
Macrolide	*mphE*	NF	F	F	NF	NF

Table 2. *Cont.*

Resistance	Gene Name	Number of Reads				
		Bageswar	Bagwan	Rasulabad Ghat	Sahidabad	Triveni Sangam
Macrolide	*mphF*	NF	NF	F	NF	NF
Nitroimidazole	*msbA*	NF	F	F	NF	NF
Erythromycin; Azithromycin; Telithromycin; Quinupristin; Pristinamycin_IA; Virginiamycin_S	*msr(D)*	NF	NF	F	NF	NF
Macrolide	*msr(E)*	F	F	F	NF	NF
Diaminopyrimidine; Fluoroquinolone; Glycylcycline; Nitrofuran; Tetracycline	*oqxA*	NF	NF	F	NF	NF
Diaminopyrimidine; Fluoroquinolone; Glycylcycline; Nitrofuran; Tetracycline	*oqxB*	NF	NF	F	NF	NF
Aminocoumarin; Aminoglycoside; Carbapenem;cephalosporin; Cephamycin; Diaminopyrimidine; Fluoroquinolone; Macrolide; Monobactam; Penem; Peptide; Phenicol; Sulfonamide; Tetracycline	*Pseudomonas aeruginosaCpxR*	NF	NF	F	NF	NF
Fluoroquinolone	*qnrD2*	NF	F	NF	NF	NF
Carbapenem; Cephalosporin; Cephamycin; Fluoroquinolone; Glycylcycline; Monobactam; Penam; Phenicol; Rifamycin; Tetracycline; Triclosan	*ramA*	NF	F	F	NF	NF
Rifamycin	*rphB*	NF	NF	F	NF	NF
Aminoglycoside	*spw*	NF	NF	F	NF	NF
Sulfonamide	*sul1*	NF	NF	F	NF	F
Sulfonamide	*sul2*	NF	NF	F	NF	F
Sulfonamide	*sul4*	NF	NF	F	F	NF
Tetracycline	*tet(36)*	NF	F	F	NF	NF
Tetracycline	*tet(39)*	F	F	F	NF	NF
Tetracycline	*tet(A)*	NF	NF	F	NF	NF
Tetracycline	*tet(G)*	NF	NF	F	NF	NF
Doxycycline; Tetracycline; Minocycline	*tet(M)*	NF	NF	F	NF	NF
Doxycycline; Tetracycline; Minocycline	*tet(O)*	NF	NF	F	NF	NF
Doxycycline; Tetracycline; Minocycline	*tet(Q)*	NF	NF	F	NF	NF

Table 2. *Cont.*

Resistance	Gene Name	Number of Reads				
		Bageswar	Bagwan	Rasulabad Ghat	Sahidabad	Triveni Sangam
Doxycycline; Tetracycline; Minocycline	*tet(X)*	NF	NF	F	NF	NF
Tetracycline	*tetC*	NF	NF	F	NF	NF
Aminocoumarin; Aminoglycoside; Carbapenem; Cephalosporin; Cephamycin; Fluoroquinolone; Glycylcycline; Macrolide; Penam; Peptide; Phenicol; Rifamycin; Tetracycline; Triclosan	*tolC*	NF	F	NF	NF	NF

2.4. Virulence Factor (VF) Abundance

Our comprehensive study examined the distribution of virulence genes and associated factors across multiple locations. Different contigs and their corresponding NCBI accession numbers, alongside the designation of virulence genes and factors, were identified in the present study and were exclusively linked to *Pseudomonas aeruginosa* (Table 3).

The analysis revealed the widespread distribution of flagella-associated genes (e.g., *flgC*, *flgG*, *flgH*, *flgI*) across various locations. The *flgC* (Flagella VF0273) was identified in Bagwan, Triveni Sangam, and Rasulabad Ghat only. The genes related to Type III and Type IV secretion systems, such as *pcrD*, *pscR*, *pcrH* in Triveni Sangam, and *pilG* in Triveni Sangam, Bagwan, and Sahidabad, were also identified. Alginate biosynthesis genes, like *algU* (Alginate VF0091) in Sahidabad and algI in Bagwan and Triveni Sangam, were detected. The presence of genes associated with pyochelin synthesis (*pchD*, *pchC*, *pchG*, *pchF*, *pchB*, *pchR*) exclusively in Rasulabad Ghat highlights the region-specific adaptation of bacteria in iron acquisition, a critical factor for bacterial survival and virulence. Moreover, *clpV1*, *hsiG1*, *dotU1*, *hcp1*, *hsiB1/vipA*, and *hsiC1/vipB* in Rasulabad Ghat, associated with a Type VI secretion system (HSI-I VF0334), were identified. This study also identified the *acpXL* gene in Bageswar, which was linked to LPS (CVF383) in *Brucella* sp.

Table 3. List of virulence factors found across sediment samples in the river Ganga. The virulence factors have been categorized across samples and virulence factors.

Contig Id	Location	NCBI Accession No.	Virulence Gene	Virulence Factor
contigs_2469; contigs_1; contigs_240	Bagwan; Triveni Sangam; Rasulabad Ghat	NP_249769	*flgC*	
contigs_45; contigs_11691; contigs_19; contigs_3945	Rasulabad Ghat; sahidabad; Triveni Sangam; Bagwan	NP_249773	*flgG*	Flagella (VF0273) (*Pseudomonas aeruginosa*)
contigs_45	Rasulabad Ghat	NP_250143	*flhA*	
contigs_45; contigs_641; contigs_19	Rasulabad Ghat; Bagwan; Triveni Sangam	NP_250137	*fliP*	
contigs_45	Rasulabad Ghat	NP_250138	*fliQ*	

Table 3. *Cont.*

Contig Id	Location	NCBI Accession No.	Virulence Gene	Virulence Factor
contigs_11691; contigs_19; contigs_3945	Sahidabad; Triveni Sangam; Bagwan	NP_249774	*flgH*	Flagella (VF0273) (*Pseudomonas aeruginosa*)
contigs_45; contigs_641; contig_19; contigs_366	Rasulabad Ghat; Bagwan; Triveni Sangam; Bagwan	NP_250134	*fliM*	
contigs_45; contigs_641; contig_19; contigs_366	Rasulabad Ghat; Bagwan; Triveni Sangam; Bagwan	NP_249793	*fliG*	
contigs_45; contigs_11691; contigs_19; contigs_3945	Rasulabad Ghat; sahidabad; Triveni Sangam; Bagwan	NP_249775	*flgI*	
contigs_45; contigs_641; contig_19; contigs_366	Rasulabad Ghat; Bagwan; Triveni Sangam; Bagwan	NP_250145	*fleN*	
contigs_45; contigs_641; contigs_19	Rasulabad Ghat; Bagwan; Triveni Sangam	NP_249795	*fliI*	
contigs_45; contigs_641	Rasulabad Ghat; Bagwan	NP_249788	*fleQ*	
contigs_4	Triveni Sangam	NP_250394	*pcrD*	Type III TTSS (VF0083) (*Pseudomonas aeruginosa*)
contigs_4	Triveni Sangam	NP_250384	*pscR*	
contigs_4	Triveni Sangam	NP_250398	*pcrH*	
contigs_68665	Sahidabad	NP_249453	*algU*	Alginate (VF0091) (*Pseudomonas aeruginosa*)
contigs_5362; contigs_1	Bagwan; Triveni Sangam	NP_252238	*algI*	
contigs_1	Triveni Sangam	NP_252231	*alg8*	
contigs_42942	Rasulabad Ghat	NP_273273	*katA*	
contigs_41	Rasulabad Ghat	NP_460110	*csgG*	
contigs_45	Rasulabad Ghat	NP_251103	*pvdH*	
contigs_45; contigs_53	Rasulabad Ghat; Triveni Sangam	NP_251116	*pvdS*	
contigs_665	Rasulabad Ghat	NP_252911	*fptA*	
contigs_76423	Bagwan	BAA94855	*astA*	
contigs_2	Rasulabad Ghat	NP_253699	*waaF*	
contigs_45; contigs_269352	Rasulabad Ghat; Sahidabad	NP_251102	*mbtH-like*	
contigs_627	Bagwan	AAF37887	*ompA*	
contigs_5362	Bagwan	NP_252241	*algA*	
contigs_665	Rasulabad Ghat	NP_252918	*pchD*	Pyochelin (VF0095) (*Pseudomonas aeruginosa*)
contigs_665	Rasulabad Ghat	NP_252919	*pchC*	
contigs_665	Rasulabad Ghat	NP_252914	*pchG*	
contigs_665	Rasulabad Ghat	NP_252915	*pchF*	
contigs_665	Rasulabad Ghat	NP_252920	*pchB*	
contigs_665	Rasulabad Ghat	NP_252917	*pchR*	

Table 3. *Cont.*

Contig Id	Location	NCBI Accession No.	Virulence Gene	Virulence Factor
contigs_4; contigs_24665; contigs_67305; contigs_39	Triveni Sangam; Bagwan; sahidabad; Bagwan	NP_249099	*pilG*	Type IV pili (VF0082) (*Pseudomonas aeruginosa*)
contigs_24665; contigs_67305; contigs_39	Bagwan; Sahidabad; Bagwan	NP_249100	*pilH*	
contigs_39	Bagwan	NP_249086	*pilT*	
contigs_622	Rasulabad Ghat	NP_248780	*clpV1*	Type VI HSI-I (VF0334) (*Pseudomonas aeruginosa*)
contigs_622	Rasulabad Ghat	NP_248778	*hsiG1*	
contigs_622	Rasulabad Ghat	NP_248768	*dotU1*	
contigs_622	Rasulabad Ghat	NP_248775	*hcp1*	
contigs_622	Rasulabad Ghat	NP_248773	*hsiB1/vipA*	
contigs_622	Rasulabad Ghat	NP_248774	*hsiC1/vipB*	
contigs_239842	Bageswar	NP_540392	*acpXL*	LPS (CVF383) (Brucella)
contigs_240	Rasulabad Ghat	NP_249768	*flgB*	Deoxyhexose linking sugar 209 Da capping structure (AI138) (*Pseudomonas aeruginosa*)
contigs_641	Bagwan	NP_250146	*fliA*	
contigs_204	Rasulabad Ghat	NP_254009	*algC*	Alginate biosynthesis (CVF522) (*Pseudomonas aeruginosa*)

2.5. KEGG Pathway Analysis

Our KEGG pathway analysis revealed a diverse range of biological processes across all six distinct locations in the river Ganga (Figure 7). Notably, antimicrobial resistance pathways were significantly represented, especially in Rasulabad Ghat and Sahidabad. Core metabolic pathways, including energy and carbohydrate metabolism, were uniformly present across all locations. The distribution of pathways related to diseases, such as cancer and endocrine disorders, varied among locations. There was a noticeable diversity in amino acid metabolism pathways, underscoring the metabolic adaptability of organisms in different environments. We also found unclassified pathways, possibly linked with genetic information processing and the metabolism process.

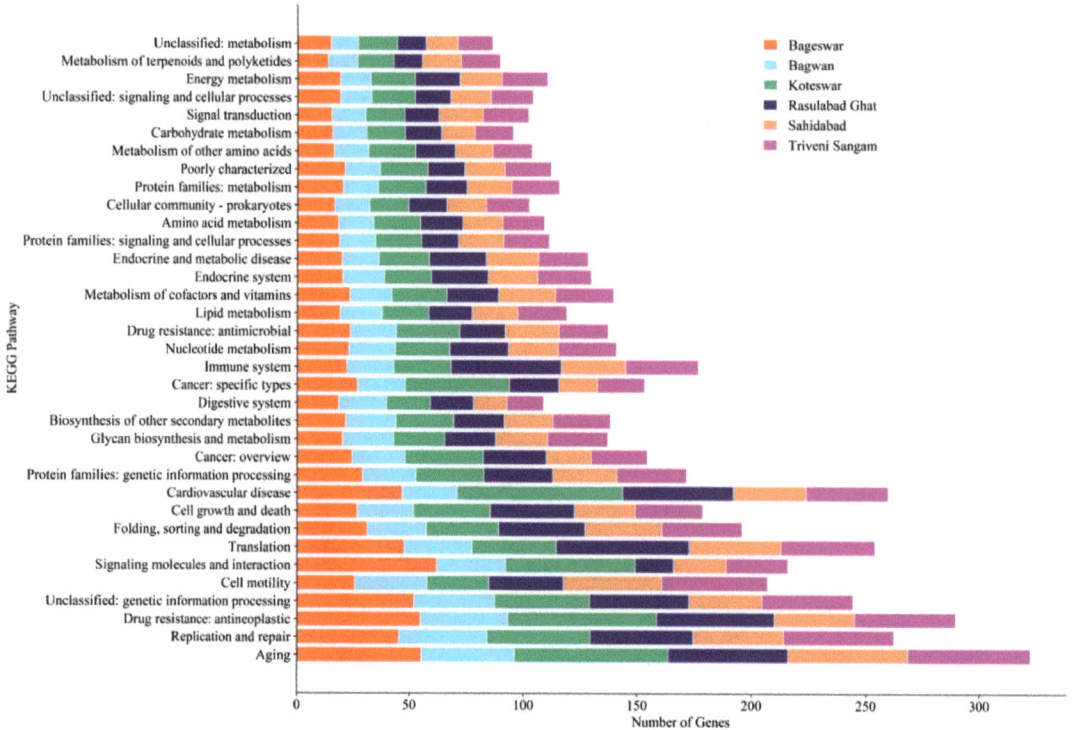

Figure 7. Graphical representation of the distribution of various biological processes in the Ganga River basin as analyzed from the KEGG. It depicts a comparative analysis across the six locations (Bageswar, Bagwan, Koteswar, Rasulabad Ghat, Sahidabad, and Triveni Sangam), showing the frequency of processes ranging from aging and replication to metabolism and drug resistance.

2.6. COG Analysis

The Cluster of Orthologous Groups (COG) analysis conducted across the six locations revealed varied distributions of functional categories (Figure 8). The categories related to "Energy production and conversion", "Amino acid transport and metabolism", and "Carbohydrate transport and metabolism" were notably prevalent. Significant representation of "Cell cycle control, cell division, chromosome partitioning" and "Replication, recombination and repair" highlights the active cellular processes occurring in these environments. The variability in "Defense mechanisms", "Signal transduction mechanisms", and "Inorganic ion transport and metabolism" across locations were found. We also found a notable number of sequences under "Function unknown".

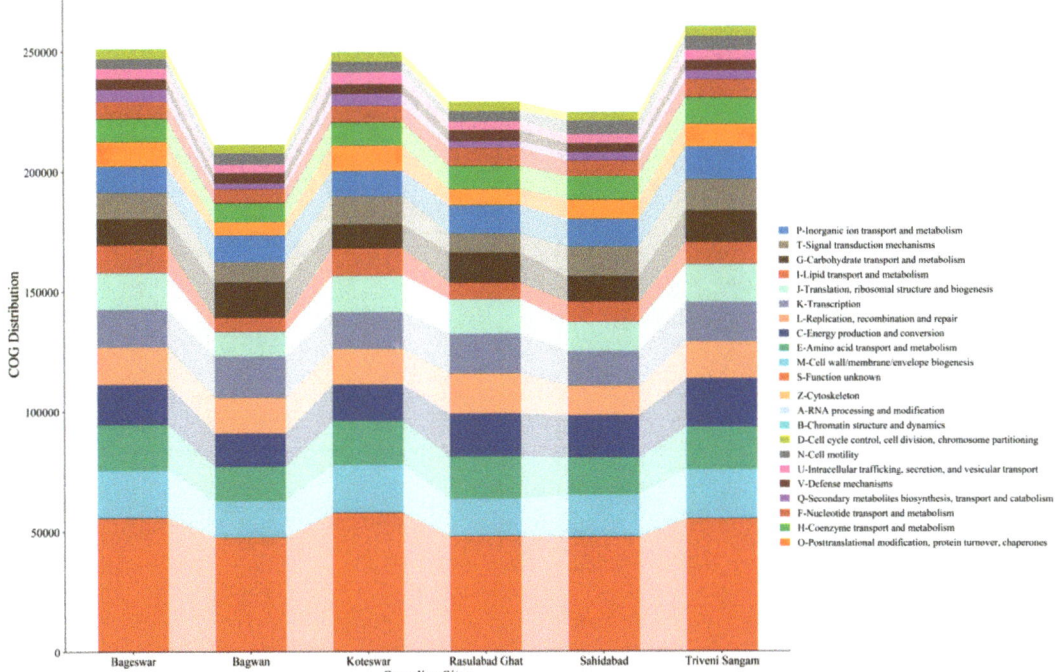

Figure 8. Bar chart displaying the Cluster of Orthologous Groups (COG) functional category distribution across the six locations in the Ganga River basin. The categories range from RNA processing and chromatin structure to metabolism and defense mechanisms, highlighting the diversity and abundance of microbial functions in these regions.

3. Materials and Methods

3.1. Sample Collection

Sediment and water samples were systematically collected from six distinct sites along the river Ganga. These locations included Koteswar (N 300.25′37.67″, E 780.52′54.77″), Bagwan (N 300.22′41.84″ E 780.68′12.99″), and Bageswar (N 300.13′90.18″ E 780.59′68.21″) near Devprayag, Uttarakhand, India, along with Rasulabad Ghat (N 250.50′24.64″ E 810.85′57.41″), Triveni Sangam (N 250.42′63.09″ E 810.88′81.93″), and Sahidabad (N 250.39′41.57″ E 810.91′61.04″) near Allahabad, Uttar Pradesh, India. Collections were conducted in the morning hours, between 8.30 and 10.30 AM, in March 2021 (Figure 9). From each location, approximately 500 g of sediment and 500 mL of water were collected. These samples were then meticulously stored in distinct autoclaved amber glass bottles (500 mL), clearly labeled as Koteswar, Bagwan, Bageswar, Rasulabad Ghat, Triveni Sangam, and Sahidabad. At every site, five sediment samples were obtained at intervals of approximately 200 m and subsequently combined to form a single representative sample for each location. The pH and temperature of each sample were measured on-site using an MT-222 Digiflexi digital thermometer (Dr. Morepen, New Delhi, India) and portable pH meter (Hanna Instrument, Sigma, St. Louis, MO, USA). All sediment samples were carefully placed in sterile plastic bags, securely sealed, and transported on ice (4 °C), and subsequently stored at −20 °C for further analysis.

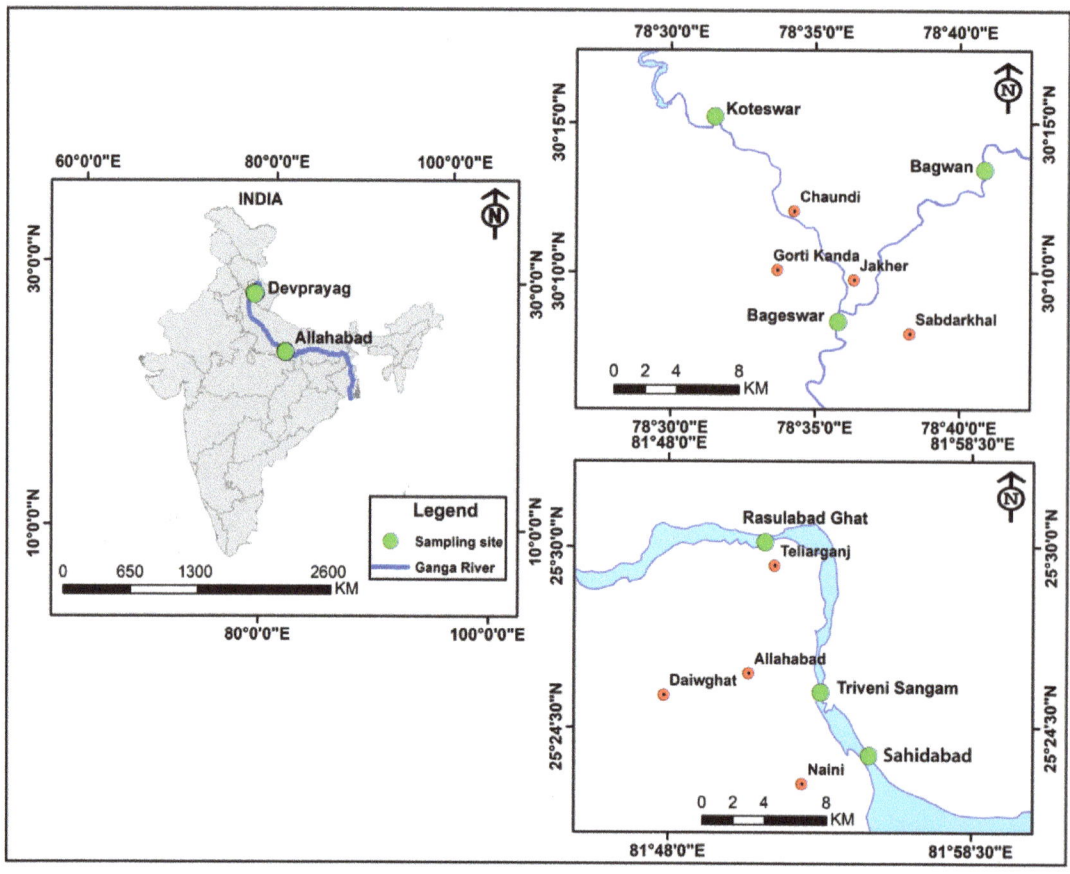

Figure 9. Map depicting the sampling sites along the Ganga River for the metagenomic study. Key locations include Bageswar, Bagwan, Koteswar, Rasulabad Ghat, Sahidabad, and Triveni Sangam spread across various geographical coordinates. Other locations near to the studied regions are marked with red circles.

3.2. Genomic DNA Isolation, Library Preparation, and Sequencing

Genomic DNA was extracted from the collected sediment samples using the Xpress-DNA Soil Kit (MagGenome, Union City, CA, USA), with certain modifications to the standard protocol. The integrity and concentration of the extracted DNA were assessed using 1% agarose gel electrophoresis and Nanodrop™ (Thermo Scientific, Waltham, MA, USA), respectively, and the samples were subsequently preserved at −20 °C for future analysis. A criterion for the DNA library construction was established, requiring an optical density (OD) absorbance between 1.8 and 2.0 at a 260/280 nm purity ratio and a minimum DNA concentration of 1 µg.

The purified DNA was sent to Genotypic Technology Pvt. Ltd. (Bangalore, India) for library preparation and sequencing. Briefly, a NEBNext Ultra DNA Library Prep Kit (Ipswich, MA, USA) was employed to prepare the paired-end sequencing library, following the manufacturer's protocol. The DNA fragments were then purified using a MinElute PCR Purification Kit (Qiagen, Ltd., Crawley, UK). Post-preparation, the libraries were subjected to DNA segmentation quantification in conjunction with HyperLadder IV (Bioline, London, UK) to ascertain the size of the DNA library. In line with Illumina's standard protocol, the libraries were pooled at equal molar concentrations for sequencing. An Illumina HiSeq

2500 (San Diego, CA, USA) quick run of 2 × 150 bp was utilized for sequencing, and duplicate samples were allocated over two lanes for comprehensive sequencing. The detailed workflow used in this study is shown in Figure 10.

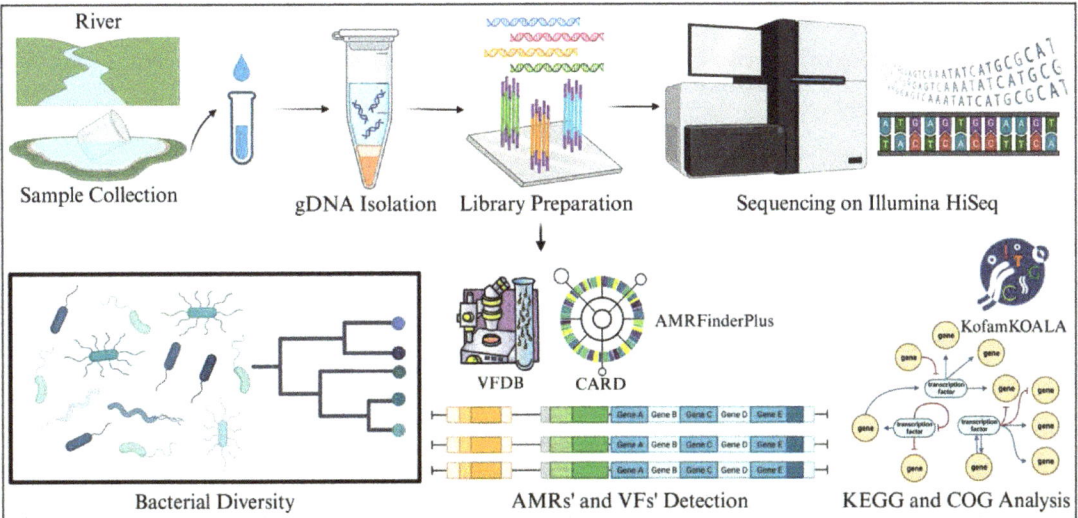

Figure 10. Illustration of the methodological framework of the present study, starting from sample collection through sequencing and analysis. It includes following methodologies like genomic DNA (gDNA) isolation, library preparation, and Illumina HiSeq sequencing. The computational workflow of bacterial diversity assessment, the identification of virulence factors (VFs) from the VFDB, and the analysis of antibiotic resistance using CARD and AMRFinderPlus are shown. The final stages involve the detection of AMR and VFs, followed by KEGG and COG analysis for comprehensive genetic evaluation.

3.3. Bacterial Diversity Detection

Taxonomic profiling of six metagenomic samples was conducted utilizing the NCBI taxonomy dataset. For each sample, a taxonomic tree was constructed by employing the neighbor-joining method facilitated by MEGAN6 [26] and Kraken2 v2.1.3 [27]. The Kraken2 report file was finally used for generating a bacterial diversity classification plot or Sankey plot using Pavian v1.0.

3.4. Functional Analysis

In the present river sediment metagenomic sample analysis, the assembly file was annotated using PROKKA v1.14.5 [28]. The annotated sequence was used in the Virulence Factors Database (VFDB) to determine virulence factors. To ascertain the presence of ARGs within the river sediment, various databases, including the Comprehensive Antibiotic Resistance Database (CARD), NCBI, and Resfinder, were employed. For the annotation of core orthologues, consensus sequences were subjected to BLAST analysis against KOfam, a database of KEGG orthologues, employing kofamKOALA [29]. Following this, the eggNOG-mapper tool [30], in conjunction with the EggNOG database [31], was utilized to systematically categorize all core orthologue sequences into clusters of orthologous groups of proteins (COGs).

4. Discussion

The observed bacterial diversity and the prevalence of specific taxa, in particular locations of the river Ganga basin, emphasize the intricate relationship between microbial communities and their environmental conditions. These findings have significant implications for understanding the ecological health and biogeochemical processes within the river system.

The predominance of Proteobacteria across all examined locations aligns with the existing literature, which often cites Proteobacteria as a dominant phylum in aquatic environments [32–34]. This ubiquity can be attributed to the diverse metabolic capabilities of Proteobacteria, allowing them to thrive in various environmental conditions. In specific sites, like Bageswar, Koteswar, and Sahidabad, the marked prevalence of *Flavobacterium* spp. is noteworthy. *Flavobacterium* is known for its role in nutrient cycling and has been previously identified in freshwater ecosystems [35]. Its abundance in these areas might indicate specific ecological functions, possibly related to the organic matter degradation or nitrogen cycle in these river segments. Furthermore, the distinct presence of *Sulfurospirillum* spp. in Bagwan and Triveni Sangam and *Pseudomonas* spp. in Sahidabad deserves attention. *Sulfurospirillum* spp. are known for their role in sulfur cycling and have been identified in environments with low oxygen levels [36], which might suggest specific anoxic conditions or sulfur-rich environments in these parts of the river Ganga. On the other hand, *Pseudomonas* spp., known for its metabolic versatility and adaptability, might indicate a high level of organic pollutants or anthropogenic influence in Sahidabad, as these bacteria are often associated with contaminated sites.

Our investigation into the distribution of antimicrobial resistance (AMR) genes across multiple geographical locations revealed a complex and diverse landscape of resistance mechanisms. This study encompassed a wide array of resistance types, including Aminoglycoside, Streptomycin, Cephalosporin, Penam, and others, across six locations in river Ganga, i.e., Bageswar, Bagwan, Koteswar, Rasulabad Ghat, Sahidabad, and Triveni Sangam.

The findings demonstrated significant variability in the presence and prevalence of specific AMR genes among the studied locations. For example, genes conferring resistance to Aminoglycosides like *aac(6')-Ib*, *aadS*, *acrD*, and *ANT(2")-Ia* were predominantly identified in Rasulabad Ghat. This suggests a localized emergence or higher usage of aminoglycoside antibiotics in this area, leading to selective pressure and subsequent development of resistance. The role of selective pressure on antibiotic resistance has been well reviewed in an earlier work [37] and well studied in *P. aeroginosa* [38]. The detection of *aadS* in Bagwan and Triveni Sangam further indicates the spread of this resistance mechanism beyond a single locality. Notably, Streptomycin resistance genes such as *aadA1*, *aadA5*, and *aadA6* showed a similar pattern of being exclusively found in Rasulabad Ghat. This further supports the hypothesis of region-specific antibiotic usage or resistance development mechanisms. The region-specific antimicrobial resistance has been described in earlier studies on *Streptococcus pneumoniae* [39], *Mycobacterium tuberculosis* [40], and *Klebsiella pneumoniae* [41]. Beta-lactam resistance genes, like *blaOXA-209*, which are unique to Bagwan and Rasulabad Ghat, and *blaOXA-119* in Triveni Sangam, underscore the heterogeneity in the distribution of resistance genes. These genes have been well studied in an earlier work on the members of genus *Tenacibaculum* [42].

Furthermore, the gene *acrB*, associated with resistance to a broad spectrum of antibiotics, was observed in Bagwan and Rasulabad Ghat, which shows the presence of multi-drug resistant strains in these areas. The *acrB* gene encodes a heterotrimeric protein that forms a component of the inner membrane and is primarily tasked with substrate recognition and energy transduction. It functions as a drug/proton antiporter, playing a pivotal role in these processes [43,44]. The occurrence of blaRm3, a gene showing resistance to a wide range of antibiotics, in Bagwan and Sahidabad, and *blaTHIN-B* in Sahidabad, points toward the emergence of high-level antibiotic resistance in these areas. This gene is one of the key genes related to antibiotic resistance and has been well studied as an indicator of antibiotic resistance in various water sources [45–47]. In addition, the minimal presence of the surveyed AMR genes in Bageswar indicates a possible lower prevalence of resistant strains or divergent antibiotic utilization patterns in this locality. A study examining AMR genes in the Ili River reported a lower occurrence of these genes, indicating minimal human intervention in certain areas [48]. So, the AMR genes analyzed in the present study would help in finding the effect of human intervention on the upper and lower river Ganga basin.

The study also revealed that the distribution of these resistance genes is not uniform across the regions, indicating a complex interplay of factors such as local antibiotic usage patterns, environmental conditions, and genetic exchange mechanisms that might contribute to this varied distribution. The distribution and diversity of AMR genes across the studied locations provide a crucial understanding of the regional dynamics of antibiotic resistance. The findings highlight the necessity for targeted surveillance and stewardship programs to monitor and manage the spread of AMR in these specific areas. Understanding the patterns of resistance gene prevalence can aid in developing strategic interventions to curb the burgeoning issue of antibiotic resistance in diverse geographical settings.

The current investigation into the distribution of virulence factors across various locations offers significant insights into the adaptive mechanisms of pathogenic bacteria, particularly *Pseudomonas aeruginosa*. This study underscores the complexity of bacterial virulence and its dependency on environmental context.

The detection of flagella-associated genes such as *flgC*, *flgG*, *flgH*, and *flgI* in multiple locations implies a widespread reliance on motility and adherence as critical virulence factors. The prevalence of these genes across diverse geographical areas signifies a common strategy employed by bacteria to establish infection and colonization. This consistency in virulence gene distribution suggests a potential universal response to similar environmental pressures or host interactions [49].

The identification of genes related to Type III and Type IV secretion systems in specific locations, like Triveni Sangam and Sahidabad, indicates the presence of advanced bacterial systems for effector protein delivery. These secretion systems are pivotal in bacterial pathogenesis, facilitating direct interactions with host cells [50,51]. The localized presence of these genes may reflect regional variations in bacterial–host dynamics or environmental factors that favor certain pathogenic strategies. Alginate biosynthesis genes, particularly *algU* and *algI*, highlight the capability of bacterial populations in these regions to form biofilms. Biofilms confer significant advantages to bacteria, including enhanced antibiotic resistance and protection from host immune responses [52]. The regional distribution of these genes suggests environmental or selective pressures favoring biofilm-forming strains, potentially due to their survival and persistence advantages in specific niches. The role of biofilm in bacterial survival in the river Ganga basin has been studied in an earlier work [53,54]. The exclusive presence of pyochelin synthesis genes in Rasulabad Ghat points to an environment where iron acquisition is a crucial survival factor. Iron is a vital nutrient for bacterial growth, and its acquisition is often a limiting factor in pathogenic success. The specificity of these genes to Rasulabad Ghat may indicate unique iron availability or competition dynamics in this site.

The presence of Type VI secretion system genes in Rasulabad Ghat suggests an environment rich in bacterial competition. This system is known for its role in bacterial warfare, allowing for the delivery of toxins into competing bacterial cells [55,56]. The concentration of these genes in one location might reflect a high-density bacterial community with intense inter-bacterial interactions.

The geographical variability in virulence gene profiles poses challenges for infection control and management strategies. Understanding the specific virulence factors in Ganga River water can aid in developing targeted therapeutic and preventive measures. This study highlights the need for the localized surveillance of pathogenic bacteria to better understand and combat region-specific infectious challenges.

The distinct distribution of genes in processes like aging, replication, repair, and cell motility across studied locations underscore the unique ecological characteristics of each site. This diversity can be attributed to a multitude of factors, including environmental conditions, the presence of specific microbial communities, and local selective pressures. The variability observed in the data reflects the adaptive responses of organisms to their respective habitats. The adaptive response of microbial communities to the environment has been studied in various research works, reflecting its importance in future drug design [57,58].

The genes related to antimicrobial resistance, particularly in regions like Rasulabad Ghat and Sahidabad, raise significant public health concerns. This observation suggests that these areas might be reservoirs of drug-resistant organisms, potentially due to the overuse of antibiotics or the presence of other selective agents. The data necessitate a more focused approach toward monitoring and managing antimicrobial resistance in these regions. The uniform distribution of primary metabolic activities, such as energy and carbohydrate metabolism across all locations, indicates the fundamental nature of these processes in sustaining life. However, the variation in amino acid metabolism across different regions highlights the metabolic flexibility and adaptability of the residing organisms, allowing them to thrive in diverse environmental conditions. The presence of disease-related categories, like cancer and endocrine disorders, in the data suggests potential environmental or genetic factors influencing disease prevalence in these regions. These findings could be instrumental in guiding further epidemiological studies to explore the environmental contributions to disease etiology.

A significant portion of the genes fell into unclassified categories, pointing to the existence of unknown or poorly understood biological processes in these regions. This observation opens avenues for future research aimed at uncovering novel biological functions and mechanisms, which could have far-reaching implications on understanding ecosystem dynamics and organismal adaptations.

The Cluster of Orthologous Groups (COG) analysis, encompassing six distinct geographical locations, unveiled a rich tapestry of functional biodiversity. This diversity, evident in the distribution of various COG categories, reflects the intricate interplay between microbial communities and their respective environments.

Central to our findings is the representation of categories related to energy production, carbohydrate metabolism, and amino acid transport across all studied regions. This uniformity in metabolic profiles suggests a fundamental role of these processes in sustaining microbial life [59–61]. It underscores the universality of certain metabolic functions, which serve as the cornerstone for microbial survival and proliferation, irrespective of geographical variances.

Further study revealed the genes involved in cellular processes, particularly cell cycle control, cell division, and chromosomal dynamics. The marked presence of these categories indicates active cellular mechanisms, potentially as a response to local environmental pressures or genomic instabilities. This observation aligns with the notion that microorganisms are in a constant state of adaptation, modifying their cellular processes to optimize survival and efficiency in diverse habitats, which supports various studies related to this [62–64].

The variation observed in defense mechanisms and signal transduction pathways among the different locations indicates the adaptive strategies employed by microbial communities. This variability could stem from the need to respond to specific local environmental conditions, such as nutrient availability, the presence of antimicrobial agents, or other ecological pressures [65]. The differential expression of these categories highlights the role of local environmental factors in shaping the functional capabilities of microbial communities.

A particularly intriguing aspect of our analysis is the substantial proportion of sequences classified under "Function unknown". This finding points to a significant gap in our understanding of microbial functional diversity and suggests the presence of novel or poorly understood biological processes within these communities. It opens avenues for future research to explore these uncharacterized functions, which could lead to groundbreaking discoveries in microbial ecology and biology.

5. Conclusions

In conclusion, this study offers critical insights into the bacterial diversity across six regions of the river Ganga through a metagenomics approach. In addition to this, the

Antibiotics **2023**, *12*, 1735

spatial distribution of AMR and virulence factors, illustrating a complex and diverse landscape of antibiotic resistance across various geographical locations on the river Ganga, has been depicted. The findings emphasize the importance of region-specific public health strategies and the need to integrate these with local environmental and socioeconomic contexts to effectively combat AMR. This study also highlights the intricate relationship between organisms and their environments, as evidenced by the diversity of biological processes observed in different locations. This emphasizes the need for local environmental considerations in both ecological and biological research and for region-specific strategies to address public health challenges, such as AMR. The research contributes significantly to our understanding of the geographical distribution of bacterial virulence factors and the importance of environmental and regional factors in bacterial pathogenesis. While the study provides valuable insights, it is limited by its focus on specific resistance genes and geographical locations. Future research should broaden to include a wider array of resistance determinants and environmental samples to fully comprehend AMR dynamics. This expansion is crucial for the global fight against the growing threat of antimicrobial resistance and for developing effective infection control and management strategies. Understanding the diverse functional profiles of microbial communities and their adaptability will be crucial to addressing ecological dynamics and ensuring environmental sustainability.

Author Contributions: Conceptualization, B.K.B.; methodology, A.K.R., P.S.T., S.D. and D.U.B.; validation, A.K.R., S.D., B.B. and D.U.B.; formal analysis, A.K.R., P.S.T., S.D. and D.U.B.; investigation, B.K.B.; resources, A.K.R., P.S.T., S.D. and D.U.B.; data curation, A.K.R., P.S.T., S.D. and D.U.B.; writing—original draft preparation, A.K.R., P.S.T., S.D., D.U.B. and B.B.; writing—review and editing, B.K.B. and B.K.D.; visualization, A.K.R., S.D., P.S.T. and D.U.B.; supervision, B.K.B., B.K.D. and B.B.; project administration, B.K.B.; funding acquisition, B.K.B. All authors have read and agreed to the published version of the manuscript.

Funding: The present study was undertaken within the framework of the CABin Scheme, located in New Delhi.

Data Availability Statement: Metagenome data derived from our study were deposited to the NCBI Sequence Read Archive (SRA), which can be accessed via SRR16085958 (Koteswar), SRR16085957 (Bagwan), SRR16085956 (Bageswar), SRR16085955 (Rasulabad Ghat), SRR16085954 (Triveni Sangam), and SRR16085953 (Sahidabad).

Acknowledgments: The authors thank Asim Kumar Jana, a Senior Technical Assistant at ICAR-CIFRI in Barrackpore, West Bengal, for his assistance in sample collection and technical support throughout this study. We express our gratitude to the Indian Council of Medical Research (ICMR), located in New Delhi, India, for providing us with their support.

Conflicts of Interest: The authors declare no conflict of interest.

References

1. Ali, S.; Singh, S.; Singh, R.; Tyagi, M.; Pandey, R. Influence of multidrug resistance bacteria in river Ganges in the stretch of Rishikesh to Haridwar. *Environ. Chall.* **2021**, *3*, 100068. [CrossRef]
2. Srivastava, A.; Verma, D. Comparative bacteriome and antibiotic resistome analysis of water and sediment of the Ganga River of India. *World J. Microbiol. Biotechnol.* **2023**, *39*, 294. [CrossRef]
3. Mittal, P.; Prasoodanan, P.K.V.; Dhakan, D.B.; Kumar, S.; Sharma, V.K. Metagenome of a polluted river reveals a reservoir of metabolic and antibiotic resistance genes. *Environ. Microbiome* **2019**, *14*, 5. [CrossRef]
4. Reddy, B.; Dubey, S.K. River Ganges water as reservoir of microbes with antibiotic and metal ion resistance genes: High throughput metagenomic approach. *Environ. Pollut.* **2019**, *246*, 443–451. [CrossRef]
5. Behera, B.K.; Chakraborty, H.J.; Patra, B.; Rout, A.K.; Dehury, B.; Das, B.K.; Sarkar, D.J.; Parida, P.K.; Raman, R.K.; Rao, A.R. Metagenomic analysis reveals bacterial and fungal diversity and their bioremediation potential from sediments of river Ganga and Yamuna in India. *Front. Microbiol.* **2020**, *11*, 556136. [CrossRef] [PubMed]
6. Behera, B.K.; Patra, B.; Chakraborty, H.J.; Sahu, P.; Rout, A.K.; Sarkar, D.J.; Parida, P.K.; Raman, R.K.; Rao, A.R.; Rai, A. Metagenome analysis from the sediment of river Ganga and Yamuna: In search of beneficial microbiome. *PLoS ONE* **2020**, *15*, e0239594. [CrossRef] [PubMed]
7. Grenni, P. Antimicrobial resistance in rivers: A review of the genes detected and new challenges. *Environ. Toxicol. Chem.* **2022**, *41*, 687–714. [CrossRef]

8. He, Y.; Yuan, Q.; Mathieu, J.; Stadler, L.; Senehi, N.; Sun, R.; Alvarez, P.J. Antibiotic resistance genes from livestock waste: Occurrence, dissemination, and treatment. *NPJ Clean Water* **2020**, *3*, 4. [CrossRef]
9. Osińska, A.; Korzeniewska, E.; Harnisz, M.; Felis, E.; Bajkacz, S.; Jachimowicz, P.; Niestępski, S.; Konopka, I. Small-scale wastewater treatment plants as a source of the dissemination of antibiotic resistance genes in the aquatic environment. *J. Hazard. Mater.* **2020**, *381*, 121221. [CrossRef] [PubMed]
10. Behera, B.K.; Patra, B.; Chakraborty, H.J.; Rout, A.K.; Dixit, S.; Rai, A.; Das, B.K.; Mohapatra, T. Bacteriophages diversity in India's major river Ganga: A repository to regulate pathogenic bacteria in the aquatic environment. *Environ. Sci. Pollut. Res.* **2023**, *30*, 34101–34114. [CrossRef] [PubMed]
11. Choudhury, N.; Sahu, T.K.; Rao, A.R.; Rout, A.K.; Behera, B.K. An Improved Machine Learning-Based Approach to Assess the Microbial Diversity in Major North Indian River Ecosystems. *Genes* **2023**, *14*, 1082. [CrossRef] [PubMed]
12. Chaturvedi, P.; Chaurasia, D.; Pandey, A.; Gupta, P. Co-occurrence of multidrug resistance, β-lactamase and plasmid mediated AmpC genes in bacteria isolated from river Ganga, northern India. *Environ. Pollut.* **2020**, *267*, 115502. [CrossRef]
13. Matta, N.; Bisht, G. Detection and enumeration of coliforms in Ganga Water Collected from different ghats. *J. Bioprocess Biotech.* **2018**, *8*, 1–10. [CrossRef]
14. Behera, B.K.; Sahu, P.; Rout, A.K.; Parida, P.K.; Sarkar, D.J.; Kaushik, N.K.; Rao, A.R.; Rai, A.; Das, B.K.; Mohapatra, T. Exploring microbiome from sediments of River Ganga using a metagenomic approach. *Aquat. Ecosyst. Health Manag.* **2021**, *24*, 12–22. [CrossRef]
15. Rout, A.K.; Dehury, B.; Parida, P.K.; Sarkar, D.J.; Behera, B.; Das, B.K.; Rai, A.; Behera, B.K. Taxonomic profiling and functional gene annotation of microbial communities in sediment of river Ganga at Kanpur, India: Insights from whole-genome metagenomics study. *Environ. Sci. Pollut. Res.* **2022**, *29*, 82309–82323. [CrossRef]
16. Srivastava, A.; Verma, D. Ganga River sediments of India predominate with aerobic and chemo-heterotrophic bacteria majorly engaged in the degradation of xenobiotic compounds. *Environ. Sci. Pollut. Res.* **2023**, *30*, 752–772. [CrossRef]
17. Kumar, N.; Gupta, A.K.; Sudan, S.K.; Pal, D.; Randhawa, V.; Sahni, G.; Mayilraj, S.; Kumar, M. Abundance and diversity of phages, microbial taxa, and antibiotic resistance genes in the sediments of the River Ganges through metagenomic approach. *Microb. Drug Resist.* **2021**, *27*, 1336–1354. [CrossRef]
18. Zhang, S.Y.; Tsementzi, D.; Hatt, J.K.; Bivins, A.; Khelurkar, N.; Brown, J.; Tripathi, S.N.; Konstantinidis, K.T. Intensive allochthonous inputs along the Ganges River and their effect on microbial community composition and dynamics. *Environ. Microbiol.* **2019**, *21*, 182–196. [CrossRef]
19. Li, W.; Su, H.; Cao, Y.; Wang, L.; Hu, X.; Xu, W.; Xu, Y.; Li, Z.; Wen, G. Antibiotic resistance genes and bacterial community dynamics in the seawater environment of Dapeng Cove, South China. *Sci. Total Environ.* **2020**, *723*, 138027. [CrossRef]
20. Shao, S.; Hu, Y.; Cheng, J.; Chen, Y. Research progress on distribution, migration, transformation of antibiotics and antibiotic resistance genes (ARGs) in aquatic environment. *Crit. Rev. Biotechnol.* **2018**, *38*, 1195–1208. [CrossRef]
21. Calero-Cáceres, W.; Balcázar, J.L. Antibiotic resistance genes in bacteriophages from diverse marine habitats. *Sci. Total Environ.* **2019**, *654*, 452–455. [CrossRef] [PubMed]
22. Karkman, A.; Pärnänen, K.; Larsson, D.J. Fecal pollution can explain antibiotic resistance gene abundances in anthropogenically impacted environments. *Nat. Commun.* **2019**, *10*, 80. [CrossRef] [PubMed]
23. Di Cesare, A.; Eckert, E.M.; D'Urso, S.; Bertoni, R.; Gillan, D.C.; Wattiez, R.; Corno, G. Co-occurrence of integrase 1, antibiotic and heavy metal resistance genes in municipal wastewater treatment plants. *Water Res.* **2016**, *94*, 208–214. [CrossRef] [PubMed]
24. Basili, M.; Techtmann, S.M.; Zaggia, L.; Luna, G.M.; Quero, G.M. Partitioning and sources of microbial pollution in the Venice Lagoon. *Sci. Total Environ.* **2022**, *818*, 151755. [CrossRef]
25. Buccheri, M.A.; Salvo, E.; Coci, M.; Quero, G.M.; Zoccarato, L.; Privitera, V.; Rappazzo, G. Investigating microbial indicators of anthropogenic marine pollution by 16S and 18S High-Throughput Sequencing (HTS) library analysis. *FEMS Microbiol. Lett.* **2019**, *366*, fnz179. [CrossRef] [PubMed]
26. Gautam, A.; Zeng, W.; Huson, D.H. MeganServer: Facilitating interactive access to metagenomic data on a server. *Bioinformatics* **2023**, *39*, btad105. [CrossRef] [PubMed]
27. Lu, J.; Rincon, N.; Wood, D.E.; Breitwieser, F.P.; Pockrandt, C.; Langmead, B.; Salzberg, S.L.; Steinegger, M. Metagenome analysis using the Kraken software suite. *Nat. Protoc.* **2022**, *17*, 2815–2839. [CrossRef]
28. Seemann, T. Prokka: Rapid prokaryotic genome annotation. *Bioinformatics* **2014**, *30*, 2068–2069. [CrossRef]
29. Aramaki, T.; Blanc-Mathieu, R.; Endo, H.; Ohkubo, K.; Kanehisa, M.; Goto, S.; Ogata, H. KofamKOALA: KEGG Ortholog assignment based on profile HMM and adaptive score threshold. *Bioinformatics* **2020**, *36*, 2251–2252. [CrossRef]
30. Cantalapiedra, C.P.; Hernández-Plaza, A.; Letunic, I.; Bork, P.; Huerta-Cepas, J. EggNOG-mapper v2: Functional annotation, orthology assignments, and domain prediction at the metagenomic scale. *Mol. Biol. Evol.* **2021**, *38*, 5825–5829. [CrossRef]
31. Jensen, L.J.; Julien, P.; Kuhn, M.; von Mering, C.; Muller, J.; Doerks, T.; Bork, P. EggNOG: Automated construction and annotation of orthologous groups of genes. *Nucleic Acids Res.* **2007**, *36*, D250–D254. [CrossRef] [PubMed]
32. Cheng, H.; Cheng, L.; Wang, L.; Zhu, T.; Cai, W.; Hua, Z.; Wang, Y.; Wang, W. Changes of bacterial communities in response to prolonged hydrodynamic disturbances in the eutrophic water-sediment systems. *Int. J. Environ. Res. Public Health* **2019**, *16*, 3868. [CrossRef] [PubMed]

33. He, Y.; Sen, B.; Zhou, S.; Xie, N.; Zhang, Y.; Zhang, J.; Wang, G. Distinct seasonal patterns of bacterioplankton abundance and dominance of phyla α-Proteobacteria and cyanobacteria in Qinhuangdao coastal waters off the Bohai sea. *Front. Microbiol.* **2017**, *8*, 1579. [CrossRef]

34. Zhao, Z.; Zhao, R.; Qiu, X.; Wan, Y.; Lee, L. Structural Diversity of Bacterial Communities and Its Relation to Environmental Factors in the Surface Sediments from Main Stream of Qingshui River. *Water* **2022**, *14*, 3356. [CrossRef]

35. Zhou, J.S.; Cheng, J.F.; Li, X.D.; Li, Y.H. Unique bacterial communities associated with components of an artificial aquarium ecosystem and their possible contributions to nutrient cycling in this microecosystem. *World J. Microbiol. Biotechnol.* **2022**, *38*, 72. [CrossRef]

36. Finster, K.; Liesack, W.; Tindall, B. *Sulfurospirillum arcachonense* sp. nov., a new microaerophilic sulfur-reducing bacterium. *Int. J. Syst. Evol. Microbiol.* **1997**, *47*, 1212–1217. [CrossRef]

37. Lupo, A.; Coyne, S.; Berendonk, T.U. Origin and evolution of antibiotic resistance: The common mechanisms of emergence and spread in water bodies. *Front. Microbiol.* **2012**, *3*, 18. [CrossRef] [PubMed]

38. Sanz-García, F.; Sánchez, M.B.; Hernando-Amado, S.; Martínez, J.L. Evolutionary landscapes of *Pseudomonas aeruginosa* towards ribosome-targeting antibiotic resistance depend on selection strength. *Int. J. Antimicrob. Agents* **2020**, *55*, 105965. [CrossRef]

39. Cornick, J.E.; Chaguza, C.; Harris, S.R.; Yalcin, F.; Senghore, M.; Kiran, A.M.; Govindpershad, S.; Ousmane, S.; Plessis, M.D.; Pluschke, G. Region-specific diversification of the highly virulent serotype 1 *Streptococcus pneumoniae*. *Microb. Genom.* **2015**, *1*, e000027. [CrossRef]

40. Advani, J.; Verma, R.; Chatterjee, O.; Pachouri, P.K.; Upadhyay, P.; Singh, R.; Yadav, J.; Naaz, F.; Ravikumar, R.; Buggi, S. Whole genome sequencing of *Mycobacterium tuberculosis* clinical isolates from India reveals genetic heterogeneity and region-specific variations that might affect drug susceptibility. *Front. Microbiol.* **2019**, *10*, 309. [CrossRef]

41. Willers, C.; Wentzel, J.F.; Du Plessis, L.H.; Gouws, C.; Hamman, J.H. Efflux as a mechanism of antimicrobial drug resistance in clinical relevant microorganisms: The role of efflux inhibitors. *Expert Opin. Ther. Targets* **2017**, *21*, 23–36. [CrossRef]

42. Satyam, R.; Ahmad, S.; Raza, K. Comparative genomic assessment of members of genus Tenacibaculum: An exploratory study. *Mol. Genet. Genom.* **2023**, *298*, 979–993. [CrossRef] [PubMed]

43. Alenazy, R. Drug efflux pump inhibitors: A promising approach to counter multidrug resistance in Gram-negative pathogens by targeting AcrB protein from AcrAB-TolC multidrug efflux pump from *Escherichia coli*. *Biol.* **2022**, *11*, 1328. [CrossRef] [PubMed]

44. Schuster, S.; Vavra, M.; Greim, L.; Kern, W.V. Exploring the contribution of the AcrB homolog MdtF to drug resistance and dye efflux in a multidrug resistant *E. coli* isolate. *Antibiotics* **2021**, *10*, 503. [CrossRef] [PubMed]

45. Plattner, M.; Gysin, M.; Haldimann, K.; Becker, K.; Hobbie, S.N. Epidemiologic, phenotypic, and structural characterization of aminoglycoside-resistance gene aac (3)-IV. *Int. J. Mol. Sci.* **2020**, *21*, 6133. [CrossRef]

46. Ranjbar, R.; Sami, M. Genetic Investigation of beta-lactam associated antibiotic resistance among *Escherichia coli* strains isolated from water sources. *Open Microbiol. J.* **2017**, *11*, 203. [CrossRef]

47. Rossolini, G.M.; Prenna, M.; Thaller, M.C.; Frère, J.-M.; Docquier, J.-D.; Lopizzo, T.; Liberatori, S. Biochemical Characterization of the THIN-B. *Antimicrob. Agents Chemother.* **2004**, *48*, 4778.

48. Yang, X.; Yan, L.; Yang, Y.; Zhou, H.; Cao, Y.; Wang, S.; Xue, B.; Li, C.; Zhao, C.; Zhang, X. The occurrence and distribution pattern of antibiotic resistance genes and bacterial community in the ili river. *Front. Environ. Sci.* **2022**, *10*, 840428. [CrossRef]

49. Zagui, G.S.; de Almeida, O.G.G.; Moreira, N.C.; Abichabki, N.; Machado, G.P.; De Martinis, E.C.P.; Darini, A.L.C.; Andrade, L.N.; Segura-Munoz, S.I. A set of antibiotic-resistance mechanisms and virulence factors in GES-16-producing *Klebsiella quasipneumoniae* subsp. similipneumoniae from hospital wastewater revealed by whole-genome sequencing. *Environ. Pollut.* **2023**, *316*, 120645. [CrossRef]

50. Christie, P.J.; Vogel, J.P. Bacterial type IV secretion: Conjugation systems adapted to deliver effector molecules to host cells. *Trends Microbiol.* **2000**, *8*, 354–360. [CrossRef]

51. Galán, J.E.; Lara-Tejero, M.; Marlovits, T.C.; Wagner, S. Bacterial type III secretion systems: Specialized nanomachines for protein delivery into target cells. *Annu. Rev. Microbiol.* **2014**, *68*, 415–438. [CrossRef] [PubMed]

52. Wang, J.; Wang, Y.; Lou, H.; Wang, W. AlgU controls environmental stress adaptation, biofilm formation, motility, pyochelin synthesis and antagonism potential in *Pseudomonas protegens* SN15-2. *Microbiol. Res.* **2023**, *272*, 127396. [CrossRef] [PubMed]

53. Shukla, B.; Singh, D.; Sanyal, S. Attachment of non-culturable toxigenic Vibrio cholerae 01 and non-01 and Aeromonas spp. to the aquatic arthropod Gerris spinolae and plants in the River Ganga, Varanasi. *FEMS Immunol. Med. Microbiol.* **1995**, *12*, 113–120. [CrossRef]

54. Watnick, P.I.; Fullner, K.J.; Kolter, R. A role for the mannose-sensitive hemagglutinin in biofilm formation by *Vibrio cholerae* El Tor. *J. Bacteriol.* **1999**, *181*, 3606–3609. [CrossRef] [PubMed]

55. Coulthurst, S.J. The Type VI secretion system—A widespread and versatile cell targeting system. *Res. Microbiol.* **2013**, *164*, 640–654. [CrossRef] [PubMed]

56. Ho, B.T.; Dong, T.G.; Mekalanos, J.J. A view to a kill: The bacterial type VI secretion system. *Cell Host Microbe* **2014**, *15*, 9–21. [CrossRef]

57. Gharechahi, J.; Vahidi, M.F.; Bahram, M.; Han, J.-L.; Ding, X.-Z.; Salekdeh, G.H. Metagenomic analysis reveals a dynamic microbiome with diversified adaptive functions to utilize high lignocellulosic forages in the cattle rumen. *ISME J.* **2021**, *15*, 1108–1120. [CrossRef]

58. Grzymski, J.J.; Murray, A.E.; Campbell, B.J.; Kaplarevic, M.; Gao, G.R.; Lee, C.; Daniel, R.; Ghadiri, A.; Feldman, R.A.; Cary, S.C. Metagenome analysis of an extreme microbial symbiosis reveals eurythermal adaptation and metabolic flexibility. *Proc. Natl. Acad. Sci. USA* **2008**, *105*, 17516–17521. [CrossRef]

59. Edirisinghe, J.N.; Weisenhorn, P.; Conrad, N.; Xia, F.; Overbeek, R.; Stevens, R.L.; Henry, C.S. Modeling central metabolism and energy biosynthesis across microbial life. *BMC Genom.* **2016**, *17*, 568. [CrossRef]

60. Jiang, X.; Yan, Y.; Feng, L.; Wang, F.; Guo, Y.; Zhang, X.; Zhang, Z. Bisphenol A alters volatile fatty acids accumulation during sludge anaerobic fermentation by affecting amino acid metabolism, material transport and carbohydrate-active enzymes. *Bioresour. Technol.* **2021**, *323*, 124588. [CrossRef]

61. Millet, C.O.; Lloyd, D.; Coogan, M.P.; Rumsey, J.; Cable, J. Carbohydrate and amino acid metabolism of *Spironucleus vortens*. *Exp. Parasitol.* **2011**, *129*, 17–26. [CrossRef] [PubMed]

62. Brooks, A.N.; Turkarslan, S.; Beer, K.D.; Yin Lo, F.; Baliga, N.S. Adaptation of cells to new environments. *Wiley Interdiscip. Rev. Syst. Biol. Med.* **2011**, *3*, 544–561. [CrossRef] [PubMed]

63. Mitchell, A.; Romano, G.H.; Groisman, B.; Yona, A.; Dekel, E.; Kupiec, M.; Dahan, O.; Pilpel, Y. Adaptive prediction of environmental changes by microorganisms. *Nature* **2009**, *460*, 220–224. [CrossRef] [PubMed]

64. Torsvik, V.; Øvreås, L. Microbial Diversity, Life Strategies, and Adaptation to Life in Extreme Soils. In *Microbiology of Extreme Soils*; Springer: Berlin/Heidelberg, Germany, 2008; pp. 15–43.

65. Huang, L.; Ahmed, S.; Gu, Y.; Huang, J.; An, B.; Wu, C.; Zhou, Y.; Cheng, G. The effects of natural products and environmental conditions on antimicrobial resistance. *Molecules* **2021**, *26*, 4277. [CrossRef]

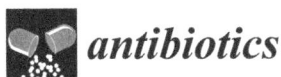

antibiotics

Article

Developing a Slow-Release Permanganate Composite for Degrading Aquaculture Antibiotics

Chainarong Sakulthaew [1], Chanat Chokejaroenrat [2,*], Sidaporn Panya [2], Apisit Songsasen [3], Kitipong Poomipuen [1], Saksit Imman [4], Nopparat Suriyachai [4], Torpong Kreetachat [4] and Steve Comfort [5]

[1] Department of Veterinary Technology, Faculty of Veterinary Technology, Kasetsart University, Bangkok 10900, Thailand; cvtcns@ku.ac.th (C.S.); kitipong.po@ku.th (K.P.)
[2] Department of Environmental Technology and Management, Faculty of Environment, Kasetsart University, Bangkok 10900, Thailand; sidaporn.pa@ku.th
[3] Department of Chemistry and Center of Excellence for Innovation in Chemistry, Faculty of Science, Kasetsart University, Bangkok 10900, Thailand; fsciass@ku.ac.th
[4] Integrated Biorefinery Excellent Center (IBC), School of Energy and Environment, University of Phayao, Phayao 56000, Thailand; saksit.im@up.ac.th (S.I.); nopparat.su@up.ac.th (N.S.); torpong.kr@up.ac.th (T.K.)
[5] School of Natural Resources, University of Nebraska-Lincoln, Lincoln, NE 68583-0915, USA; scomfort1@unl.edu
* Correspondence: chanat.c@ku.ac.th; Tel.: +66-2579-3877

Abstract: Copious use of antibiotics in aquaculture farming systems has resulted in surface water contamination in some countries. Our objective was to develop a slow-release oxidant that could be used in situ to reduce antibiotic concentrations in discharges from aquaculture lagoons. We accomplished this by generating a slow-release permanganate (SR-MnO_4^-) that was composed of a biodegradable wax and a phosphate-based dispersing agent. Sulfadimethoxine (SDM) and its synergistic antibiotics were used as representative surrogates. Kinetic experiments verified that the antibiotic-MnO_4^- reactions were first-order with respect to MnO_4^- and initial antibiotic concentration (second-order rates: 0.056–0.128 s^{-1} M^{-1}). A series of batch experiments showed that solution pH, water matrices, and humic acids impacted SDM degradation efficiency. Degradation plateaus were observed in the presence of humic acids (>20 mgL^{-1}), which caused greater MnO_2 production. A mixture of $KMnO_4$/beeswax/paraffin (SRB) at a ratio of 11.5:4:1 (w/w) was better for biodegradability and the continual release of MnO_4^-, but MnO_2 formation altered release patterns. Adding tetrapotassium pyrophosphate (TKPP) into the composite resulted in delaying MnO_2 aggregation and increased SDM removal efficiency to 90% due to the increased oxidative sites on the MnO_2 particle surface. The MnO_4^- release data fit the Siepmann–Peppas model over the long term (t < 48 d) while a Higuchi model provided a better fit for shorter timeframes (t < 8 d). Our flow-through discharge tank system using SRB with TKPP continually reduced the SDM concentration in both DI water and lagoon wastewater. These results support SRB with TKPP as an effective composite for treating antibiotic residues in aquaculture discharge water.

Keywords: antibiotic removal; binding agents; dispersing agents; permanganate oxidation; release kinetics; slow-release formulations

Citation: Sakulthaew, C.; Chokejaroenrat, C.; Panya, S.; Songsasen, A.; Poomipuen, K.; Imman, S.; Suriyachai, N.; Kreetachat, T.; Comfort, S. Developing a Slow-Release Permanganate Composite for Degrading Aquaculture Antibiotics. *Antibiotics* **2023**, *12*, 1025. https://doi.org/10.3390/antibiotics12061025

Academic Editors: Jonathan Frye, Anusak Kerdsin and Jinquan Li

Received: 14 May 2023
Revised: 27 May 2023
Accepted: 1 June 2023
Published: 7 June 2023

1. Introduction

Veterinary antibiotics are indispensable inputs for aquaculture practices. While both prophylactic and therapeutic uses of antibiotics are very effective in promoting aquacultural yields, the subsequent effects of antibiotics on water quality have largely been ignored [1–3]. Antibiotic-contaminated discharge water usually receives zero or insufficient treatment prior to being released into downgradient watersheds. Subsequently, these untreated antibiotics may affect the environment by introducing antibiotic-resistant pathogens or killing waterborne microorganisms [4].

In this study, sulfadimethoxine (SDM) was selected as a representative antibiotic because it is the most commonly used sulfonamide antibiotic in veterinary medicine and is administered solely or synergistically with ormetoprim (OMP) and trimethoprim (TMP) [5]. Moreover, previous researchers have documented that SDM-contaminated water can pollute drinking water supplies and may cause environmental threats. For example, Yuan et al. [6] collected samples from natural receiving water and sediment from the Hangzhou Bay area of China and found SDM in the range of 0.59–1.21 ng L^{-1}; SDM concentrations in the range 1.73–2.5 ng L^{-1} were detected in drinking water sources for Guilin area, China [7]. Zhou et al. [8] found that SDM was toxic to four aquatic organisms (microalgae, freshwater *Chlorella vulgaris*, marine *Isochrysis galbana*, and *Daphnia magna*). Finally, SDM and other sulfonamide antibiotics are not readily biodegradable; thus, they require a longer time for conventional biological treatment [9]. Therefore, it may be necessary to oxidize the SDM into smaller molecules before applying a biodegradation process.

Removing antibiotics from aquaculture systems presents numerous challenges. Frequently employed technologies, such as chlorination, exhibit limited efficacy and could lead to unexpected ecological consequences from byproduct toxicity [10]. Recently, several techniques have been devised for the removal of antibiotic pollutants from aqueous solutions, including adsorption, photocatalysis, persulfate oxidation, and advanced oxidation processes (AOPs) [11–15]. However, a significant challenge to these techniques mostly pertains to the high levels of dissolved organic carbon concentrations present in the wastewater generated by aquaculture farming. As a result, a large quantity of MnO$_4^-$ is necessary to address this issue. The configurations of the discharge zones in aquaculture lagoons also create chemical application issues, such as how to apply the oxidant and how often.

The efficacy of a slow-release oxidant has been demonstrated in providing a gradual and prolonged release over a period of time, which negates the need for oxidant replenishment. The two most suitable oxidants include persulfate (S$_2$O$_8^{2-}$) and permanganate (MnO$_4^-$). Although slow-release persulfate has shown potential as a remediation option for subsurface contaminants, it typically necessitates an activation method to produce more potent radicals (i.e., SO$_4^{\cdot-}$) [16,17]. Therefore, the selection of slow-release permanganate (SR-MnO$_4^-$) appears to be more appealing due to its potential for facile implementation [18,19].

Various composites have been developed to produce SR-MnO$_4^-$. The type of binding agent in the formulation, such as paraffin wax, polymer, or cement, is an important factor in MnO$_4^-$ release [19–22]. Where possible, a biodegradable binding agent material is preferable to a synthetic one [23]. In addition, the manganese dioxide (MnO$_2$) that forms during the release of MnO$_4^-$ can block pores used for permanganate diffusion from the SR surface [24]. To date, only a few studies have investigated the releasing mechanisms of SR-MnO$_4^-$ using modeling [25].

Our objective was to develop a slow-release permanganate composite using biowax and a phosphate-based dispersing agent that could be used in situ to reduce antibiotic concentrations in aquaculture lagoons. In this study, we determined changes in the physicochemical properties on the slow-release surfaces, the releasing patterns of permanganate, the optimum composite for maintaining the continual release of permanganate, the influential effects on antibiotic degradation, and the impact environmental conditions had on antibiotic degradation rates.

2. Results and Discussion

2.1. Antibiotic Kinetic Experiments

Results showed that antibiotic concentrations (SDM, OMP, and TMP) proportionally decreased faster at higher MnO$_4^-$ concentrations or lower initial antibiotic concentrations (Supplementary Materials Figure S1). Quick drops in SDM concentrations were observed, unlike those of OMP and TMP, which displayed a continual decrease (Figure S1A vs. Figure S1B,C). Here, the difference in antibiotic degradation efficiency was solely attributable to where MnO_4^- would tend to attack preferentially, such as the S-N bond of sulfonamide and aniline-SO_2 [26,27].

Laszakovits et al. [28] reported that MnO_4^- was in excess when the molar ratio of MnO_4^- to contaminant was 5–10, and then the antibiotic destruction rates (k_{obs}) can be determined as pseudo 1st order rates ($k_{obs\text{-}SDM}$ = 0.017–3.893 h^{-1}, $k_{obs\text{-}OMP}$ = 0.033–0.514 h^{-1}, and $k_{obs\text{-}TMP}$ = 0.029–0.307 h^{-1}). According to the general rate equation (Equation (1)), the 2nd order rate constant (k^n) can be calculated from Equations (2) and (3):

$$r = k^n [Antib]^\alpha [MnO_4^-]^\beta \tag{1}$$

$$r = k_{obs}[Antib]^\alpha \tag{2}$$

$$k^n = \frac{k_{obs}}{[MnO_4^-]^\beta} \tag{3}$$

where r is the reaction rate, α is the reaction order with respect to antibiotics, and β is the reaction order with respect to MnO_4^-.

By using these equations, these antibiotic-MnO_4^- reactions resulted in second-order rates of 0.128 ± 0.062 s^{-1} M^{-1} for SDM, 0.097 ± 0.005 s^{-1} M^{-1} for OMP, and 0.056 ± 0.008 s^{-1} M^{-1} for TMP (Figure 1). These rates were consistent with the ranges for other antibiotics under similar conditions, such as ciprofloxacin (0.61 s^{-1} M^{-1}) [29]. Hassan et al. [30] have suggested that the accelerated degradation rate observed in the presence of MnO_4^- could also be attributed to the presence of other active manganese oxide species (MnO_x) that may have acted concurrently with MnO_4^-, especially at lower solution pH levels. In our case, the organic solvent was not involved in the experimental setup and so could not cause the auto-decomposition of MnO_4^- to produce MnO_2, as the MnO_4^- concentration ratio was quite high [31]. Therefore, any effect from MnO_x during our oxidation process was unlikely.

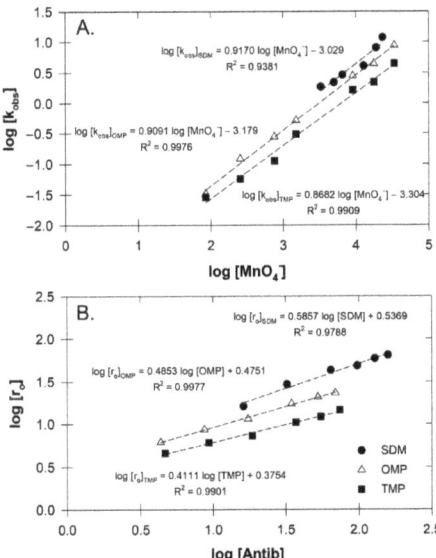

Figure 1. (**A**) Plot of pseudo-order rate constants and various concentrations of MnO_4^- for antibiotics three antibiotics (Sulfadimethoxine, SDM; ormetoprim, OMP; or trimethoprim, TMP) treated with MnO_4^- (**B**) Plot of initial rates and various concentrations of antibiotics when treated with MnO_4^- at 1.133 mM.

2.2. Effect of Co-Contaminants

The presence of OMP or TMP with SDM resulted in a 3-fold decreased rate of SDM degradation (Figure S2A). Likewise, adding SDM to OMP slowed OMP degradation by 8-fold, and adding SDM to TMP slowed TMP degradation by 6.5-fold (Figure S2B,C). This confirmed our previous results that SDM was preferentially oxidized over OMP and TMP and that the sensitivity of the core molecules to MnO_4^- was the limiting factor for antibiotic degradation.

Here, the sulfonamide structure was more prone to disruption than the diaminopyridine ring of OMP and TMP. Albeit these three aquaculture antibiotics could be ultimately removed, the required time was quite extended compared to other well-known antibiotics, such as oxytetracycline. The presence of the N atom on the heterocyclic ring of SDM, OMP, and TMP, can minimize the electron density on the rings and deflect the attack by MnO_4^- to initiate the ring cleavage [32].

2.3. Effect of Initial pH

We observed changes from the initial pH level toward a neutral pH and a slight decrease of MnO_4^- (inset of Figure 2A). Using twice as much MnO_4^- (3.34 mM) also produced similar changes in MnO_4^- and pH. As the MnO_4^- reaction proceeds, the Mn–byproduct (MnO_2) will naturally form, and the pH will more likely be in the range of 4–6. This would allow the MnO_2 to enhance the oxidative performance, resulting in a faster reaction in this pH range [27]. Although MnO_2 can catalyze oxidative reactions, it could negatively impact our slow-release MnO_4^-. MnO_2 can also block MnO_4^- releasing passage from the slow-release composite, which would delay contaminant degradation. Therefore, minimizing MnO_2 during treatment was an important research niche for developing a slow-release oxidant composite for aquacultural systems.

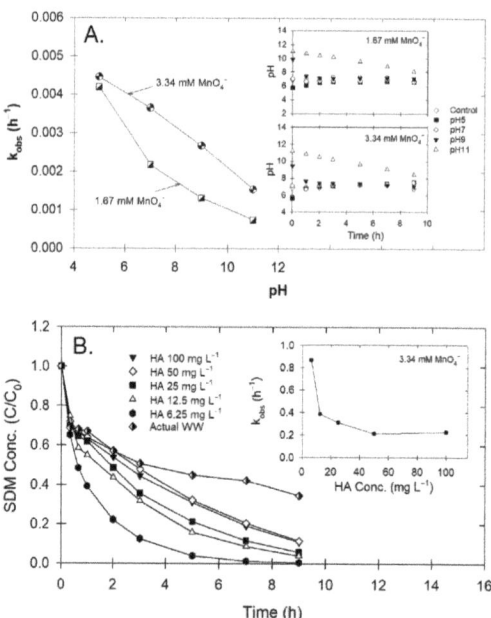

Figure 2. (**A**) Observed kinetic rate constant (k_{obs}) of SDM degradation with different initial pH levels following treatment with MnO_4^-. Inset graph shows temporal changes of pH of corresponding MnO_4^- concentration. (**B**) Temporal changes of SDM concentration following treatment with MnO_4^- under varying humic acid concentrations or actual wastewater discharge. Inset graph shows comparison of k_{obs} at corresponding HA concentration.

2.4. Effect of Humic Acids and Real Wastewater

Results showed that the k_{obs} decreased with increasing humic acid, indicating the strong influence of HM on SDM degradation (Figure 2B). Conversely, Sun et al. [33] reported that the presence of HM increased contaminant removal efficiency via the formation of a secondary oxidant (MnO_2) during the MnO_4^- reaction. However, the increased k_{obs} did not appear in our experiments, perhaps due to several reasons: (1) the operating pH (unbuffered pH) did not facilitate MnO_2 formation; (2) the SDM-MnO_4^- rate was quite slow compared to the tentative reaction time of MnO_2 with other contaminants, which usually occurred within the first 30 min; and (3) over time, the MnO_4^- concentration was unchanged, indicating that if MnO_2 did form, it might be insufficient to initiate MnO_2 oxidation. Notably, k_{obs} values were unchanged at high HM concentrations; in addition, the SDM relative concentration seemed to reach a plateau sooner with the wastewater compared to the 100 mg L^{-1} HM solution (Figure 2B). Here, MnO_2 may have been readily liberated as the MnO_4^- was surrounded by organic constituents that are prone to react with any oxidative substance.

Given these possibilities, previous reports also demonstrated that the interaction of organic matter with oxidative molecules was quite complex; thus, different types of impact may be expected depending on the oxidant. For example, phenolic moieties in organic matter may also act as an activator for persulfate oxidation, which would result in a much faster degradation rate [34]. However, our results showed that humic substances could have a major inhibitory effect on SDM degradation, delaying it by as much as 50% compared to the control (no HM; Figure S1 vs. Figure 2B). Similar observations showed that, at only 5 mg L^{-1} of HM, the degradation of sulfamethoxazole was inhibited during MnO_4^- oxidation (Gao et al., 2014). Therefore, prolonging the contact time of the oxidant and having a slightly higher MnO_4^- concentration must be considered for real-world applications. The aforementioned statements provide sufficient proof to support the beneficial application of slow-release MnO_4^-.

2.5. Release Concentration of SR Permanganate

2.5.1. Release Concentration

Using paraffin and no biowax, a rigid cylindrical shape was produced that provided the continual release of MnO_4^- up to ~500 mg L^{-1}, which was nearly 95% of MnO_4^- in one SR (Figure S3B). Because paraffin mostly contains saturated long-chain hydrocarbons (C18–C60), its biodegradation can take some time. Furthermore, Carrilloa et al. [35] reported that the accumulation of paraffin wax can cause severe health effects on aquatic life and their habitat, which could also threaten human health.

During the preparation of slow-release samples, we found that the soy wax-paraffin-MnO_4^- mixture was unlikely to form. The mixture's homogeneity was so sparse that the material was crumbly with an obvious covering of wax. These crumbs provided individual encapsulation that would have served as many SR-MnO_4^- sites and therefore provided higher MnO_4^- release (Figure S3C). The deformation of soy wax may have been due to its being more branched with short-chain fatty acids, hydroxyl groups, and containing more ester compounds, making it very difficult to form a rigid SR [23,36]. In addition, soy wax thermographs from differential scanning calorimetry support its ability to melt at a lower temperature compared to paraffin and beeswax [37]. We believe that these abilities may cause deformity of the mixture and its failure to re-solidify into the desired shape at room temperature, resulting in undesirable shredding. However, our current results showed that the releasing concentration was quite low (<350 mg L^{-1}) as most $KMnO_4$ granules were entirely covered with unmixed waxes that minimized the surface diffusion channel, worsening the release of MnO_4^- (Figure S3C).

As discussed earlier, the physicochemical properties of waxes play an important role in the releasing ability of MnO_4^-. The rice bran wax chemical composition was ester compounds (up to 73.4%), triacylglycerols (21.9%), and free aliphatic alcohol (4.6%) [38]. Here, rice bran wax failed to form a rigid shape with any of the mixtures as the MnO_4^- releasing concentrations were inconsistent for both short-term (<7 d) and long term (>7 d) release, resulting in large variations in the MnO_4^- concentration (Figure S3D). In addition, the rice bran wax tended to swell in water in our separate swelling test experiment. Therefore, rice bran wax was not suitable as a binding agent for $SR-MnO_4^-$.

On the other hand, beeswax performed very similarly to using paraffin alone, despite lessening the amount of paraffin in the wax proportion, resulting in a spongier surface. In terms of releasing MnO_4^- concentration, large concentration discrepancies were observed between samples from 0.25 d to 7 d and from 28 d to 56 d. In contrast, the releasing concentration was quite consistent from 7 d to 28 d (Figure S3E). Compared to the paraffin, the initial phase of beeswax provided 1-fold more releasing concentration, indicating that beeswax was a better binding agent than paraffin alone (Figure S3B vs. Figure S3E). With time, oxidation of MnO_4^- on the beeswax slowly occurred, with the possible formation of MnO_2, resulting in blockage of the diffusing channel of MnO_4^- during 7 d to 28 d. We observed more obvious cracks on the SR surface on day 28, which created new diffusing channels, resulting in more MnO_4^- concentration being released. At 56 d, the highest concentrations of beeswax at all ratios were still 17% lower than from using paraffin alone (Figure S3E).

In terms of chemical composition, beeswax consists of longer chain carbons compared to soy wax. One of the major components of beeswax is esters, which contain up to 52 carbons and a series fraction of internal chain methylene (int-(CH_2)) [39]. Therefore, the beeswax can degrade more easily than paraffin.

2.5.2. SR-MnO$_4^-$ Surface Properties

We initially selected beeswax $SR-MnO_4^-$ (SRB) to further characterize its changes in surface properties using FTIR (Figure 3). The double peaks at 2912–2845 cm^{-1} were attributed to the presence of fatty acid chains, while peaks at 1320 and 729 cm^{-1} were ascribed to C-H stretching in symmetry with aliphatic hydrocarbons and the amide group. These spectra resembled the major component of natural beeswax [40]. The signals at 1467 and 1794 cm^{-1} belonged to the C=C stretching band of saturated hydrocarbons and the C=O stretching vibration in the wax polymer.

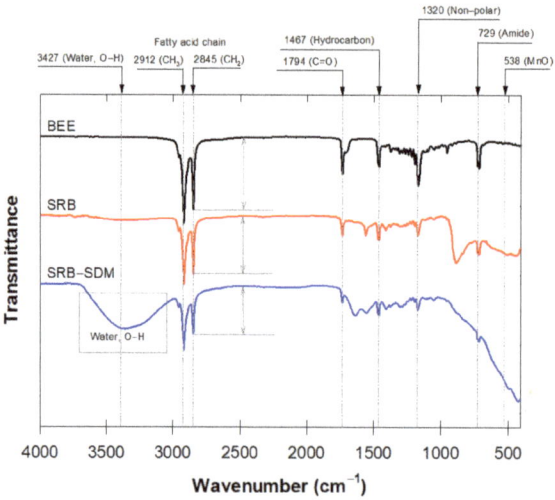

Figure 3. Fourier-transform infrared spectroscopy spectra of three different SRs: pure beeswax (BEE), slow-release permanganate consisted beeswax in the mixture (SRB), and SRB after soaked in SDM solution.

The peak intensities decreased with a decreased portion of beeswax in the SRB and SRB-SDM, while still showing the original components of beeswax (Figure 3). This decrease may imply that the short longevity of SRB improved its suitability for being biodegradable. The absence of the CH_2 rocking bands at 800 cm^{-1} on the SRB-SDM indicated the loss of the crystal structure of the hydrocarbon chain due to MnO_4^- oxidation on the SR surface during the batch experiment. Shaabani et al. [41] reported that MnO_4^- oxidation was responsible for shortening the aliphatic hydrocarbon chain, causing the disappearance of the FTIR bands. The 538 cm^{-1} band corresponded to the stretching vibration of the adsorption band of MnO on the MnO_2 molecular structure that resulted from the SDM-MnO_4^- reaction [42]. Therefore, it could be concluded that the MnO_2 rind that appeared on the SRB surface during oxidation could later block the MnO_4^- diffusing passage. This meant that chemical additions, such as dispersing agents, were needed to prevent the aggregation of MnO_2 and simultaneously enlarge the release passage.

2.5.3. Chemical Addition/MnO_4^- Residual on Surface

In this releasing experiment of mixture set B, we selectively presented the controls (XC0) and ones denoted as XT1, XT2, XS1, and XS2 where X represents the type of wax—S, R, B, or P—in the successive releasing experiment (Figure S4). Despite adding the TKPP or SHMP to benefit the emulsifying activity and support gel formation in the mixture [43], at higher amounts (>0.04 g), our SR failed to achieve the desired cylindrical shape after one week (Table S4). This is because increasing the dispersing agent by more than 2.5% of the total SR weight—the total of binding agents was then less than 24.7%—could easily dissolve in water and leave voids in the SR surface, making it unstable to maintain the original shape (Table S4).

We found that in the short term, chemical addition made only minor differences in the MnO_4^- release compared to previous experiments with no chemical addition (Figure S3 vs. Figure S4). Soy wax and rice bran wax still presented oscillated concentrations due to unsuitability between the binding agent and MnO_4^-, while beeswax and paraffin provided more stable release. Among these various tests, BT2 and BS2 provided the best releasing concentration (Figure S4), which was approximately 20% better than without chemical addition (Figure S3). This was due to the phosphate ions binding with the colloidal manganese oxide, resulting in the creation of repulsive forces that later delayed MnO_2 aggregation.

2.5.4. Releasing Empirical Formula

Generally, release MnO_4^- concentration showed fresh dissolution in the initial phase, followed by continual release until reaching the saturation plateau (Figure S6). Although most of the MnO_4^- release patterns had similar trends, the release kinetics differed depending on various types of mixtures and amounts of binding agent (Table 1). The MnO_4^- release pattern can be varied depending on the uniformity of the mixture and the granule-aligning configuration of the SR. Biphasic graph types of the release kinetics were observed in all the SR formulations, confirming the common pattern for oxidant release, as our research group previously demonstrated (Table 1; Figures S6–S10). We evaluated a full range of experimental times (60 d) for all the theoretical models, except the Higuchi models, in which the partial time (~60% of released concentration; ~8 d) was separately evaluated, as suggested by Passot et al. [44]. The results indicated that beeswax and paraffin had longer steady state time spans (11 d vs. 15 d) than those of soy wax and rice bran wax (~5 d; Figure S7). Therefore, linear regression for the shorter timespan (<8 d) for the Higuchi model provided a better fit (Figure S8).

Table 1. Release model parameters for selected types of SR (paraffin and beeswax) with different chemical additions (TKPP or SHMP).

Model	Siepman-Peppas				Higuchi; t < 60 d			Higuchi; t ≤ 8 d			Noyes-Whitney			Weibull			
Generalized Eq.	$R_t = \alpha t^\beta$				$R_t = k\sqrt{t}$			$R_t = k\sqrt{t}$			$-\ln(1-R_t) = kt$			$\ln[-\ln(1-R_t/100)] = \ln\alpha + \beta\ln t$			
Graphs	Figure S5				Figure S6			Figure S7			Figure S8			Figure S9			
Parameters	α	β	R²	r²adj	k	R²	r²adj	k	R²	r²adj	k	R²	r²adj	α	β	R²	r²adj
SC0	186.9	0.216	0.815	0.736	65.75	0.113	N/A	163.1	0.932	0.898	0.0361	N/A	N/A	0.3555	0.4325	0.8661	0.809
ST1	195.7	0.189	0.801	0.716	56.64	N/A	N/A	144.8	0.894	0.841	0.0276	N/A	N/A	0.3119	0.4536	0.8476	0.782
ST2	214.2	0.170	0.822	0.746	57.24	N/A	N/A	151.6	0.907	0.861	0.0296	N/A	N/A	0.3816	0.4015	0.8557	0.794
SS1	183.7	0.212	0.797	0.710	63.24	0.055	N/A	161.4	0.93	0.895	0.0359	N/A	N/A	0.3335	0.5269	0.8673	0.810
SS2	171.3	0.221	0.826	0.751	62.30	0.194	N/A	142.3	0.926	0.889	0.0304	N/A	N/A	0.3067	0.4877	0.8740	0.820
RC0	199.7	0.212	0.824	0.749	55.66	N/A	N/A	140.9	0.87	0.805	-0.0265	N/A	N/A	0.3639	0.3899	0.8171	0.739
RT1	207.0	0.189	0.804	0.720	52.79	N/A	N/A	152.4	0.86	0.790	-0.0266	N/A	N/A	0.3548	0.3924	0.8432	0.776
RT2	222.6	0.174	0.820	0.743	52.68	N/A	N/A	146.6	0.842	0.763	-0.0272	N/A	N/A	0.3243	0.4192	0.8786	0.827
RS1	196.4	0.209	0.797	0.710	53.27	N/A	N/A	135.8	0.929	0.894	-0.0243	N/A	N/A	0.3431	0.4012	0.8891	0.842
RS2	187.8	0.212	0.809	0.727	55.53	N/A	N/A	134.6	0.885	0.828	-0.0274	N/A	N/A	0.3713	0.3667	0.8923	0.846
BC0	137.4	0.313	0.933	0.904	73.47	0.791	0.739	97.40	0.984	0.976	-0.0396 (-0.0995)	0.371 (0.980)	0.214 (0.975)	0.8823	0.4831	0.9667	0.952
BT1	142.8	0.296	0.95	0.929	71.78	0.743	0.679	101.2	0.994	0.991	-0.0365 (-0.9901)	0.171 (0.978)	N/A (0.973)	0.2556	0.5198	0.9698	0.957
BT2	114.1	0.343	0.957	0.939	66.27	0.862	0.828	91.90	0.989	0.984	-0.0325 (-0.0727)	0.518 (0.952)	N/A (0.940)	0.2306	0.4737	0.9805	0.972
BS1	169.9	0.250	0.854	0.791	70.06	0.545	0.431	124.8	0.974	0.961	-0.0349 (-0.1162)	N/A (0.896)	N/A (0.870)	0.8908	0.4774	0.9281	0.897
BS2	216.3	0.189	0.85	0.786	64.85	0.119	N/A	153.5	0.966	0.949	-0.0355 (-0.1306)	N/A (0.631)	N/A (0.539)	0.4012	0.4398	0.8958	0.851
PC0	238.6	0.199	0.944	0.920	74.47	0.238	0.048	154.6	0.939	0.909	-0.0563 (-0.1603)	N/A (0.829)	N/A (0.786)	0.5897	0.3955	0.9732	0.962
PT1	241.2	0.186	0.934	0.906	70.18	0.083	N/A	166.7	0.935	0.903	-0.0465 (-0.1472)	N/A (0.480)	N/A (0.350)	0.5432	0.3993	0.9431	0.919
PT2	247.3	0.185	0.93	0.900	71.45	0.069	N/A	168.3	0.942	0.913	-0.0499 (-0.1747)	N/A (0.786)	N/A (0.733)	0.5666	0.4048	0.9291	0.899
PS1	234.5	0.201	0.933	0.904	73.64	0.229	0.036	160.0	0.961	0.942	-0.0509 (-0.1746)	N/A (0.859)	N/A (0.824)	0.5650	0.4044	0.9311	0.902
PS2	237.9	0.189	0.937	0.910	70.38	0.118	N/A	161.8	0.943	0.915	-0.0470 (-0.1594)	N/A (0.764)	N/A (0.705)	0.5638	0.3809	0.9382	0.912

All of the r^2_{adj} values obtained using the Noyes-Whitney model were unsatisfactory due to the slight increase toward the end of releasing experiments and its possessing biphasic behavior (Table 1; Figure S9). The Noyes-Whitney model calculation is based on a uniform layer, while our SR was manufactured from a mixture of binding agents, which may not have uniformly encapsulated both granules of MnO_4^- and the dispersing agents. In addition, we observed that only beeswax with dispersing agents (BT1, BT2, and BS1) could provide a better fit within the first 15 d of the experiment ($r^2_{adj} > 0.87$). This might have been due to the texture of the beeswax itself, which allowed for more uniform mixing from the circumferential surface toward the center of the SR cylinder. In addition, TKPP and biowax were better distributed in the SR mixture than SHMP. Unlike the Higuchi model, it was clear that the Noyes-Whitney model would only be suitable for slow-release types that had reached 80% of the released concentration.

The lack of correlation using the Weibull model was observed for soy wax and rice bran wax (r^2_{adj} values of 0.73–0.84; Table 1; Figure S10). Because of the obvious biphasic feature of the release pattern in these two types of biowax, it was unlikely to achieve a well-fitted pattern with a Weibull model. Unlike the beeswax and paraffin SR, the r^2_{adj} was better described with the Weibull model. Furthermore, the shape parameters (β values) of 0.3667–0.5269 in all formulations implied that the SR released MnO_4^- according to Fickian diffusion [45].

Among the other models, the Higuchi model could better provide phenomenological analysis of releasing data, but only within the recommended timeline [44]. None of the r^2_{adj} values for SR manufacturing with soy wax and rice bran wax were acceptable in the full timespan range (Table 1), confirming that these SR types did not correlate well with this model using the entire timespan and that these waxes contributed to the random release of MnO_4^-, even in the initial phase. These physical wax characteristics were so inconsistent that the wax texture prevented the mixture uniformity. The uneven mixture was probably the main reason causing the rind and wax blockage on the MnO_4^- dissolution front.

Considering only $t < 8$ d, the r^2_{adj} values using soy wax and rice bran wax were still unsatisfactory, with the paraffin and beeswax applications providing much better fits (r^2_{adj} 0.944–0.991; Table 1). In addition, when paraffin was used with TKPP or SHMP addition, the k values were more consistent compared to those using beeswax, indicating that paraffin could provide a likely controllable release (Table 1). The beeswax was more likely controllable with TKPP addition than SHMP addition.

Overall, in the beeswax formulations, TKPP addition produced a better fit and slightly lower k values than SHMP addition. By extending to the full range of release analysis, the Siepmann-Peppas model, based on the power law model, was better suited with much higher r^2_{adj} values and could better predict the release of MnO_4^- from the SR mixture formulation. Similar to the Higuchi model, only formulations with beeswax or paraffin only provided relatively high r^2_{adj} values > 0.9. The only exception was the SHMP addition in the beeswax formulation that provided a relatively low r^2_{adj} value, indicating that SHMP might not be a good candidate to provide constant MnO_4^- release.

The results obtained by applying the Siepmann-Peppas model showed that this model was most suitable for full-range analysis of the release of MnO_4^-. The release longevity revealed that the MnO_4^- reached its maximum capacity no later than 20 d (Figure S6). It also revealed that the MnO_4^- releasing trends were deliberate when the α and β values were lower than 200 and relatively close to 0.300 (Table 1). In other words, a high amount of chemical addition would either produce an out-of-shape SR cylinder or make the release pattern unpredictably random.

In addition, from a structural wax standpoint, both paraffin and beeswax contain up to 90% CH_2 carbons, but beeswax also contains larger amounts of polar compounds, such as alcohols, free acids, and esters, [46]. When SRB meets water, part of the beeswax would swell and possibly hinder the release of MnO_4^- by partially blocking the diffusion channel. This would be unlikely to occur with paraffin as it contains mostly alkane groups, which are hydrophobic. Therefore, there could have been several pores on the SR surface once MnO_4^- started to diffuse, making it easier to control chemical release.

2.5.5. Comparison of SDM Degradations by MnO_4^- Solution and SR-MnO_4^-

Results showed that the MnO_4^- solution alone removed SDM better than the composites in the short term ($\sim$0.08 d), while the SR composites performed much better over the long term (up to 48 d) (Figure 4). A dispersing agent in SR-MnO_4^- revealed up to 20–30% better SDM removal efficiency (Figure 4). This indicated that both TKPP and SHMP could perfectly delay MnO_2 aggregation.

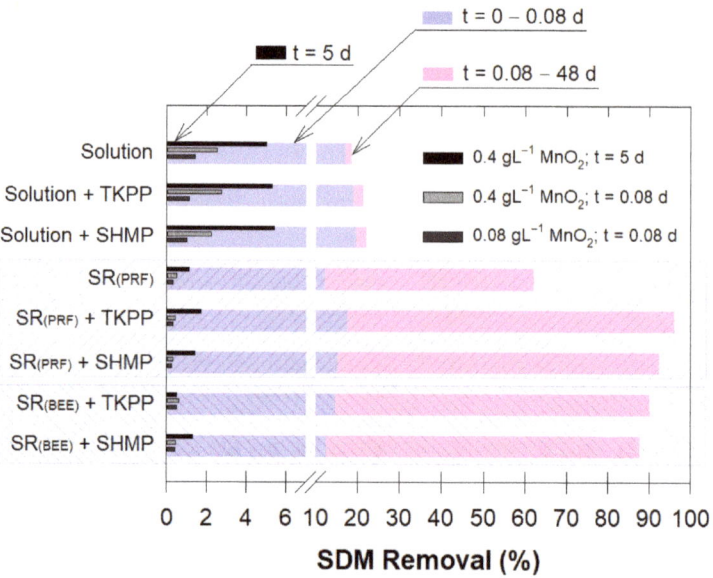

Figure 4. SDM removal percentage with different treatments of permanganate (solution or SR) for short-term (0.08 d) and long-term (48 d). Embedded bar graphs represent SDM removal percentages for different treatments of MnO_2 at varying MnO_2 amounts. The MnO_2 treatment used a similar configuration (solution or SR) to that of the corresponding MnO_4^- bar graph.

The oxidation of MnO_2 alone with SDM showed that the SDM removal was proportional to the amount of MnO_2, but to a lesser extent than for MnO_4^- and that the presence of chemical addition did not change the SDM removal efficiency (see embedded bars in Figure 4). In addition, no adsorption of SDM on the MnO_2 surface was observed; rather, it has been shown to easily degrade with the initiation of electron transfer (Gao et al., 2012). Furthermore, the available oxidative sites on the MnO_2 surface could be hindered by binding agent embedment on the MnO_2 particles. The formation of rind on the SR surface could be minimized by using a dispersing agent, which allowed more MnO_4^- to be released into the solution.

The paraffin SR-MnO_4^- was better at releasing MnO_4^- and degrading SDM compared to the beeswax SR-MnO_4^- (Figure 4, Figures S3 and S4). However, adding TKPP was a better combination with beeswax than adding SHMP, regardless of these two SR types. This was due to the smaller phosphate group attached to the TKPP molecules (diphosphate or pyrophosphate) (Table S2) that allowed better chelating ability on metal ions and the shorter chained polyphosphates of TKPP, giving it approximately two-fold greater water solubility than SHMP [47].

To ensure the absence of MnO_2 on the SR surface of SRB with TKPP addition, we proved the MnO_2 formation using XRD. By comparing the results of four different types of SRB with the various polymorphs of the MnO_2 standard (pyrolusite, ramsdellite, and hollandite), there was no matching of any MnO_2 formation on the surface, indicating that TKPP could successfully prevent self-aggregation of MnO_2 (Figure S5). Notably, there was also no clear evidence of colloidal or other precipitates in the solution.

2.6. SR Permanganate Use in Contact Tank

Results showed that the MnO_4^- solution could not decrease the SDM concentration in both matrices and may even have slightly increased the overall SDM concentration with time because of the continuous flow of newly flushed SDM-contaminated water into the system (Figure 5). This indicated a possible adverse effect when $KMnO_4$ was selected as the sole treatment. Although there was a slight decrease in the SDM concentration in the first cycle, the available MnO_4^- in the contact tank may have been insufficient for successive flushing cycles.

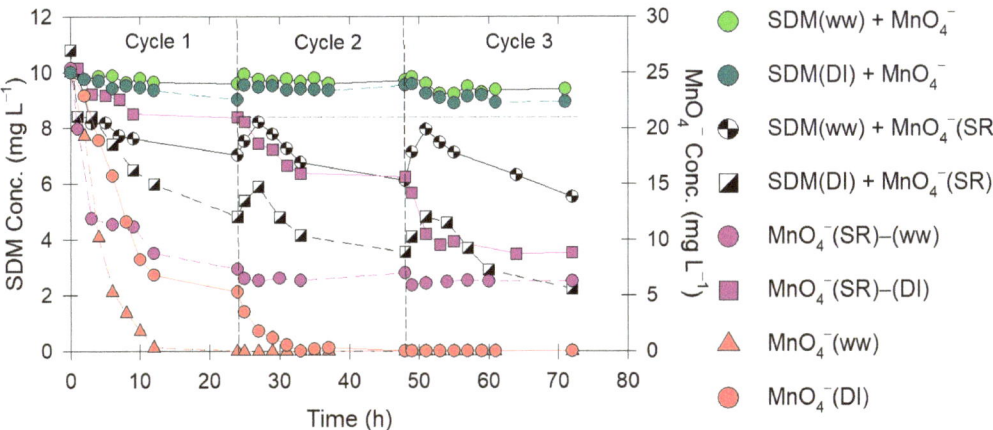

Figure 5. Temporal changes in SDM concentration (C/C_o) and MnO_4^- concentration observed in contact tank following treatment with different water matrices (DI water or actual wastewater).

When SRB (i.e., with TKPP) was used, the results showed that both the SDM concentration and the MnO_4^- residual concentration continually decreased with time (Figure 5). Again, a slight increase in the SDM concentration was observed. The MnO_4^- concentration was less than the total concentration in the releasing experiment because of the sizing difference. However, with this low concentration of MnO_4^- prior to entering the effluent reservoir, we suggest that numerous SRB types could be used and the contact time could be extended to facilitate system efficiency.

Because we expected that other organic contents would affect our system and our SRB, we mimicked the previous experiment with the actual aquaculture discharge water (ww). Similar decreasing trends in both the SDM and MnO_4^- concentrations were observed. However, after the first cycle, the overall removal percentage of SDM reached ~27% and ~55% for DI water and actual wastewater and continued to decrease with time (Figure 5). The addition of TKPP proved to prolong the slow release of MnO_4^-, delay the formation of MnO_2, and negate the need for frequent replenishment of the SRB.

Based on the SDM removal efficiency and the MnO_4^- concentration, the contact tank experiment showed less SDM removal and a lower MnO_4^- concentration than the batch experiment (Figure 5 vs. Figure S1). This could have been due to differences in the contact tank volume, indicating that regular cleaning practices and environmental conditions on the farm may need to be further evaluated with our developed SR to efficiently remove these contaminants from farming wastewater. Overall, we proved that SRB+TKPP was more effective than using MnO_4^- solution alone, provided that the existence of organic constituents in the wastewater was taken into consideration.

3. Materials and Methods

3.1. Chemicals and Analyses

The chemicals used in experiments were purchased from several vendors. Sulfadimethoxine ($C_{12}H_{14}N_4O_4S$: 122-11-2, SDM), ormetoprim ($C_{14}H_{18}N_4O_2$: 6981-18-6, OMP), and trimethoprim ($C_{14}H_{18}N_4O_3$: 738-70-5, TMP; Table S1) were obtained from Dr. Ehrenstorfer GmbH (Wesel, Germany). Manganese dioxide (MnO_2) was purchased from BDH (Poole, England). Potassium permanganate ($KMnO_4$), ascorbic acid, tetrapotassium pyrophosphate (TKPP), and sodium Hexametaphosphate (SHMP; Table S2) were of analytical reagent (AR) grade and purchased from Ajax Finechem (Oakland, New Zealand). Humic acid was obtained from Sigma-Aldrich (St. Louis, MO, USA). All SR binding agents (synthetic paraffin, paraffin, soy wax, beeswax, and rice bran wax) were acquired from Chemipan (Bangkok, Thailand), a local wax manufacturing company in Bangkok, Thailand.

Changes in antibiotic concentration were determined based on high-performance liquid chromatography (HPLC) with an e2695 unit using a diode-array UV detector no. 2998 (Waters, Milford, MA, USA). For the isocratic elution of acetonitrile, 0.1% acetic acid (60:40) was used as the mobile phase at a flow rate of 1 mL min^{-1}. The detection wavelength was set at 270 nm for SDM analysis and at 200 nm for OMP or TMP analysis. After injecting 20 µL of samples, antibiotics were separated using a Mightysil RP-18GP column (250 × ∅ 4.6 mm, 5 µm) coupled with a guard column. The MnO_4^- concentration was measured using a Cary60 Agilent UV-Vis spectrophotometer (Santa Clara, CA, USA) at a wavelength of 525 nm.

The SR samples made of selected binding agents were selectively analyzed for surface properties. Fourier-transform infrared spectroscopy (FTIR; Bruker Tensor 27; Billerica, MA, USA) was used to analyze the surface functional groups of the unheated beeswax (BEE), SR-MnO_4^- made of beeswax (SRB), and 7 d SDM-soaked solution SRB (SRB-SDM). To further confirm the absence of MnO_2 following adding chemical addition (TKPP), a 2θ scan (15–80°) was performed using X-ray diffraction (XRD; Bruker D2 Phaser; Billerica, MA, USA). Comparisons were made after using the SRB with and without TKPP on testing with SDM by soaking in SDM solution for 7 d.

3.2. Antibiotic Kinetic Experiments

The first experiment was to determine the MnO_4^- degradation efficiency of antibiotics in a series of batch experiments. A 250 mL Erlenmeyer flask was used as an experimental unit for a 100 mL aqueous solution. Unless stated otherwise, all experiment units were covered with aluminum foil to prevent photodegradation of MnO_4^-. All experiments were performed under agitation using an orbital shaker at 150 rpm. Treated samples were quenched to further prevent antibiotic transformation following treatment with MnO_4^-. We used ascorbic acid as a quenching agent instead of using manganese salts to avoid interference with the properties of aliquot samples. The typical quenching procedure involved transferring a 1 mL sample at preselected times into a 1.5 mL centrifuge tube that contained 0.1 mL of freshly prepared ascorbic acid (20,000 mg L^{-1}), centrifuging at 14,000 rpm for 10 min, removing the supernatant to an HPLC vial, and storing samples until analysis based on HPLC.

Although SDM was the main focus of this research, OMP and TMP were also selected for antibiotic kinetic experiments as they act synergistically with SDM at a 5:1 ratio in real-world medicinal applications [5]. To determine antibiotic reaction rates, we performed batch experiments where the SDM initial concentration was fixed at 161.12 µM and the MnO_4^- concentrations ranged from 0.315 to 5.033 mM. Based on the applicable ratio, OMP or TMP was fixed at 36.45 µM and 34.44 µM, and the MnO_4^- concentrations ranged from 0.189 to 27.181 mM. These high concentration ranges of MnO_4^- allowed us to evaluate the reaction rates when the MnO_4^- was in excess.

Likewise, using the initial MnO_4^- concentration at 1.133 mM, we treated varying concentrations of either SDM (16.11 to 161.12 µM) or OMP (4.56 to 72.91 µM) or TMP (4.56 to 72.91 µM) individually. The initial rate method modified from Sakulthaew and Chokejaroenrat [19] was selected to determine the kinetic order rates of the antibiotic and MnO_4^-.

In addition, we conducted a series of experiments that compared degradation rates when antibiotics were treated alone and in combination (i.e., as co-contaminants) to quantify SDM degradation in the presence of other synergistic antibiotics (OMP and TMP).

3.3. Influential Effects on Antibiotic Degradation

3.3.1. Effect of pH

The ambient pH of aquaculture water can fluctuate due to the excreted ammonia from fish following protein feeds, which can cause a slightly higher pH in the discharge water [48]. Therefore, it would be more difficult to degrade antibiotics because MnO_4^- is more efficient in acidic solutions. Therefore, we conducted a series of batch experiments to verify that the SDM destruction rates by MnO_4^- (1.67 and 3.32 mM) were similar at differing levels of the initial pH. The experiment was investigated over a pH range of 3–11 to cover a vital range (4–11). The solution pH was adjusted to the designated pH using either 0.1 M NaOH or 0.1 M HCl. A stock solution of SDM was spiked into the solution to obtain the final concentration of 161.12 µM. Samples were collected periodically following the monitoring of SDM concentrations and pH measurement of the solution.

3.3.2. Effect of Humic Acids and Real Wastewater

Aside from the micropollutant contamination in the discharge water from aquaculture farming, high levels of organic constituents can be a major contributing factor in scavenging for available MnO_4^-. In separate sets of vessels, we used a 3.32 mM solution of MnO_4^- and varied the humic acid concentration ranging from 6.25 to 100 mg L^{-1}, which was used as a representative of natural organic matter (NOM). To test the treatability of MnO_4^- on-site treatment for SDM, we used real discharge water as the solution matrix in the batch experiment. This wastewater was provided from local prawn farms in Kampangsaen district, Nakhon Pathom province, Thailand, and was collected during the harvesting period. Its water characteristics are presented in Table S3. Similar to most aquaculture farming in rural areas, this water had received insufficient treatment prior to disposal in the adjacent lagoon watershed.

3.4. Slow-Release Permanganate

A series of ratios between solid wax (acting as a binding agent), $KMnO_4$, and stabilization aids are discussed later in this section. The mixture was heated until the liquid was on a hotplate at 75 °C and continuously stirred to achieve textural homogeneity prior to pouring it into a cylindrical mold (∅ 0.6 cm). Each SR sample was trimmed and weighed to 0.75 ± 0.05 g to ensure minimal fluctuation in the release of the MnO_4^- concentration. These samples were kept in a desiccator at room temperature prior to use within 5 d.

3.4.1. Manufacturing Mixture Ratio

To determine the most optimal mixture for $SR\text{-}MnO_4^-$, two types of mixture ratios (A and B) were used for different purposes. The set A mixture was used to evaluate the best slow-but-sustained release of MnO_4^- using different kinds of binding agents (i.e., synthetic paraffin and three types of biowax), whereas the set B mixture was used to evaluate the most suitable type and the amount of dispersing agent (TKPP or SHMP) in the SR mixture. Other research proved that SHMP facilitated a more consistent release of MnO_4^- [24], and both SHMP and TKPP allowed MnO_4^- to enter low permeable zones much deeper than without using these chemical agents in the transport experiments [49].

For mixture set A, we used different amounts of each composition while maintaining the same total weight (3.3 g per batch). In general, biowax was more difficult to solidify compared to paraffin. In each batch, we varied the amount of biowax (0.2–1.0 g per batch) and the paraffin (intervals of 20% or 0–0.8 g per batch) while maintaining the same amount of $KMnO_4$ (Figure S3A). We selected this mixture ratio for the succeeding experiments based on two criteria: (1) the best slow-but-sustained release of MnO_4^- and (2) the ability of $SR-MnO_4^-$ to retain its cylindrical shape.

Mixture set B involved the addition of stabilization aids or dispersing agents. The TKPP and SHMP were reported to reduce MnO_2 rind formation substantially during the sweeping of MnO_4^- flushing in the subsurface [49]. The new mixtures were investigated using varying amounts of the stabilization aid (0.01, 0.02, 0.04, or 0.08 g) (Table S4). To elucidate the effect of the dispersing agents, we maintained the weight of each $SR-MnO_4^-$ at 0.75 ± 0.05 g and the constant amount of paraffin at 0.09 g. Therefore, we compensated for the addition of either TKPP or SHMP by reducing the amount of biowax (Table S4). Here, each type of SR is abbreviated and written as wax·chemical additive·additive amount (Figure S4; Table S4). For example, ST2 was used as the abbreviation for soy wax mixed with 0.02 g of TKPP (per SR). The additional criterion for selecting the most suitable proportion was that the SR should be able to continually release MnO_4^- in the aqueous solution while preventing rind formation.

3.4.2. MnO_4^- Releasing Experiments

Batch experiments were conducted for MnO_4^- releasing to evaluate the optimum ratio for each mixture set. Typical experiments involved placing the $SR-MnO_4^-$ into individual 1.5 L flasks that contained 1 L of water. Each container was thoroughly covered with aluminum foil to prevent MnO_4^- photodegradation. The $SR-MnO_4^-$ was suspended 10 cm from the top of the water surface using cheesecloth bags that allowed 100% MnO_4^- diffusion. Each unit was done in quadruplicate. Sampling for MnO_4^- concentrations occurred immediately after the $SR-MnO_4^-$ had been removed from the flasks. The deformity of SR was recorded as not applicable and was not considered in the succeeding experiments.

3.4.3. Slow-Release Applicability Test

By flushing SR with fresh water, the MnO_4^- concentration is quickly released via diffusion mechanisms because rind formation and different binding agents could interfere with the release of MnO_4^-. In an individual container, each SR sample from mixture set B was soaked in 1 L of water for 2 h to imitate the flushing event on aquaculture farms. The MnO_4^- concentration was monitored 12 times during 28 d. Then, we removed the SR from the soaking unit and left it at room temperature until the next sampling time. Four empirical formulas (Siepmann-Peppas, Higuchi, Noyes-Whitney, and Weibull) were selected to quantify the releasing mechanism and better understand the MnO_4^- release. Both the coefficient of determination (R^2), obtained using the graphical software, and the adjustable coefficient (r^2_{adj}) (Equation (4)) [50] were applied to evaluate the best fitting model for MnO_4^- release.

$$r^2_{adj} = \frac{(1 - R^2)(N - 1)}{(N - m - 1)} \tag{4}$$

where N is the number of samples in each run and m is the number of parameters in each empirical model. As one of the criteria of SR selection was to maintain its cylindrical shape, we only selected ones with sufficient binding agent (dispersing agent < 2.5%) for further discussion on the releasing model.

To compare the SDM removal using MnO_4^- solution and $SR-MnO_4^-$, we conducted additional experiments that monitored SDM concentrations up to 48 d. Either TKPP or SHMP was included in both treatments (i.e., MnO_4^- solution and $SR-MnO_4^-$). For $SR-MnO_4^-$, we compared only two types of binding agents: (1) paraffin and (2) beeswax. To further evaluate if MnO_2 could serve as an oxidative surface for SDM in our treatment configuration, we added either 0.08 g L^{-1} or 0.4 g L^{-1} MnO_2 to the experimental unit.

3.5. Contact Tank Experiment

In the final part of this research, a contacting system was constructed to investigate the ability of SR-MnO$_4^-$ to effectively treat intermittent discharge water (Figure 6).

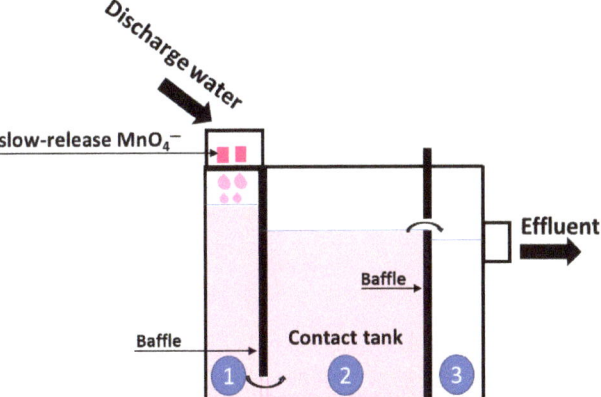

Figure 6. Contact tank diagram for SR-MnO$_4^-$ treatment system. Number 1 to 3 represents each chambers in the tank.

3.5.1. Construction of Contact Tank

The specifically designed tank (45 cm × 30 cm × 30 cm) was rectangular and made of acrylic, which is a non-SDM absorbable material. The release of MnO$_4^-$ started in the first chamber when the SR-MnO$_4^-$ met water just 5 cm above the water surface. Baffles were used to divide the chambers. The first baffle attached to the first chamber forced water to pass only from the bottom of the tank to ensure that the reaction commenced within this chamber. The second chamber was the contact area, where mixing of the water allowed the accumulation and reaction with diffused MnO$_4^-$. Therefore, the second baffle height was adjusted depending on the time required for the MnO$_4^-$ to treat the SDM. The contact area was in the second and last chambers, which allowed precipitates to settle prior to wastewater release into the receiving watershed.

3.5.2. Remediation Experiment

Spiked-SDM in the discharge water was prepared to determine if the SR could treat multiple discharge events. We used a peristaltic pump model no. BT 100 2J (Baoding City, Hubei, China) connected with Masterflex Viton® tubing (Coleparmer, IL, USA) to introduce water from an SDM solution reservoir at 50 mg L^{-1}. Sampling was collected in the three chambers and at the end of the ditch to determine the overall removal efficiency of SDM in the effluent during each cycle. This allowed us to quantify the effect of residence times under dynamic conditions. Only the treatment of SRB+TKPP is selectively presented, along with the addition of MnO$_4^-$ solution in the matrices of either SDM-spiked DI water or wastewater. We imitated the use of SRB+TKPP by placing it in the holder so that the release of MnO$_4^-$ would only occur when needed (Figure 6).

4. Conclusions

In this study, we developed a slow-release oxidant consisting of permanganate (MnO$_4^-$), biodegradable wax, and a phosphate-based dispersing agent to degrade aquaculture antibiotics (SDM, OMP, and TMP). The details of our findings are provided in the following:

- The second-order degradation rates for these antibiotics were 0.128 s^{-1} M^{-1} for SDM, 0.097 s^{-1} M^{-1} for OMP, and 0.056 s^{-1} M^{-1} for TMP, proving that the MnO$_4^-$ efficiency for a variety of antibiotics depends upon their molecular structure.

- Manganese dioxide (MnO_2) formed during treatment and enhanced SDM degradation by promoting surface-coordinated oxidization, but it also acted like a low permeable rind that reduced MnO_4^- release.
- Solution pH beyond neutral (pH > 4–6) and the presence of natural scavengers, such as organic constituents, slowed and sometimes halted oxidative degradation.
- While the oxidant composite was effective in treating SDM, the biodegradable wax component still required some synthetic paraffin in the mixture (>12%) to provide structural integrity. Among the several biowax and mixing ratios tested, 80% beeswax in the SR composite (SRB) produced the most consistent permanganate release patterns.
- Both dispersing agents (TKPP, SHMP) mixed in the composite produced delayed MnO_2 rind formation. By increasing this addition to more than 2.5% (>0.02 g) per SR weight, the cylindrical shape was compromised. Within this upper limit as a suitable amount, the addition of TKPP (SRB+TKPP) provided the best releasing concentration (up to 20% greater release) in the beeswax formulation. The Siepmann-Peppas model provided the best fit of MnO_4^- release rates over 60 d.
- Using SRB+TKPP in the contact tank receiving the SDM-contaminated discharge water removed 80% of the SDM over three flushing cycles. These results confirmed that our SRB+TKPP formulation could provide sustained release of MnO_4^- and warrant the proposed oxidant composite as a low-cost treatment technology suitable for treating antibiotic-contaminated discharge water.

Supplementary Materials: The following supporting information can be downloaded at: https://www.mdpi.com/article/10.3390/antibiotics12061025/s1, Figure S1: Temporal changes in antibiotic relative concentrations (A; SDM 161.12 μM, B; OMP 36.45 μM, C; TMP 34.44 μM) following treatment with varying MnO_4^- concentrations (0.315 to 5.033 mM for SDM or 0.189 to 27.181 mM for OMP or TMP) and loss of initial concentrations of antibiotics (D; SDM 16.11 to 161.12 μM, E; OMP 4.56 to 72.91 μM, F; TMP 4.56 to 72.91 μM) when treated with MnO_4^- at 1.133 mM.; Figure S2: Observed kinetic rate constant (k_{obs}) of each antibiotic degradation (A; SDM, B; OMP, or C; TMP) with presence of different synergetic antibiotics (as individual, SDM+OMP, or SDM+TMP) following treatment with MnO_4^- at 180 mg L^{-1}; Figure S3: Permanganate release concentration [Mixing ratio: Set A]; (A) Weight composition of SR-MnO_4^- per batch (3.3 g) at different natural wax percentages. (B–E) Permanganate concentrations of each type of SR-MnO_4^- at different natural wax percentages (20–100%) and at different timelines (0.25, 7, 28, and 56 d). Graphs (B–E) represent different types of natural wax in the mixture: (B) synthetic paraffin, (C) soy wax, (D) rice bran wax, and (E) beeswax; Figure S4: Permanganate concentrations of each type of SR-MnO_4^- with different formulations of natural wax, synthetic paraffin, and chemical addition (TKPP or SHMP) for different timelines: (A) 0.25 d, (B) 15 d, and (C) 56 d. (D) Temporal changes of MnO_4^- releasing concentration from selected types of SR; Figure S5: X-ray diffraction analysis of different types of SRB before and after soaking in SDM solution for 7 d; Figure S6: Temporal changes in MnO_4^- concentration from each type of SR-MnO_4^-: (A) soy wax; (B) rice bran wax (C) beeswax; and (D) paraffin; Figure S7: Release pattern of MnO_4^- concentration of each type of SR-MnO_4^- plotted for Higuchi releasing model with all selected data (t < 60 d): (A) soy wax; (B) rice bran wax (C) beeswax; and (D) paraffin. Hatched boxes represented range of time that data may be fitted in linear regression; Figure S8: Linear regression of each type of SR-MnO_4^- using Higuchi releasing model with selected data from t < 8 d: (A) soy wax; (B) rice bran wax (C) beeswax; and (D) paraffin; Figure S9: Release pattern of MnO_4^- concentration of each type of SR-MnO_4^- plotted for Noyes-Whitney releasing model: (A) soy wax; (B) rice bran wax (C) beeswax; and (D) paraffin. Hatched boxes represent range of time that data may be fitted in linear regression; Figure S10: Linear regression of each type of slow-release permanganate using Weibul releasing model: (A) soy wax; (B) rice bran wax (C) beeswax; and (D) paraffin; Table S1: Physiochemical characteristics of antibiotics; Table S2: Properties of TKPP and SHMP (Chokejaroenrat et al., 2014); Table S3: Physicochemical properties of aquaculture discharge wastewater; Table S4: Weight composition of SR-MnO_4^- with chemical addition (TKPP or SHMP) per SR (0.75 g) [Mixing ratio: Set B]. References [51–55] are cited in the Supplementary Materials.

Author Contributions: Conceptualization, C.S. and C.C.; formal analysis, C.S. and C.C.; methodology, C.S., S.P., K.P. and C.C.; supervision, C.C.; resources, C.S. and A.S.; visualization, C.S. and C.C.; data curation, C.C.; validation, C.C.; project administration, C.C.; funding acquisition, C.C.; writing—original draft, C.S. and C.C.; writing—review and editing, C.S., N.S., S.I., N.S., T.K., S.C. and C.C. All authors have read and agreed to the published version of the manuscript.

Funding: This work was financially supported by the Office of the Ministry of Higher Education, Science, Research and Innovation; and the Thailand Science Research and Innovation through Kasetsart University Reinventing University Program 2021, and Kasetsart University Research and Development (KURDI), (grant number FF(KU)18.66).

Institutional Review Board Statement: Not applicable.

Informed Consent Statement: Not applicable.

Data Availability Statement: The authors confirm that the data supporting the findings of this study are available within the article.

Acknowledgments: This work was financially supported by the Office of the Ministry of Higher Education, Science, Research and Innovation and the Thailand Science Research and Innovation through the Kasetsart University Reinventing University Program 2021, and Kasetsart University Research and Development (KURDI), (grant number FF(KU)18.66). The Faculty of Veterinary Technology provided facility support and access to analytical instruments. The authors also thank Warachayagorn Isarapakdee for technical assistance.

Conflicts of Interest: The authors declare no conflict of interest.

References

1. Alarcon, P.; Wieland, B.; Mateus, A.L.; Dewberry, C. Pig farmers' perceptions, attitudes, influences and management of information in the decision-making process for disease control. *Prev. Veter. Med.* **2014**, *116*, 223–242. [CrossRef] [PubMed]
2. Rico, A.; Oliveira, R.; McDonough, S.; Matser, A.; Khatikarn, J.; Satapornvanit, K.; Nogueira, A.J.; Soares, A.M.; Domingues, I.; Brink, P.J.V.D. Use, fate and ecological risks of antibiotics applied in tilapia cage farming in Thailand. *Environ. Pollut.* **2014**, *191*, 8–16. [CrossRef] [PubMed]
3. Speksnijder, D.; Jaarsma, A.; Van Der Gugten, A.; Verheij, T.J.; Wagenaar, J. Determinants associated with veterinary antimicrobial prescribing in farm animals in the Netherlands: A qualitative study. *Zoonoses Public Health* **2015**, *62*, 39–51. [CrossRef] [PubMed]
4. Hatosy, S.M.; Martiny, A.C. The Ocean as a Global Reservoir of Antibiotic Resistance Genes. *Appl. Environ. Microbiol.* **2015**, *81*, 7593–7599. [CrossRef]
5. Boison, J.; Turnipseed, S.B. A Review of Aquaculture Practices and Their Impacts on Chemical Food Safety from a Regulatory Perspective. *J. AOAC Int.* **2015**, *98*, 541–549. [CrossRef]
6. Yuan, J.; Ni, M.; Liu, M.; Zheng, Y.; Gu, Z. Occurrence of antibiotics and antibiotic resistance genes in a typical estuary aquaculture region of Hangzhou Bay, China. *Mar. Pollut. Bull.* **2018**, *138*, 376–384. [CrossRef]
7. Qin, L.-T.; Pang, X.-R.; Zeng, H.-H.; Liang, Y.-P.; Mo, L.-Y.; Wang, D.-Q.; Dai, J.-F. Ecological and human health risk of sulfonamides in surface water and groundwater of Huixian karst wetland in Guilin, China. *Sci. Total Environ.* **2019**, *708*, 134552. [CrossRef]
8. Zhou, J.; Yun, X.; Wang, J.; Li, Q.; Wang, Y. A review on the ecotoxicological effect of sulphonamides on aquatic organisms. *Toxicol. Rep.* **2022**, *9*, 534–540. [CrossRef]
9. Wang, Q.; Guo, M.; Yates, S.R. Degradation kinetics of manure-derived sulfadimethoxine in amended soil. *J. Agric. Food Chem.* **2006**, *54*, 157–163. [CrossRef]
10. Park, K.-Y.; Choi, S.-Y.; Lee, S.-H.; Kweon, J.-H.; Song, J.H. Comparison of formation of disinfection by-products by chlorination and ozonation of wastewater effluents and their toxicity to *Daphnia magna. Environ. Pollut.* **2016**, *215*, 314–321. [CrossRef]
11. Alvarez-Torrellas, S.; Rodríguez, A.; Ovejero, G.; García, J. Comparative adsorption performance of ibuprofen and tetracycline from aqueous solution by carbonaceous materials. *Chem. Eng. J.* **2016**, *283*, 936–947. [CrossRef]
12. Bi, X.; Huang, Y.; Liu, X.; Yao, N.; Zhao, P.; Meng, X.; Astruc, D. Oxidative degradation of aqueous organic contaminants over shape-tunable MnO_2 nanomaterials via peroxymonosulfate activation. *Sep. Purif. Technol.* **2021**, *275*. [CrossRef]
13. Chokejaroenrat, C.; Sakulthaew, C.; Satchasataporn, K.; Snow, D.D.; Ali, T.E.; Assiri, M.A.; Watcharenwong, A.; Imman, S.; Suriyachai, N.; Kreetachat, T. Enrofloxacin and Sulfamethoxazole Sorption on Carbonized Leonardite: Kinetics, Isotherms, Influential Effects, and Antibacterial Activity toward *S. aureus* ATCC 25923. *Antibiotics* **2022**, *11*, 1261. [CrossRef] [PubMed]
14. Jutarvutikul, K.; Sakulthaew, C.; Chokejaroenrat, C.; Pattanateeradetch, A.; Imman, S.; Suriyachai, N.; Satapanajaru, T.; Kreetachat, T. Practical use of response surface methodology for optimization of veterinary antibiotic removal using UV/H_2O_2 process. *Aquac. Eng.* **2021**, *94*, 102174. [CrossRef]
15. Yao, N.; Wang, X.; Yang, Z.; Zhao, P.; Meng, X. Characterization of solid and liquid carbonization products of polyvinyl chloride (PVC) and investigation of the PVC-derived adsorbent for the removal of organic compounds from water. *J. Hazard. Mater.* **2023**, *456*. [CrossRef]

16. Kambhu, A.; Gren, M.; Tang, W.; Comfort, S.; Harris, C.E. Remediating 1,4-dioxane-contaminated water with slow-release persulfate and zerovalent iron. *Chemosphere* **2017**, *175*, 170–177. [CrossRef]

17. Liang, C.; Chen, C.-Y. Characterization of a Sodium Persulfate Sustained Release Rod for in Situ Chemical Oxidation Groundwater Remediation. *Ind. Eng. Chem. Res.* **2017**, *56*, 5271–5276. [CrossRef]

18. Evans, P.J.; Dugan, P.; Nguyen, D.; Lamar, M.; Crimi, M. Slow-release permanganate versus unactivated persulfate for long-term in situ chemical oxidation of 1,4-dioxane and chlorinated solvents. *Chemosphere* **2019**, *221*, 802–811. [CrossRef]

19. Sakulthaew, C.; Chokejaroenrat, C. Oxidation of 17β-Estradiol in Water by Slow-Release Permanganate Candles. *Environ. Eng. Sci.* **2016**, *33*, 224–234. [CrossRef]

20. Hastings, J.L.; Lee, E.S. Optimization and Analysis of a Slow-Release Permanganate Gel for Groundwater Remediation in Porous and Low-Permeability Media. *Water* **2021**, *13*, 755. [CrossRef]

21. Liang, S.; Kao, C.; Kuo, Y.; Chen, K.; Yang, B. In situ oxidation of petroleum-hydrocarbon contaminated groundwater using passive ISCO system. *Water Res.* **2011**, *45*, 2496–2506. [CrossRef] [PubMed]

22. O'Connor, D.; Hou, D.; Ok, Y.S.; Song, Y.; Sarmah, A.K.; Li, X.; Tack, F.M. Sustainable in situ remediation of recalcitrant organic pollutants in groundwater with controlled release materials: A review. *J. Control. Release* **2018**, *283*, 200–213. [CrossRef]

23. Rezaei, K.; Wang, T.; Johnson, L.A. Combustion characteristics of candles made from hydrogenated soybean oil. *J. Am. Oil Chem. Soc.* **2002**, *79*, 803–808. [CrossRef]

24. Christenson, M.; Kambhu, A.; Reece, J.; Comfort, S.; Brunner, L. A five-year performance review of field-scale, slow-release permanganate candles with recommendations for second-generation improvements. *Chemosphere* **2016**, *150*, 239–247. [CrossRef] [PubMed]

25. Ma, Y.; Feng, Y.; Feng, Y.; Liao, G.; Sun, Y.; Ma, J. Characteristics and mechanisms of controlled-release KMnO4 for groundwater remediation: Experimental and modeling investigations. *Water Res.* **2020**, *171*, 115385. [CrossRef] [PubMed]

26. Gao, J.; Hedman, C.; Liu, C.; Guo, T.; Pedersen, J.A. Transformation of Sulfamethazine by Manganese Oxide in Aqueous Solution. *Environ. Sci. Technol.* **2012**, *46*, 2642–2651. [CrossRef]

27. Zhuang, J.; Wang, S.; Tan, Y.; Xiao, R.; Chen, J.; Wang, X.; Jiang, L.; Wang, Z. Degradation of sulfadimethoxine by permanganate in aquatic environment: Influence factors, intermediate products and theoretical study. *Sci. Total Environ.* **2019**, *671*, 705–713. [CrossRef]

28. Laszakovits, J.; Patterson, A.; Hipsher, C.; MacKay, A.A. Diethyl phenylene diamine (DPD) oxidation to measure low concentration permanganate in environmental systems. *Water Res.* **2018**, *151*, 403–412. [CrossRef]

29. Hu, L.; Martin, H.M.; Strathmann, T.J. Oxidation Kinetics of Antibiotics during Water Treatment with Potassium Permanganate. *Environ. Sci. Technol.* **2010**, *44*, 6416–6422. [CrossRef]

30. Hassan, M.; Alhemiary, N.A.; Albadani, A.S. Kinetics of Oxidation of dl-Tartaric Acid by Potassium Permanganate in Aqueous and Aqueous Micellar Media. *Arab. J. Sci. Eng.* **2012**, *37*, 1263–1270. [CrossRef]

31. Chokejaroenrat, C.; Comfort, S.D.; Harris, C.E.; Snow, D.D.; Cassada, D.; Sakulthaew, C.; Satapanajaru, T. Transformation of Hexahydro-1,3,5-trinitro-1,3,5-triazine (RDX) by Permanganate. *Environ. Sci. Technol.* **2011**, *45*, 3643–3649. [CrossRef] [PubMed]

32. Ji, Y.; Shi, Y.; Wang, L.; Lu, J.; Ferronato, C.; Chovelon, J.-M. Sulfate radical-based oxidation of antibiotics sulfamethazine, sulfapyridine, sulfadiazine, sulfadimethoxine, and sulfachloropyridazine: Formation of SO2 extrusion products and effects of natural organic matter. *Sci. Total Environ.* **2017**, *593–594*, 704–712. [CrossRef] [PubMed]

33. Sun, B.; Zhang, J.; Du, J.; Qiao, J.; Guan, X. Reinvestigation of the role of humic acid in the oxidation of phenols by permanganate. *Environ. Sci. Technol.* **2013**, *47*, 14332–14340. [CrossRef]

34. Fang, G.-D.; Dionysiou, D.D.; Zhou, D.-M.; Wang, Y.; Zhu, X.-D.; Fan, J.-X.; Cang, L.; Wang, Y.-J. Transformation of polychlorinated biphenyls by persulfate at ambient temperature. *Chemosphere* **2013**, *90*, 1573–1580. [CrossRef]

35. Carrillo, J.-C.; Danneels, D.; Woldhuis, J. Relevance of animal studies in the toxicological assessment of oil and wax hydrocarbons. Solving the puzzle for a new outlook in risk assessment. *Crit. Rev. Toxicol.* **2021**, *51*, 418–455. [CrossRef] [PubMed]

36. Yao, L.; Lio, J.; Wang, T.; Jarboe, D.H. Synthesis and Characterization of Acetylated and Stearylyzed Soy Wax. *J. Am. Oil Chem. Soc.* **2013**, *90*, 1063–1071. [CrossRef]

37. Rezaei, K.; Wang, T.; Johnson, L.A. Hydrogenated vegetable oils as candle wax. *J. Am. Oil Chem. Soc.* **2002**, *79*, 1241–1247. [CrossRef]

38. Wijarnprecha, K.; Aryusuk, K.; Santiwattana, P.; Sonwai, S.; Rousseau, D. Structure and rheology of oleogels made from rice bran wax and rice bran oil. *Food Res. Int.* **2018**, *112*, 199–208. [CrossRef]

39. Garnier, N.; Cren-Olivé, C.; Rolando, C.; Regert, M. Characterization of Archaeological Beeswax by Electron Ionization and Electrospray Ionization Mass Spectrometry. *Anal. Chem.* **2002**, *74*, 4868–4877. [CrossRef]

40. Luo, W.; Li, T.; Wang, C.; Huang, F. Discovery of Beeswax as binding agent on a 6th-century BC Chinese Turquoise-inlaid Bronze sword. *J. Archaeol. Sci.* **2012**, *39*, 1227–1237. [CrossRef]

41. Shaabani, A.; Tavasoli-Rad, F.; Lee, D.G. Potassium Permanganate Oxidation of Organic Compounds. *Synth. Commun.* **2005**, *35*, 571–580. [CrossRef]

42. Xará, S.M.; Delgado, J.N.; Almeida, M.F.; Costa, C.A. Laboratory study on the leaching potential of spent alkaline batteries. *Waste Manag.* **2009**, *29*, 2121–2131. [CrossRef] [PubMed]

43. Nagyová, G.; Buňka, F.; Salek, R.; Černíková, M.; Mančík, P.; Grůber, T.; Kuchař, D. Use of sodium polyphosphates with different linear lengths in the production of spreadable processed cheese. *J. Dairy Sci.* **2014**, *97*, 111–122. [CrossRef]

44. Passot, C.; Pouw, M.F.; Mulleman, D.; Bejan-Angoulvant, T.; Paintaud, G.; Dreesen, E.; Ternant, D. Therapeutic drug monitoring of biopharmaceuticals may benefit from pharmacokinetic and pharmacokinetic–pharmacodynamic modeling. *Ther. Drug Monit.* **2017**, *39*, 322–326. [CrossRef] [PubMed]
45. Kobryń, J.; Sowa, S.; Gasztych, M.; Dryś, A.; Musiał, W. Influence of hydrophilic polymers on the factor in weibull equation applied to the release kinetics of a biologically active complex of aesculus hippocastanum. *Int. J. Polym. Sci.* **2017**, *2017*, 3486384. [CrossRef]
46. Bucio, A.; Moreno-Tovar, R.; Bucio, L.; Espinosa-Dávila, J.; Anguebes-Franceschi, F. Characterization of Beeswax, Candelilla Wax and Paraffin Wax for Coating Cheeses. *Coatings* **2021**, *11*, 261. [CrossRef]
47. Cornforth, D.; West, E. Evaluation of the Antioxidant Effects of Dried Milk Mineral in Cooked Beef, Pork, and Turkey. *J. Food Sci.* **2002**, *67*, 615–618. [CrossRef]
48. Famoofo, O.O.; Adeniyi, I.F. Impact of effluent discharge from a medium-scale fish farm on the water quality of Odo-Owa stream near Ijebu-Ode, Ogun State, Southwest Nigeria. *Appl. Water Sci.* **2020**, *10*, 68. [CrossRef]
49. Chokejaroenrat, C.; Comfort, S.; Sakulthaew, C.; Dvorak, B. Improving the treatment of non-aqueous phase TCE in low permeability zones with permanganate. *J. Hazard. Mater.* **2014**, *268*, 177–184. [CrossRef]
50. Sakulthaew, C.; Watcharenwong, A.; Chokejaroenrat, C.; Rittirat, A. Leonardite-Derived Biochar Suitability for Effective Sorption of Herbicides. *Water Air Soil Pollut.* **2021**, *232*, 1–17. [CrossRef]
51. Sanders, S.; Srivastava, P.; Feng, Y.; Dane, J.; Basile, J.; Barnett, M. Sorption of the Veterinary Antimicrobials Sulfadimethoxine and Ormetoprim in Soil. *J. Environ. Qual.* **2008**, *37*, 1510–1518. [CrossRef] [PubMed]
52. Straub, J.O. An Environmental Risk Assessment for Human-Use Trimethoprim in European Surface Waters. *Antibiotics* **2013**, *2*, 115–162. [CrossRef] [PubMed]
53. Gros, M.; Petrović, M.; Barceló, D. Development of a multi-residue analytical methodology based on liquid chromatography-tandem mass spectrometry (LC-MS/MS) for screening and trace level determination of pharmaceuticals in surface and wastewaters. *Talanta* **2006**, *70*, 678–690. [CrossRef] [PubMed]
54. Qiang, Z.; Adams, C. Potentiometric determination of acid dissociation constants (pKa) for human and veterinary antibiotics. *Water Res.* **2004**, *38*, 2874–2890. [CrossRef]
55. Samuelsen, O.B.; Lunestad, B.T.; Ervik, A.; Fjelde, S. Stability of antibacterial agents in an artificial marine aquaculture sediment studied under laboratory conditions. *Aquaculture* **1994**, *126*, 283–290. [CrossRef]

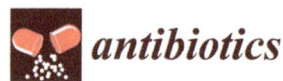

MDPI

Article

Enrofloxacin and Sulfamethoxazole Sorption on Carbonized Leonardite: Kinetics, Isotherms, Influential Effects, and Antibacterial Activity toward *S. aureus* ATCC 25923

Chanat Chokejaroenrat [1], Chainarong Sakulthaew [2,*], Khomson Satchasataporn [2], Daniel D. Snow [3], Tarik E. Ali [4,5], Mohammed A. Assiri [4], Apichon Watcharenwong [6,7], Saksit Imman [8], Nopparat Suriyachai [8] and Torpong Kreetachat [8]

[1] Department of Environmental Technology and Management, Faculty of Environment, Kasetsart University, Bangkok 10900, Thailand
[2] Department of Veterinary Technology, Faculty of Veterinary Technology, Kasetsart University, Bangkok 10900, Thailand
[3] Water Sciences Laboratory, Nebraska Water Center/School of Natural Resources, University of Nebraska—Lincoln, Lincoln, NE 68583-0844, USA
[4] Department of Chemistry, Faculty of Science, King Khalid University, Abha 62529, Saudi Arabia
[5] Department of Chemistry, Faculty of Education, Ain Shams University, Cairo 11566, Egypt
[6] School of Environmental Engineering, Institute of Engineering, Suranaree University of Technology, Nakhon Ratchasima 30000, Thailand
[7] Center of Excellence in Advanced Functional Materials, Suranaree University of Technology, Nakhon Ratchasima 30000, Thailand
[8] Integrated Biorefinery Excellent Center (IBC), School of Energy and Environment, University of Phayao, Tambon Maeka, Amphur Muang, Phayao 56000, Thailand
* Correspondence: cvtcns@ku.ac.th; Tel.: +66-2942-8200 (ext. 616018)

Citation: Chokejaroenrat, C.; Sakulthaew, C.; Satchasataporn, K.; Snow, D.D.; Ali, T.E.; Assiri, M.A.; Watcharenwong, A.; Imman, S.; Suriyachai, N.; Kreetachat, T. Enrofloxacin and Sulfamethoxazole Sorption on Carbonized Leonardite: Kinetics, Isotherms, Influential Effects, and Antibacterial Activity toward *S. aureus* ATCC 25923. *Antibiotics* 2022, 11, 1261. https://doi.org/10.3390/antibiotics11091261

Academic Editors: Anusak Kerdsin, Jinquan Li and Jonathan Frye

Received: 20 July 2022
Accepted: 7 September 2022
Published: 16 September 2022

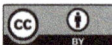
Abstract: Excessive antibiotic use in veterinary applications has resulted in water contamination and potentially poses a serious threat to aquatic environments and human health. The objective of the current study was to quantify carbonized leonardite (cLND) adsorption capabilities to remove sulfamethoxazole (SMX)- and enrofloxacin (ENR)-contaminated water and to determine the microbial activity of ENR residuals on cLND following adsorption. The cLND samples prepared at 450 °C and 850 °C (cLND450 and cLND550, respectively) were evaluated for structural and physical characteristics and adsorption capabilities based on adsorption kinetics and isotherm studies. The low pyrolysis temperature of cLND resulted in a heterogeneous surface that was abundant in both hydrophobic and hydrophilic functional groups. SMX and ENR adsorption were best described using a pseudo-second-order rate expression. The SMX and ENR adsorption equilibrium data on cLND450 and cLND550 revealed their better compliance with a Langmuir isotherm than with four other models based on 2.3-fold higher values of q_{mENR} than q_{mSMX}. Under the presence of the environmental interference, the electrostatic interaction was the main contributing factor to the adsorption capability. Microbial activity experiments based on the growth of *Staphylococcus aureus* ATCC 25923 revealed that cLND could successfully adsorb and subsequently retain the adsorbed antibiotic on the cLND surface. This study demonstrated the potential of cLND550 as a suitable low-cost adsorbent for the highly efficient removal of antibiotics from water.

Keywords: adsorption isotherm; adsorption kinetics; antibiotic adsorption; carbonization; elovich; enrofloxacin; growth inhibition zone; intraparticle diffusion; leonardite; sulfamethoxazole

1. Introduction

An exponential increase in medicinal technology development has resulted in excessive antibiotic use in veterinary practices. In many countries, farmers use antibiotics not only therapeutically but also prophylactically (as growth promoters) in livestock, poultry farming, and aquaculture in an effort to gain a substantial additional yield in a relatively shorter time frame [1–3]. The excess antibiotic may enter the environment via animal waste excretion or in discharge water and may even exist in active forms, as it can be partially metabolized by animals [4–7]. These residuals (estimated at 30–90% of the initial load) are mostly still considered to be pharmaceutically active compounds. Without proper waste and discharge water treatment, these chemicals can potentially contaminate soils, surface water, and ground water and pose a serious threat to the environment [8–12]. Long-term exposure to these contaminated antibiotics is considered to be directly interrelated to the proliferation of antibiotic resistance genes, which can be genetically transferred among local microorganisms [13,14].

The sulfonamide, macrolide, and tetracycline antibiotic families have been mostly detected at microgram-per-liter levels in tropical Asian countries [15]. Among these chemicals, sulfamethoxazole (SMX) has been detected at up to 1720 ng L^{-1}, which is higher than the detected levels in China and Western countries. Antibiotic residuals in conventional wastewater treatment plants (WWTPs) have been regularly reported throughout the world. The fluoroquinolone and sulfonamide families have been frequently detected in WWTPs and natural receiving water, such as canals, and rivers in Thailand [16]. Following chlorination and UV irradiation, SMX has proven to be the most difficult antibiotic to remove among the sulfonamides [17]. Up to 21 µg L^{-1} of ampicillin was detected in the effluent water from an Indian city municipal WWTP [18]. Even with the strict regulation of drug manufacturers in India, up to 31,000 µg L^{-1} of ciprofloxacin—from enrofloxacin degradation—was discovered in the effluent [19]. This evidence signifies the potential inadequacy of regular, conventional unit operations, such as chlorination, biological treatment, filtration, and coagulation. Hydroxyl radical (•OH) generation in advanced oxidation processes provides an efficient approach for mitigating antibiotics [20]. However, this treatment usually requires a large amount of oxidant and has high operational and application costs, as well as possibly leading to secondary contamination [21,22].

Adsorption was proven to be an efficient treatment meeting both economic values and environmental requirements. Although carbon nanomaterial is usually applied as a decent antibiotics adsorbent, these materials are not economical for large-scale treatments [9,23,24]. To overcome this problem, pyrolyzed material is preferentially selected, as it generally enriches with carbon, which is naturally suitable for removing organic contaminants. The pyrolyzed materials tend to possess a more porous structure, high surface area, and high cation exchange capacity that are more compatible with antibiotics capable of presenting in different ionic forms. The magnitude of antibiotic sorption is based on various mechanisms such as the hydrophobic interaction, π–π interaction, H bonding, and even electrostatic interaction [25,26]. Example of pyrolyzed material that efficiently adsorb antibiotics included animal manure, rice straw, etc. [27,28].

Uncarbonized leonardite (LND)—a byproduct from a lignite coal reaction in a power plant—is naturally abundant in humic substances, consisting of a wide variety of both carboxylic and hydroxylic sites, making it a promising material as a soil conditioner and an extremely porous material after pyrolysis (as carbonized LND or cLND). Recently, leonardite char (cLND) was used as a suitable adsorbent for both organic and inorganic pollutants, such as atrazine, organic dyes, and heavy metals [29–31]. The cLND not only had abundant C=C structures on the surface but also had numerous fractures on its planar surface, making it very suitable for adsorbing both hydrophobic and hydrophilic materials [31]. While cLND chemical and physical properties are well-understood, only limited information has been reported on cLND adsorptive application with emerging contaminants such as antibiotics.

In this study, we selected two frequently used veterinary antibiotics—sulfamethoxazole (SMX) and enrofloxacin (ENR)—as adsorbate antibiotic representatives, because they were the most frequently found antibiotics in aquacultural discharge wastewater and natural flowing streams [32]. The objectives were: (1) to quantify the ENR and SMX removal efficiencies using cLND based on adsorption kinetics and adsorption isotherms under different experimental conditions and (2) to determine the microbial activities on the adsorbed ENR on cLND using *Staphylococcus aureus* ATCC 25923 during the adsorption and desorption processes.

2. Material and Methods

2.1. Chemicals and Chemical Analyses

The representative antibiotics used in this study—enrofloxacin (ENR) and sulfamethoxazole (SMX)—were purchased from Merck. Sodium hydroxide, hydrochloric acid, sodium bicarbonate, acetic acid, and potassium chloride were used as purchased from Carlo Erba. Acetonitrile and methanol were of high-performance liquid chromatography (HPLC) grade obtained from Honeywell Burdick & Jackson. Low-grade coal (leonardite; LND) was donated from the Mae Moh lignite mine in Lampang Province, Thailand.

The antibiotics were analyzed using HPLC in a 600E unit coupled with a 2487 UV detector (Waters). The mobile phase used for the ENR analysis was a mixture of 0.1% acetic acid (v/v) and acetonitrile at 80:20, while that used for the SMX analysis was at 60:40. Peak separation was achieved using a Mightysil HPLC column (RP-18GP; 250 × Ø4.6 mm, particle size 5 μm, pore size 12.5 nm; Kanto Chemical) under a flow rate of 1 mL min^{-1} at room temperature. The injection volume was set at 20 μL, and the detection wavelengths were set at 265 and 280 nm for SMX and ENR, respectively.

We compared the cLND physical and chemical characteristics at different carbonized temperatures. The cLND morphological properties were obtained from scanning electron microscopy (SEM; JEOL JSM-6010). The surface functional groups were analyzed using Fourier-transform infrared spectroscopy (FTIR; Bruker Tensor 27).

2.2. cLND Preparation

Initially, we discarded distinctively large and darkened debris from the obtained LND before drying the remainder in a hot air oven at 105 °C for 3 h. Since the LND varied in size, we mechanically sieved using an AS200 sieve shaker (Retsch GmbH) and sorted only the <2 nm particles. Then, the LND was carbonized at a 5 °C min^{-1} heat rate to the desired carbonized temperatures of 450 °C, 550 °C, 650 °C, 750 °C, and 850 °C (denoted as cLND450 for the 450 °C carbonizations). To maintain the cLND pyrolysis conditions, the heating system was maintained for 5 h at each designated temperature under an N$_2$ flow stream. The cLND powder was kept in a desiccator at room temperature until use.

2.3. Adsorption Kinetics

The ENR and SMX stock solution was freshly prepared before use to ensure its stability at room temperature. A sample of 30 mL of 100 mg L^{-1} antibiotic solution was placed individually in a 40-mL amber vial with a Teflon-lined screw cap. An experimental unit was done in triplicate. Each vial received 30 mg cLND and was shaken on a reciprocating shaker at 200 rpm. The cLND carbonized at varying temperatures (i.e., 450, 550, 650, 750, and 850 °C) was tested individually. Samples were periodically collected, placed in separate 1.5-mL centrifuge tubes, centrifuged at 5000 rpm for 10 min, transferred to an HPLC vial, and stored at 4 °C before analysis using HPLC.

2.4. Adsorption Isotherm

The isotherm experiments were conducted in a 40-mL Teflon tube. Only cLND450 and cLND550 were selected as an absorbent for both ENR and SMX. Each antibiotic solution of 30 mL with an initial concentration ranging between 5 and 50 mg L^{-1} was separately poured into each vial. The isotherm experiment commenced when the pre-weighed cLND at 30 ± 0.2 mg was added to each vial. The cLND exact weights were recorded for further adsorbed concentration calculations. The sample collection protocol was similar to the previous experiment. However, we only collected samples twice (at 24 h and 48 h) to confirm that an equilibrium between the cLND and antibiotic had been reached. Then, the adsorbed concentration (q_e) and equilibrium concentration (C_e) were plotted and determined for the best fit adsorption isotherms.

2.5. Point of Zero Charges Determination

Since the point of zero charge (pH_{zpc}) can explain the material adsorption capacity under the presence of ionic constituents, we determined the pH_{zpc} using changes in the pH before and after adding cLND. Eleven flasks containing 50 mL of sodium chloride solution (0.01 M) were prepared. Each flask was pH-adjusted to designate pH (2–12) using 0.1 M of either HCl or NaOH. A small amount (0.12 g) of cLND was placed in each flask, and the pH was immediately measured. The first pH curve was plotted between the before and after adjusted pH. Then, all flasks were agitated at 180 rpm for 48 h. The final pH was recorded and plotted against the initial pH. The pH_{zpc} can be obtained from the intersection of both pH curves.

2.6. Influential Effect Experiments

Since other environmental parameters are known to directly affect the adsorbent surface charge, we individually varied the parameters such as solution pH, humic acid (HA), HCO_3^-, and Cl^- and measured the temporal changes in the antibiotic concentrations. The ranged concentrations of these values were based on the normal values that could be observed under natural conditions. The solution pH ranged from 3 to 11, the humic acid concentrations ranged from 2.5 to 40 mg L^{-1}, and the HCO_3^- and Cl^- concentrations ranged from 50 and 800 mg L^{-1}.

2.7. ENR Bacterial ACTIVITY after Treatment

Six ENR concentrations ranging between 10 and 100 mg L^{-1} were tested in this experiment to differentiate the cLND adsorption and desorption activities from the adsorption treatments between two cLNDs (cLND450 and cLND550) at the two cLND amounts (30 and 300 mg). The experimental setup was arranged similarly to the adsorption kinetic experiments discussed earlier. We investigated the bacterial activities of cLND-adsorbed ENR against Gram-negative *Staphylococcus aureus* (ATCC 25923) bacteria using the agar diffusion technique based on the Kirby–Bauer method. In brief, colonies of bacteria-grown culture were adjusted to an opacity equivalent to 0.5 McFarland (~1.5×10^8 CFU mL^{-1}), seeded on Mueller–Hinton agar in a petri dish, and grown overnight under aerobic conditions at 37 °C.

After the cLND-ENR reaction reached an adsorption equilibrium at 24 h, two separate samples were taken from the adsorption experimental units: (1) filtrated water and (2) used cLND (the retentate). We passed the filtrated watered using a vacuum filter through a 0.22-μm PES Corning filter membrane (Glendale, AZ, USA). Ten microliters of filtrated sample were dropped directly on a sterile blank disc (Ø = 6 mm, Whatman, USA), dried in the dark for 30 min, and placed on the bacterial inoculated agar. A standard ENR antibiotic disc (5 μg; Oxoid, UK) was used as the positive control. The culture plates were further incubated at 37 °C for 24 h. At the designated time following incubation, a symmetrical inhibition ellipse was measured using a reflected lightbox and digital calipers. To evaluate how cLND strongly adsorb ENR, we gently placed a sterile blank disc over the retentate cLNDs and dried them in the dark for 30 min. Each disc was placed in a separate bacterial inoculated agar and incubated at 37 °C for 24 h. Then, the increase in inhibition zones was compared between day 1 and day 3.

3. Results and Discussion

3.1. cLND Characteristics

A carbonized LND (cLND) morphological analysis was performed using SEM and FTIR. The cLND SEM images of two carbonization temperatures at 450 °C and 850 °C (cLND450 and cLND850) were viewed at 3000 and 15,000 magnification (Figure 1). These images indicated clear heterogeneity crowded with irregular lamella-shaped flakes overlaying each other. While irregular surface pores were observed in both carbonization temperatures, those in the cLND850 were more evident, indicating that the molecular pore-filling mechanism may be prominent at higher carbonization temperatures (Figure 1C,D). This was the initial proof that the cLND was a suitable adsorbent for both organic and inorganic compounds. High carbonization temperatures at > 550 °C eliminated the organic compounds (the carboxylic group), resulting in a rougher surface, greater hydrophobicity and porosity, and a large surface area, which provided a greater surface area and consequently provided more binding sites with adsorbate, making it a docile adsorbent, particularly with organic pollutants [29–31,33]. With lower carbonization temperatures (< 550 °C), the biochar typically had smaller pore sizes with oxygen-containing functional group residuals on the surface, rendering them well-suited for inorganic pollutant adsorption [30]. Nonetheless, the higher pyrolysis temperature did not necessarily ensure better adsorption, and this was also the case for cLND.

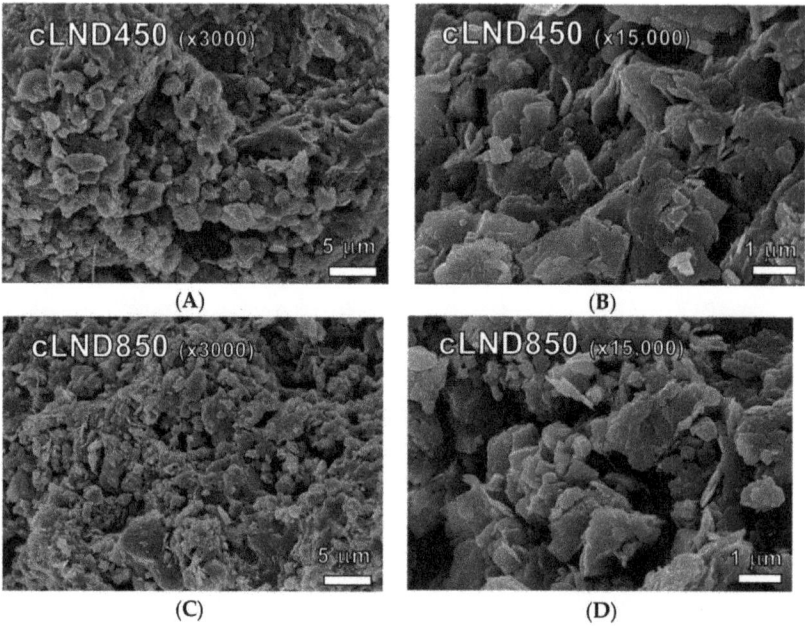

Figure 1. (**A–D**) cLND scanning electron micrograph images at 450 °C and 850 °C carbonization temperature (cLND450 and cLND850) at 3000 magnification and 15,000 magnification.

The cLND FTIR spectra were recorded in the range 600–3800 cm^{-1} to characterize the surface functional group changes between the two carbonization temperatures. Some of these changes reflected the cLND adsorptive effectiveness toward organic molecules. The higher carbonization temperature caused the loss of a stronger and broader band at 3200–3600 cm^{-1}, which was associated with the stretching vibration of the –OH groups (Figure 2). These changes in the functional groups initially confirmed that the cLND adsorption behavior could be categorized as both hydrophobic and hydrophilic interactions. The cLND450 FTIR spectra showed stronger bands of symmetrical and asymmetrical aromatic and aliphatic C-H bonding (CH_3-CH_2) at 2923–2854 cm^{-1}, while these bands almost disappeared during higher carbonization (Figure 2). A strong adsorption band at 3450 cm^{-1}, corresponding to the –OH groups, was more evident at the lower carbonization temperature similar to other hydrophilic functional groups, such as H-bonded OH, C = O, and Si-O-Si located at 3620, 1670, and 1100 cm^{-1}, respectively (Figure 2). The peak at 3620 cm^{-1} could be attributed to the H-bonded OH of the Si-OH group or other H bonding with water molecules that almost completely dissipated at the higher carbonization temperature. These results indicated that cLND850 was less polar than cLND450, supporting the beneficial use of cLND450 for hydrophilic/hydrophobic interactions and cLND850 for hydrophobic interactions.

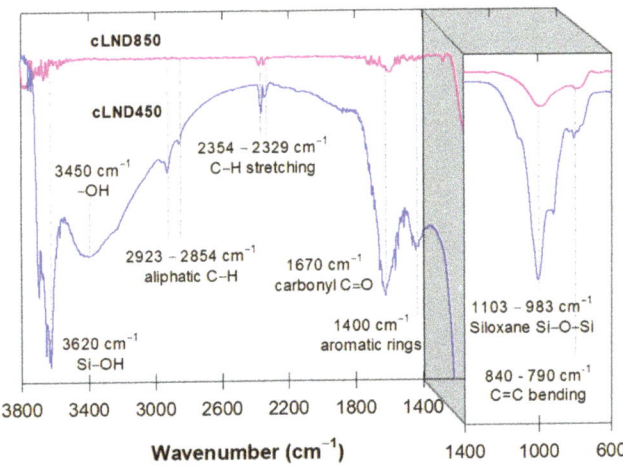

Figure 2. FTIR spectra comparisons between cLND450 and cLND850.

3.2. Adsorption Kinetics

In the kinetic experiments of both antibiotics and each cLND at different carbonization temperatures (450–850 °C), both the adsorbed concentration (q_e) and relative adsorption concentration (C/C_o) were plotted against time (Figure 3). For cLND that carbonized at 450–650 °C, a rapid decrease in antibiotic adsorption was observed (SMX < 3 h, ENR < 1 h), as shown in Figure 3C,D, respectively. At the higher carbonization temperature, slower SMX adsorption rates were observed, while the ENR adsorption rates were slightly different. Although the increase in contact time increased the adsorption performance, it mainly depended on the cLND type for SMX adsorption (Figure 3A,C). Each SMX adsorption result tended to reach a plateau at a specific adsorbed amount, indicating that the carbonization temperature directly affected the SMX adsorption performance. The ENR adsorption was substantially different compared to that of SMX (Figure 3B,D). All of them reached a plateau at relatively close q_e values, supporting the adsorbate molecular structure as the main contributing factor for better adsorption. However, a larger cLND amount tended to agglomerate into a bulkier size, decreasing the adsorptive sites in the cLND microspores [31]. Here, we did not observe such a case, as there was not enough cLND to initiate such an agglomeration. Overall, the results initially proved that cLNDs were an efficient adsorbent for both antibiotics, but the SMX and ENR adsorption rates were substantially different due to (1) the SMX and ENR chemical perspectives and (2) the differences in the carbonization temperatures.

We used four kinetic models to explain the adsorption process between each antibiotic and cLND at varying temperatures (450–850 °C). These four models were: pseudo-first-order kinetics, pseudo-second-order kinetics, Elovich, and intraparticle diffusion (Equations (1)–(4), respectively) [34].

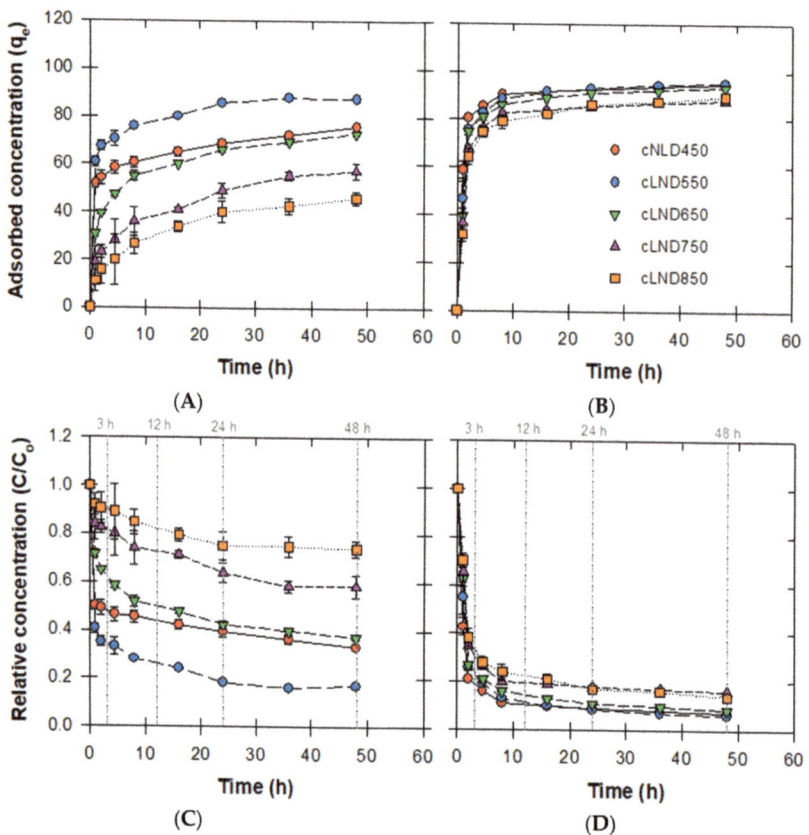

Figure 3. Adsorption kinetic studies of varying cLND with SMX or ENR. (**A,B**) Temporal changes in the antibiotic concentrations. (**C,D**) Temporal changes in the adsorbed concentrations in cLND.

$$\text{Pseudo} - \text{first} - \text{order kinetic model}: \; q_t = q_e\left(1 - e^{-K_1 t}\right) \text{ or } (q_e - q_t) = q_e e^{-K_1 t} \quad (1)$$

$$\text{Pseudo} - \sec\text{ond} - \text{order kinetic model}: \; \frac{t}{q_t} = \frac{1}{K_2 q_e^2} + \frac{1}{q_e}t \quad (2)$$

$$\text{Elovich model}: \; q_t = \left(\frac{1}{b}\right)\ln(ab) + \left(\frac{1}{b}\right)\ln t \quad (3)$$

$$\text{Intraparticle diffusion}: \; q_t = K_d t^{\frac{1}{2}} + C \quad (4)$$

where q_e and q_t (mg g^{-1}) are the cLND adsorption capacity at equilibrium and at any given time t (h), respectively, K_1 (h^{-1}) is the rate constant of the pseudo-first-order model, K_2 (g mg^{-1}h^{-1}) is the rate constant of the pseudo-second-order model, a (mg g^{-1}h^{-1}) is the Elovich chemisorption rate, b (g mg^{-1}) is the desorption rate constant, K_d (mg g^{-1}h$^{-1/2}$) is the intraparticle diffusion coefficient, and C (mg g^{-1}) is the intraparticle diffusion constant.

Two correlation values were selected to evaluate the validity of each model: the coefficient of determination (R^2) obtained from SigmaPlot software and the adjustable coefficient (r_{adj}^2) calculated from Equation (5) [35]:

$$r_{adj}^2 = 1 - \frac{(1 - R^2)(N - 1)}{(N - m - 1)} \quad (5)$$

where N is the number of data points, and m is the total number of independent variables. By comparing these two values, the small difference implies that these independent variables have less impact on the dependent variables.

By comparing the correlation values, the pseudo-second-order kinetics had a better fit than all the other models at any carbonization temperature (Table 1). In addition, SMX adsorption was a good fit only with pseudo-second-order kinetics while the ENR was a good fit with the pseudo-first- and -second-order models. The differences in R^2 and r^2_{adj} were quite large (6–33%) for the SMX pseudo-first-order kinetics, while these differences were <0.13% with the pseudo-second-order kinetics, confirming the greater usefulness of all the parameters for ENR adsorption than for SMX (Table 1). This also indicated that the chemisorption was dominant and possibly involved the primitive valence forces from the electron exchange between the antibiotic molecules and adsorbent surface functional groups [36].

Table 1. Kinetic parameters for SMX and ENR adsorption onto varying types of cLND.

Kinetic Model Parameters		Sulfamethoxazole (SMX)					Enrofloxacin (ENR)				
		cLND 450	cLND 550	cLND 650	cLND 750	cLND 850	cLND 450	cLND 550	cLND 650	cLND 750	cLND 850
Experimental q_e											
q_{exp}	mg g^{-1}	75.812	87.603	75.519	47.832	45.992	94.939	95.431	93.710	88.447	89.107
First-order kinetic model											
q_{cal}	mg g^{-1}	71.331	80.543	62.940	43.376	40.399	94.441	95.149	92.166	88.304	89.497
K_1	h^{-1}	0.737	0.893	0.161	0.847	0.086	0.916	0.681	0.637	0.604	0.498
R^2	-	0.820	0.906	0.880	0.957	0.961	0.987	0.982	0.974	0.983	0.967
r^2_{adj}	-	0.618	0.791	0.737	0.902	0.911	0.970	0.958	0.940	0.961	0.924
Second-order kinetic model											
q_{cal}	mg g^{-1}	76.336	89.286	78.125	61.38	50.000	95.238	97.087	95.238	89.286	91.043
K_2	g mg^{-1}h^{-1}	8.7 × 10^{-3}	10.6 × 10^{-3}	4.4 × 10^{-3}	3.4 × 10^{-3}	3.4 × 10^{-3}	18.7 × 10^{-3}	12.5 × 10^{-3}	11.2 × 10^{-3}	11.9 × 10^{-3}	8.1 × 10^{-3}
R^2	-	0.997	0.999	0.995	0.994	0.995	0.999	0.999	0.999	0.999	0.999
r^2_{adj}	-	0.993	0.998	0.988	0.986	0.988	0.998	0.998	0.998	0.998	0.998
Elovich model											
a	mg g^{-1}h^{-1}	21,552	39,988	161.8	22.1	23.9	57,835	3526.7	1756.9	1342.5	568.5
b	g mg^{-1}	0.163	0.141	0.088	0.099	0.107	0.129	0.096	0.090	0.092	0.081
R^2	-	0.973	0.983	0.996	0.991	0.980	0.775	0.794	0.754	0.699	0.819
r^2_{adj}	-	0.938	0.961	0.991	0.979	0.954	0.534	0.569	0.497	0.403	0.616
Intraparticle diffusion											
K_{d1}	mg g^{-1}h$^{-1/2}$	3.891	4.391	7.109	6.648	5.850	54.463	70.132	83.980	70.993	78.532
C_1	mg g^{-1}	49.344	60.910	29.834	5.979	8.287	3.551	23.186	43.631	19.242	46.47
K_{d2}	mg g^{-1}min^{-1}	-	-	-	-	-	1.641	2.367	2.439	1.067	3.011
C_2	mg g^{-1}	-	-	-	-	-	84.219	80.520	78.110	91.257	69.972
R^2	-	0.988	0.932	0.949	0.967	0.977	0.815	0.817	0.802	0.627	0.822
r^2_{adj}	-	0.972	0.847	0.884	0.924	0.947	0.608	0.612	0.584	0.292	0.622

Changes in the pseudo-first-order rates (K_1) and pseudo-second-order rates (K_2) for ENR adsorption on cLND had the same trend, with both having high values of r^2_{adj} for any cLND (0.924–0.998%), corresponding to the good fit of the adsorption data for both models, as discussed earlier (Table 1 and Figures 4 and S1). However, the changes in the reaction rates for SMX adsorption fluctuated more for K_1 and only had a high r^2_{adj} (>0.902%) for the high carbonization temperature (>750 °C), indicating that these temperatures had a high impact on the adsorption behavior of higher hydrophilic molecules under our experimental conditions (Figure S1). As the ENR correlations were close to 1 with all the cLND types, these calculated parameters were reliable and could be used to explain the adsorbate adsorption behaviors in the aqueous phase, confirming the chemisorption process.

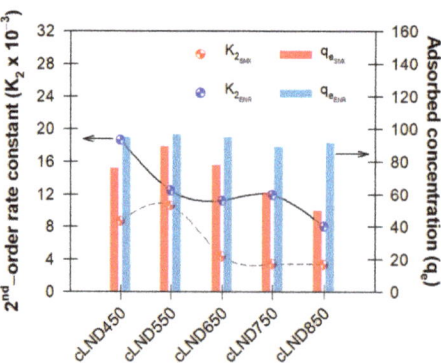

Figure 4. Changes in the pseudo-second-order reaction rates (K_2) and adsorbed concentrations (q_e).

Considering the K_2 values of SMX adsorption, cLND550 had the highest adsorption rates, confirming that the higher carbonization temperature might not be necessary (Figure 4). However, adsorbent carbonization was still needed to allow cLND to provide interactions between both the hydrophilic functional group (-COOH, -OH, and Si-OH) and the hydrophobic functional group (CH_3-CH_2 and C = C), as well as generating numerous pore structures for the better adsorption of organic substances.

All the q_e values indicated the cLND had better adsorption for ENR than for SMX (~50–89-mg SMX g^{-1}-cLND versus ~89–97-mg ENR g^{-1}-cLND), indicating that cLND was a suitable adsorbent for the hydrophobic compound at any carbonization temperature (Table 1). Notably, for ENR, an adsorbed amount almost showed complete adsorption (100 mg g^{-1}) at the lower carbonization temperature (Figure 4), because ENR was prone to being adsorbed at a lower carbonization temperature. With the SMX, q_e was the highest with cLND550 (~89 mg g^{-1}) in the pseudo-second-order rates and continued to decrease with higher carbonization temperatures, which corresponded to the highest kinetic order rates (Figure 4).

The difference between q_e obtained from the experiments (q_{exp}) and that obtained from the calculated equations (q_{cal}) could also explain the best fit model. The results showed that all q_{exp} values were higher than the ones obtained from the equations (Table 1). The differences were larger for SMX adsorption, especially for the pseudo-first-order kinetic models (6–20%); however, this was much smaller for ENR adsorption for both models (<1.6%). These calculations supported using both models to explain the ENR adsorption mechanism.

The results from fitting the Elovich model produced a bet fit for SMX adsorption (r^2_{adj} = 0.938–0.991%) compared to ENR adsorption (r^2_{adj} = 0.403–0.616%) (Table 1). Although the suitably fit with the Elovich model lends credence to the adsorbent having a heterogeneous surface, the adsorbed amount variation between sampling points could lead to an incorrect evaluation of the adsorbent surface. This could be further explained by the rapid ENR adsorption in the early stage, which approached >70% after 4 h of sampling, regardless of the carbonization temperature, thus resulting in a smaller adsorption variation afterward (ln T > 0.7). However, the adsorption surface cannot be entirely ruled out for homogeneity, as the SEM images showed its nonuniformity for the selected two carbonization temperatures (Figure 1).

Both Elovich parameters (a and b) for the antibiotic adsorption varied with the SMX adsorption more than for the ENR (Figure S2). The a and b values were high at the lower carbonization temperature (450 °C) and continued to decrease when the carbonization temperature increased. Notably, the Elovich parameter (a) can vary extremely (from 4.4×10^{18} to 1.52 mg $g^{-1}min^{-1}$) based on the calculated changes in the approaching equilibrium parameters (R_E) [37].

We used the equation model modified from Weber and Morris to determine the adsorption behavior between antibiotics and active sites and whether intraparticle diffusion governed the overall adsorption process [38,39]. The results showed that none of the y-intercepts (C) for the linear intraparticle diffusion equations (Equation (4)) were zero. However, SMX and ENR adsorption produced different patterns that resulted in single-linearity characterization for SMX and double-linearity characterization for the ENR (Figure 5). These stages represented the diffusion type order (external followed by internal diffusion).

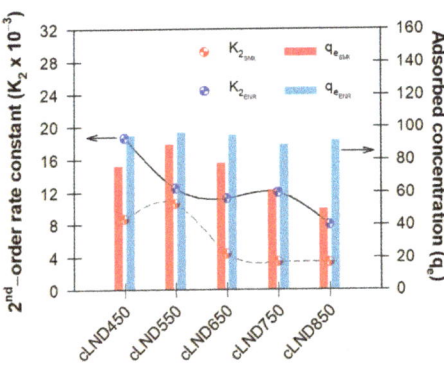

Figure 5. Intraparticle diffusion mechanism plots with varying cLND for (**A**) SMX or (**B**) ENR.

The results for SMX adsorption showed that more than one stage possibly occurred for cLND with a carbonization temperature <650 °C (Figure 5A). The R^2 was high (>0.93) at all carbonization temperatures (Table 1 and Figure 5A). Here, the diffusion behavior may have occurred simultaneously once the adsorbent met the antibiotic molecules; however, with this relatively high initial concentration, instant adsorption may have occurred before our first sampling (2 h). Therefore, instant adsorption can be easily overshadowed, and consequently, ruling out intraparticle diffusion as the rate-limiting step might be inexact.

For ENR adsorption, the fitted curves showed two distinctive slopes (i.e., K_{d1} and K_{d2}) divided at the second sampling ($t^{1/2}$ = 1.414), followed by gradually smaller adsorption variations between the samples until the end of the runs for all carbonization temperatures (Figure 5B). This rapid change in the adsorption rates indicated instant adsorption on the adsorbent surface and that the following slower adsorption rates indicated diffusional phenomenon inside the adsorbent particles [40]. However, the low R^2 values (<0.85%) and a larger difference between R^2 and r^2_{adj} indicated that this model may not be suitable to explain the adsorbent diffusion mechanisms and also implied that there were other diffusional phenomena controlling the adsorption rates.

3.3. Adsorption Isotherms

The aim for the adsorption isotherm analysis between the cLND and antibiotics is to evaluate their adsorption affinity and describe the equilibrium relationships between them. Adsorption isotherm determination is of importance, as it can provide supported data for designing an efficient adsorption system and for improving the adsorption pathways. In this study, we used five isotherm models to characterize the antibiotic molecular distribution at varying equilibrium concentrations obtained from the equilibrium adsorption experiment. The five models used in this study were: Freundlich, Langmuir (linear form Type 1), Langmuir (linear form Type 2), Temkin, Dubinin-Radushkevich (D-R), and Jovanovic (Equations (6)–(16), respectively) [35,41–43].

$$\text{Freundlich isotherm}: \ q_e = K_f C_e^{\frac{1}{n}} \tag{6}$$

$$\text{Linearized Freundlich equation}: \ \ln[q_e] = \ln\left[K_f\right] + \frac{1}{n}\ln[C_e] \tag{7}$$

$$\text{Langmuir isotherm}: \ q_e = \frac{q_m \cdot b \cdot C_e}{1 + b \cdot C_e} \tag{8}$$

$$\text{Linearized Langmuir Type 1 equation}: \ \frac{1}{q_e} = \left[\frac{1}{q_m b}\right]\frac{1}{C_e} + \frac{1}{q_m} \tag{9}$$

$$\text{Linearized Langmuir Type 2 equation}: \ \frac{C_e}{q_e} = \left[\frac{1}{q_m}\right]C_e + \frac{1}{q_m b} \tag{10}$$

$$\text{Temkin isotherm}: \ q_e = \left(\frac{RT}{b_T}\right)\ln(A_T C_e) \tag{11}$$

$$\text{Linearized Temkin equation}: \ q_e = \left(\frac{RT}{b_T}\right)\ln A_T + \left(\frac{RT}{b_T}\right)\ln C_e \tag{12}$$

$$\text{Dubinin} - \text{Radushkevich (D} - \text{R)}: \ q_e = Q_m e^{-(B\varepsilon^2)}; \ \varepsilon = RT\ln\left(1 + \frac{1}{C_e}\right) \tag{13}$$

$$\text{Linearized Dubinin} - \text{Radushkevich equation}: \ \ln q_e = \ln Q_m - B\varepsilon^2 \tag{14}$$

$$\text{Jovanovic isotherm}: \ q_e = \frac{q_m}{e^{K_j C_e}} \tag{15}$$

$$\text{Linearized Jovanovich equation}: \ \ln q_e = \ln q_m - K_j C_e \tag{16}$$

where C_e (mg L^{-1}) is the antibiotic equilibrium concentration, q_e (mg g^{-1}) is the cLND adsorption capacity at the equilibrium, q_m (mg g^{-1}) is the cLND theoretical maximum adsorption capacities, b (L mg^{-1}) is the Langmuir energy constant related to the adsorption heat, K_f (mg g^{-1}(L mg^{-1})$^{1/n}$) is the Freundlich constant, $\frac{1}{n}$ is the Freundlich adsorption intensity, R (8.314 J mol^{-1}K^{-1}) is the universal gas constant, T (K) is the temperature, b_T (J mol^{-1}) is the Temkin constant, A_T (L mol^{-1}) is the Temkin Equilibrium binding constant, Q_m is the adsorption saturation capacity, B is a Dubinin-Radushkevich constant, and K_j is the Jovanovich constant. Again, we used R^2 and r_{adj}^2 to evaluate the best fit isotherm model.

We selected cLND550 to evaluate further adsorption mechanisms, because the adsorption kinetic experiments indicated that it was a better adsorbent for two different antibiotic families. Both antibiotics were again used in this experiment, because their different chemical properties may have affected the adsorption results. In addition, we selected cLND450 to compare the adsorption behavior with the cLND550 results as, at this carbonization temperature, some hydrophilic functional groups still existed.

Based on the R^2 and r_{adji}^2 values, the adsorption process followed the order of Langmuir, Temkin, and D-R, indicating that antibiotic molecules formed multilayer coverage on the cLND heterogeneous surface (Table 2). The high R^2 values indicated that the Langmuir isotherm better described the SMX adsorption with both cLNDs similar to the ENR (Table 2). The Langmuir maximum monolayer adsorption capacity (q_m) was different between the SMX and ENR. The $q_{mENR,450}$ and $q_{mENR,550}$ values were relatively close (100.01 versus 104.16 mg g^{-1}), indicating that ENR was prone to be adsorbed with cLND regardless of the carbonization temperature due to its hydrophobicity. The $q_{mSMX,450}$ and $q_{mSMX,550}$ values differed by 17% (Table 2), indicating that cLND550 was a much better adsorbent for SMX than cLND450, corresponding with the previous experiments that showed a better adsorption for cLND550.

Table 2. SMX or ENR kinetic parameter comparisons for two types of cLND (cLND450 and cLND550).

Adsorption Isotherm Parameters		Sulfamethoxazole (SMX)		Enrofloxacin (ENR)	
		cLND 450	cLND 550	cLND 450	cLND 550
Freundlich isotherm					
K_f	mg g^{-1}(L mg^{-1})$^{1/n}$	11.987	16.211	25.554	18.460
$\frac{1}{n}$	-	0.394	0.330	0.423	0.512
R^2	-	0.822	0.844	0.818	0.877
r_{adj}^2	-	0.622	0.664	0.614	0.731
Langmuir isotherm(Linearized Langmuir Type 1 equation)					
q_m	mg g^{-1}	46.083	50.761	120.482	129.870
b	L mg^{-1}	0.179	0.239	0.014	0.094
R^2	-	0.951	0.958	0.934	0.953
r_{adj}^2	-	0.888	0.904	0.851	0.893
R_L	-	0.101–0.691	0.077–0.626	0.588–0.966	0.175–0.810
Langmuir isotherm(Linearized Langmuir Type 2 equation)					
q_m	mg g^{-1}	38.610	45.249	100.003	104.167
b_T	L mg^{-1}	0.309	0.366	0.229	0.147
R^2	-	0.974	0.985	0.956	0.946
r_{adj}^2	-	0.940	0.965	0.900	0.877
R_L	-	0.061–0.564	0.052–0.522	0.080–0.636	0.120–0.731
Temkin isotherm					
b	J mol^{-1}	275.893	251.898	101.803	95.889
A_T	L mol^{-1}	2.511	3.573	1.717	1.113
R^2	-	0.847	0.866	0.836	0.911
r_{adj}^2	-	0.670	0.708	0.649	0.802
Dubinin-Radushkevich isotherm					
Q_m	mg g^{-1}	13.330	14.013	14.879	14.441
B	-	2.92×10^{-6}	3.53×10^{-6}	4.09×10^{-6}	-4.17×10^{-6}
R^2	-	0.831	0.847	0.872	0.854
r_{adj}^2	-	0.639	0.670	0.720	0.684
Jovanovich isotherm					
q_m	mg g^{-1}	17.764	23.729	42.636	32.858
K_j	-	0.041	0.033	0.041	0.052
R^2	-	0.596	0.639	0.62	0.724
r_{adj}^2	-	0.248	0.310	0.292	0.445

Notably, the Langmuir isotherms can be linearized into four types of equations, depending on the variables plotted for the X- and Y-axis [31]. Selected linearized Langmuir equations were the only ones that had R^2 values >0.9. As it can be seen, both linearized equations provided a high correlation coefficient, supporting the well-described with Langmuir isotherm. Having said that, it does not necessarily mean all linearized Langmuir equations will always provide best fit. The difference in the linearized Y-axis and X-axis caused these fit discrepancies. Among them, Langmuir type 2 (C_e/q_e versus C_e) generally provide minimal error distributions between sampling points, hence giving a better fit than the others [25]. The Langmuir isotherm was further calculated for the reaction favorability and the isotherm type (Equation (17)).

$$R_L = \frac{1}{1 + bC_o} \tag{17}$$

where R_L is a dimensionless equilibrium parameter, and C_o (mg L^{-1}) is the antibiotic initial concentration. The results showed that all R_L values for any cLND adsorption were between 0 and 1 (0.052–0.966), indicating that the adsorption was a favorable process under the conditions applied. These numbers also coincided with the $1/n$ values (<1 for complete antibiotic adsorption) obtained from the Freundlich isotherm model, which also indicated the favorability of SMX and ENR adsorption onto cLND.

3.4. Influential Effect Experiments

3.4.1. Effect of pH

Typical environmental parameters that could potentially affect the adsorption efficiency were investigated using cLND550 against the presence of SMX or ENR. The parameters considered were: solution pH, organic matter, represented by humic acids (HA), bicarbonate (HCO$_3^-$), and chloride (Cl$^-$). We reported the changes in antibiotic removal efficiency at different timelines (3, 12, 24, and 48 h) to demonstrate how these effects influenced their adsorption mechanisms (Figures 6 and 7).

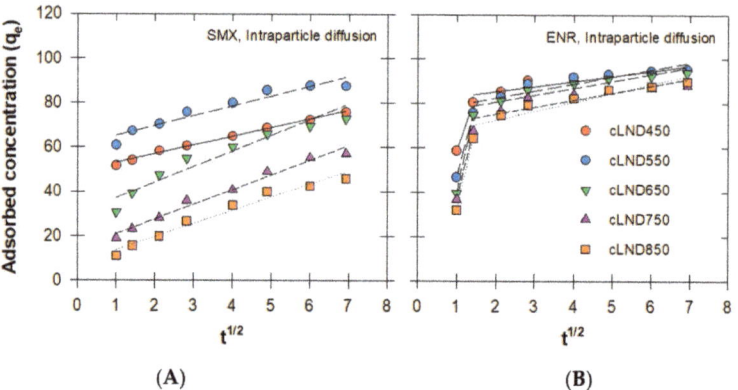

Figure 6. Effect of (**A**) initial pH and (**B**) humic acid concentrations on SMX or ENR removal efficiency using cLND550.

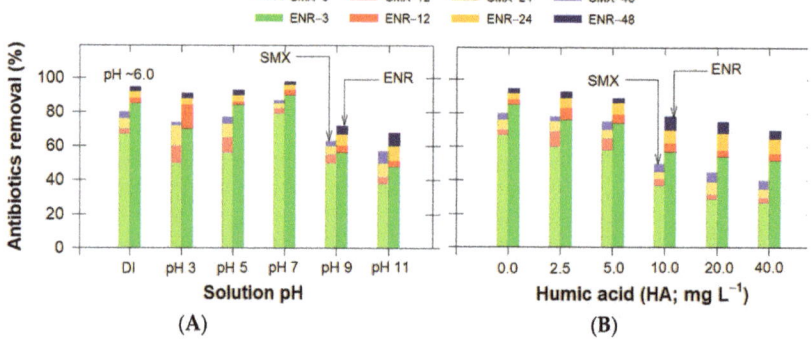

Figure 7. Effect of (**A**) bicarbonate and (**B**) chloride concentrations on SMX or ENR removal efficiency using cLND550.

Although the typical antibiotic-containing discharge water from animal farming is slightly alkaline, the pH from typical wastewater treatment plants can range between 2 and 10. The results showed that the adsorption efficiency decreased for alkaline conditions (Figure 6A). The adsorbate–adsorbent equilibrium was reached at approximately 24 h, as only slight changes were observed at 48 h. Compared with the control (adsorption in DI; pH~6.0), the SMX adsorption efficiency decreased up to 23% at pH 11, while that of ENR decreased up to 27%, indicating that the antibiotic adsorption was pH-dependent (Figure 6A). This also depended on the antibiotic chemical characteristics, as an antibiotic can be present in cationic, anionic, and neutral forms under different pH conditions. Since the important key role in the adsorption process was based on the catalyst surface, we determined the cLND550 point of zero charges (pH_{pzc}) was approximately 8.5. When the experimental pH > pH_{pzc}, the cLND550 surface became negatively charged, favoring cationic species adsorption and vice versa; when the experimental pH < pH_{pzc}, the positively charged cLND550 surface favored anionic species adsorption.

SMX and ENR had two pKa (1.85 and 5.29 for SMX and 6.19 and 7.91 for ENR) [44,45]. For pH < pKa1, the antibiotic forms were positively charged (SMX^+ and ENR^+), while, for pH > pKa2, the antibiotic forms were negatively charged (SMX^- and ENR^-). Therefore, the antibiotic zwitterionic forms ($SMX^{+/-}$ and $ENR^{+/-}$) were present when the pH was between pKa1 and pKa2.

The antibiotic rapid adsorption in the first stage (3 h) was due to these opposite charges between the adsorbate and adsorbent. As discussed earlier in the adsorption kinetic experiment, the adsorption efficiency between ENR and SMX was substantially different (Figure 3). Notably, ENR adsorption on cLND550 was high (~91%), even though both ENR and cLND550 had a positive charge. This can be explained by the ENR's low water solubility, facilitating the hydrophobic adsorption and the π–π interaction between the ENR and aliphatic functional groups on cLND550 (Figure 2) [46–48]. In addition, the ENR adsorption could have been due to the H bonding occurring between fluorine atoms in the ENR structure and -OH functional groups on the cLND surface (Figure 2) [49]. These were possibly the main reasons for the better ENR adsorption under acidic conditions despite both ENR and cLND550 having a positive charge.

Since ENR has a lower water solubility than SMX (~146 mg L^{-1} versus 281 mg L^{-1}), SMX hydrophobic adsorption and the π–π interaction could be less, resulting in a lower adsorption efficiency than for ENR [50]. In addition, under acidic conditions, the SMX water solubility was much lower than for alkaline conditions, facilitating a greater adsorption for SMX with this pH [51].

When 3 < pH < 6, the same ENR adsorption behavior was expected, as discussed earlier. By increasing the pH from 5 to 7, the SMX adsorption efficiency increased from 77 to 87% (Figure 6A), mainly due to the electrostatic attraction occurring from the increased SMX charge distribution toward SMX^- from the SMX deprotonation, making it more prone to being adsorbed on the cLND550 positively charged surface ($cLND^+$). At pH 7, the ENR adsorption reached its maximum adsorption capacity of 98% (Figure 6A). Here, the hydrophobic interaction, π–π interaction, and H bonding were more pronounced with aromatic-containing molecules -OH and Si-OH on the cLND550 surface (Figure 2) [47]. A similar observation for a neutral pH was reported for ENR adsorption on highly pyrolytic corn stalk materials [52].

For strong alkaline conditions (pH 9–11), both antibiotics had negative charges, increasing the electrostatic repulsion with $cLND^-$ [53,54]. Therefore, the SMX removal efficiencies decreased to 63% and 57% for pH 9 and 11, respectively, while those of ENR decreased to 72% and 68%, respectively (Figure 6A). The ongoing adsorption for this pH range was observed, which could be attributed to the interaction between the antibiotic molecule and the existing cLND550 functional groups, as discussed earlier.

3.4.2. Effect of Humic Acids (HAs)

Since real antibiotic-containing discharge water usually contains natural organic matter, we investigated this influential effect on the antibiotic adsorption efficiency by varying the HA content between 2.5 mg L^{-1} and 40 mg L^{-1}. Compared to the control (no HA), the results showed that HA potentially suppressed the removal efficiency by up to 40% for SMX and by up to 25% for ENR (Figure 6B).

HA is usually rich in numerous functional groups embedded on the particle surface of the HA, such as carboxylic acid and aromatic and phenolic groups [55]. This functional group existence enabled stronger interactions with other foreign chemicals on the cLND surface via either H bonding or π–π interactions. Among these, carboxylic acid is naturally deprotonated, making the HA negatively charged for most environmental pH ranges. Once presented together with cLND under normal pH conditions, cLND$^+$ (pH$_{pzc}$ = 8.5) spontaneously became available at adsorptive sites that favored HA adsorption, giving fewer sites for antibiotic adsorption. In addition, the existence of nonpolar functional groups can further adsorb HA, which can potentially compete with target antibiotic contaminants with a higher HA content. Hou et al. [10] showed that HA possibly combined with the available antibiotics and formed a more soluble complex compound that can potentially minimize the adsorption performance. However, antibiotic adsorption still occurred, indicating that the cLND surface could still provide unbound functional groups with antibiotic molecules. The better adsorption by ENR than SMX could have been due to the electrostatic attraction between ENR$^+$ and HA$^-$ for these normal pH conditions. Although most suspended solids would be removed during the preliminary process in the WWTP, other organic constituents may be of concern. This information suggested other means to initially separate abnormally high humic colloids or other organic-containing contents from the water before it entered the adsorption unit.

3.4.3. Effect of Anionic Constituents

Since bicarbonate (HCO$_3^-$) and chloride (Cl$^-$) are some of the most prominent anionic compounds in nature, we individually varied these two anionic concentrations up to 800 mg L^{-1} for neutral pH conditions. The results showed that the increase in these two ions slightly decreased the antibiotic adsorption efficiency (Figure 7). HCO$_3^-$ had fewer negative effects on antibiotic adsorption than Cl$^-$. This can be explained by the increase in the anionic concentration simultaneously filling the aqueous solution with anionic molecules that later underwent electrostatic attraction with cLND$^+$, consequently blocking the sorption sites for antibiotic adsorption.

Other than competing with the sites with cLND$^+$, the interference was more pronounced with SMX adsorption. Since this reaction occurred under neutral pH conditions, the repulsion interaction between anionic ions and SMX$^-$ also occurred, suppressing its electrostatic attraction with cLND$^+$. This anionic existence in the adsorption process may not be problematic due to the lower magnitude of interference. While our highest tested concentration was far less than the natural possible conditions (Cl$^-$ ~19,800 mg L^{-1} for seawater; [56]), the ENR-adsorbed concentrations on bamboo biochar in the presence of 3000 mg L^{-1} Cl$^-$ were reduced by only 25% [57]. Overall, the results confirmed that the negative influence of anions on the SMX/ENR adsorption should not be neglected at high anionic concentrations (>200 mg·L^{-1}).

3.5. Bacterial Activity

As stated earlier in the adsorption kinetics section, chemisorption plays a dominant role during the adsorption process, and so, the desorption processes can be ignored. To validate this statement, we used a growth inhibition zone experiment and testing Gram-negative *Staphylococcus aureus* (ATCC 25923) bacteria with treated water (filtrated water) and cLND (retentate after filtration). We selected only ENR as the target representative, as it was more frequently detected [58], and it has greater absorptivity on cLND at any carbonization temperature. The clear zone difference percentage after 24 h of adsorption (C$_{\Delta-24h}$) was calculated and plotted against the ENR initial concentration (Figure 8A).

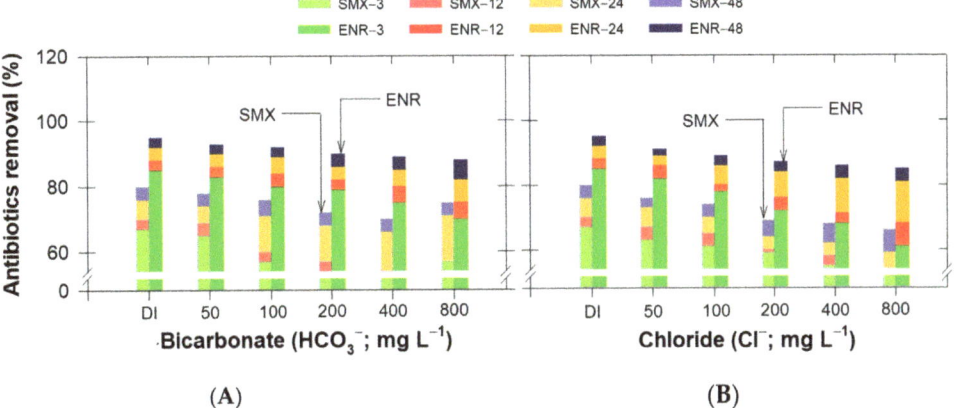

Figure 8. (A) Clear zone difference of *Staphylococcus aureus* ATCC 25923 after 24-h adsorption ($C_{\Delta\text{-}24h}$) of ENR onto each type of cLND (cLND450 and cLND550), and **(B,C)** clear zone examples at two ENR concentrations (20 and 40 mg L^{-1}) onto cLND550.

Using cLND at 300 mg, ~100% of $C_{\Delta\text{-}24h}$ at 20 mg L^{-1} ENR was observed, indicating that there was no clear zone after cLND adsorption, and thus, the cLND completely removed the ENR (Figure 8B). Conversely, at the lower cLND amount (30 mg), the ENR residue was still in the solution, resulting in ~7–~11% $C_{\Delta\text{-}24h}$ (Figure 8A). As such, regardless of the cLND type or amount, the increase in the ENR initial concentration substantially increased $C_{\Delta\text{-}24h}$ (Figure 8B,C). This can be explained by the reduced availability of the adsorptive sites on the cLND surface to adsorb ENR, as the available ENR molecules had already been chemisorbed on the surface. The cLND550 $C_{\Delta\text{-}24h}$ was slightly higher than for cLND450, signifying that the cLND550 could better adsorb antibiotics than cLND450 (Figure 8A).

Banana peel biochar can serve as a growth inhibitor for *E. coli*, because the natural potassium chloride in the biochar can hinder the bacterial cellular activities [59]. Our cLND had no such effect on the *S. aureus* ATCC 25923 strains, indicating that the clear zone occurrence was solely from the existing adsorbed ENR, not from the cLND itself, and that any cLND leached into the environment would not interfere with any local organisms.

A key to being a compatible adsorbent for real applications is that the adsorbent should retain the adsorbate without releasing it into the aqueous solution. Again, we used this sensitive bacterial growth inhibition experiment on the retentate cLND obtained from both the cLND adsorption experiments (cLND450 and cLND550) with various initial ENR concentrations. A comparison was made between day 1 and day 3 and presented as an increase in *S. aureus* growth (change percentages in the clear zone, $C_{\Delta\text{-}3d}$) at different ENR initial concentrations (Figure 9).

With the different cLND amounts or different carbonization temperatures, both cLNDs had the same clear zone trend, where an increase in the ENR initial concentration increased the $C_{\Delta\text{-}3d}$. Although $C_{\Delta\text{-}3d}$ was the highest at 100 mg L^{-1} ENR concentration in any of the experimental setups, the $C_{\Delta\text{-}3d}$ value was ~9.6% (Figure 9). This indicated that the cLND was still beneficial, as it retained (less desorption) most of the adsorbed ENR.

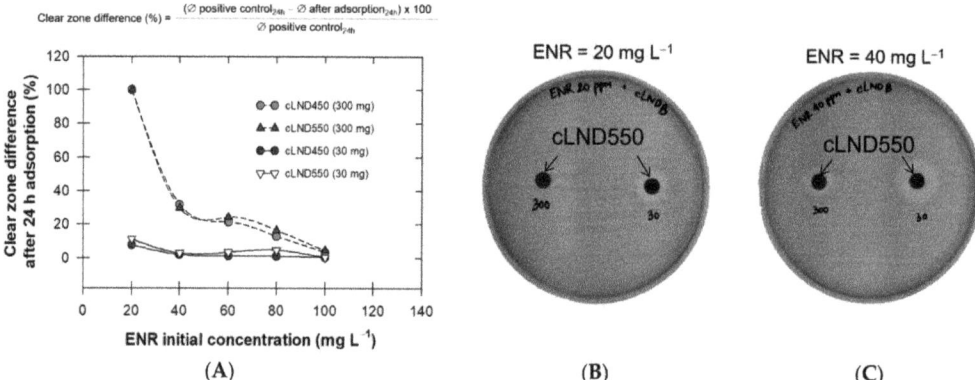

Figure 9. Changes in the clear zone after day 3 ($C_{\Delta\text{-}3d}$) of *Staphylococcus aureus* ATCC 25923 following ENR adsorption onto cLNDs.

The cLND550 retained better microbial activity than the cLND450 at any ENR initial concentration based on the value of $C_{\Delta\text{-}3d}$ (2.35% for 30 mg cLND and 1.01% for 300 mg cLND), as shown in Figure 9. The ENR stronghold on cLND can be explained by both physical adsorption and chemisorption, with more than one interaction potentially occurring, such as the π–π interaction, hydrophobic adsorption, H bonding, and pore filling between antibiotics on the biochar surface [60]. The unchanged $C_{\Delta\text{-}3d}$ value for cLND450 at 30 mg indicated little microbial activity could be expected that might interfere with the cLND adsorption activity under adsorptive competition between adsorbates. Notably, we used a much higher ENR concentration in this experiment compared to the frequently detected concentration, thus confirming that cLND could efficiently adsorb ENR even at exceptionally high concentrations, which could compromise the effectiveness of the other adsorbate organic constituents.

4. Conclusions

Carbonized leonardite (cLND) was successfully prepared from a byproduct generated from lignite coal that was carbonized at a constant heat rate to the desired temperatures between 450 °C and 850 °C under a N_2 flow stream. Of these carbonization temperatures, the cLND550 product had the highest adsorption capability for SMX and ENR, because the cLND550 had both hydrophobic and hydrophilic active functional groups on the cLND surface. The nonlinear kinetics fitting results showed that the pseudo-second-order kinetics model was more suitable for describing the cLND and SMX or ENR adsorption. Among the several isotherm models, both the SMX and ENR adsorption equilibrium data fitted well with Langmuir isotherms. The cLND yielded maximum adsorption capacities of 104.167 mg g^{-1} (ENR) and 45.249 mg g^{-1} (SMX). For neutral pH conditions, antibiotic adsorption revealed the highest removal efficiency due to the electrostatic interaction and H bonding between the antibiotic and cLND. Anionic and organic constituents suppressed the antibiotic adsorption, mostly resulting from the charge attraction between cLND and these ions, which competed with the available antibiotics. Microbial activities confirmed that cLND450 and cLND550 successfully adsorbed ENR at varying ENR initial concentrations, and the percentage desorption difference after 3 d was relatively low (1.70–35%). Overall, this work showed the potential good utilization of low-ranked coals to efficiently adsorb emerging contaminants, such as antibiotics, and the study also provided proof that cLND was a suitable adsorbent for antibiotics and could be applied to combat various kinds of water pollutants.

Supplementary Materials: The following supporting information can be downloaded at https://www. mdpi.com/article/10.3390/antibiotics11091261/s1: Figure S1: Changes in the pseudo-first-order reaction rates (K_1) and adsorbed concentrations (q_e) following varying types of cLND adsorption. Figure S2: Changes in the Elovich parameters (a and b) following varying types of cLND adsorption.

Author Contributions: Conceptualization, C.C. and C.S.; methodology, C.C., K.S., A.W. and C.S.; validation, C.C. and C.S.; formal analysis, C.C. and C.S.; investigation, C.C., C.S. and K.S.; resources, C.S.; data curation, C.C. and C.S.; writing—original draft preparation, C.C. and C.S.; writing—review and editing, C.C., C.S., S.I., N.S. and T.K.; visualization, C.C. and C.S.; supervision, D.D.S.; project administration, C.S.; and funding acquisition, C.S., T.E.A. and M.A.A. All authors have read and agreed to the published version of the manuscript.

Funding: This work was financially supported by the Office of the Ministry of Higher Education, Science, Research and Innovation and the Thailand Science Research and Innovation through the Kasetsart University Reinventing University Program 2021. The authors also extend their appreciation to the Deanship of Scientific Research at King Khalid University for funding this work through a large research groups program under grant number RGP.2-8-43.

Data Availability Statement: The authors confirm that the data supporting the findings of this study are available within the article.

Acknowledgments: This work was financially supported by the Office of the Ministry of Higher Education, Science, Research and Innovation and the Thailand Science Research and Innovation through the Kasetsart University Reinventing University Program 2021. Our appreciation is expressed to Kanitta Wongyai, Level 10th Scientist from the Electricity Generating Authority of Thailand (EGAT) at the Mae Moh lignite mine for providing the leonardite.

Conflicts of Interest: The authors declare no conflict of interest.

References

1. Coyne, L.; Arief, R.; Benigno, C.; Giang, V.N.; Huong, L.Q.; Jeamsripong, S.; Kalpravidh, W.; McGrane, J.; Padungtod, P.; Patrick, I.; et al. Characterizing Antimicrobial Use in the Livestock Sector in Three South East Asian Countries (Indonesia, Thailand, and Vietnam). *Antibiotics* **2019**, *8*, 33. [CrossRef] [PubMed]
2. Landers, T.F.; Cohen, B.; Wittum, T.E.; Larson, E.L. A review of antibiotic use in food animals: Perspective, policy, and potential. *Public Health Rep.* **2012**, *127*, 4–22. [CrossRef] [PubMed]
3. Spellberg, B.; Bartlett, J.G.; Gilbert, D.N. The future of antibiotics and resistance. *N. Engl. J. Med.* **2013**, *368*, 299–302. [CrossRef] [PubMed]
4. Chen, Y.; Chen, H.; Zhang, L.; Jiang, Y.; Gin, K.Y.-H.; He, Y. Occurrence, Distribution, and Risk Assessment of Antibiotics in a Subtropical River-Reservoir System. *Water* **2018**, *10*, 104. [CrossRef]
5. Du, L.; Liu, W. Occurrence, fate, and ecotoxicity of antibiotics in agro-ecosystems. A review. *Agron. Sustain. Dev.* **2012**, *32*, 309–327. [CrossRef]
6. Poapolathep, S.; Giorgi, M.; Chaiyabutr, N.; Chokejaroenrat, C.; Klangkaew, N.; Phaochoosak, N.; Wongwaipairote, T.; Poapo-lathep, A. Pharmacokinetics of enrofloxacin and its metabolite ciprofloxacin in freshwater crocodiles (*Crocodylus siamensis*) after intravenous and intramuscular administration. *J. Vet. Pharmacol. Ther.* **2020**, *43*, 19–25. [CrossRef]
7. Ruennarong, N.; Wongpanit, K.; Sakulthaew, C.; Giorgi, M.; Kumagai, S.; Poapolathep, A.; Poapolathep, S. Dispositions of enrofloxacin and its major metabolite ciprofloxacin in Thai swamp buffaloes. *J. Vet. Med. Sci.* **2016**, *78*, 397–403. [CrossRef]
8. Boleda, M.R.; Alechaga, É.; Moyano, E.; Galceran, M.T.; Ventura, F. Survey of the occurrence of pharmaceuticals in Spanish finished drinking waters. *Environ. Sci. Pollut. Res.* **2014**, *21*, 10917–10939. [CrossRef]
9. Carabineiro, S.A.; Thavorn-Amornsri, T.; Pereira, M.F.; Figueiredo, J.L. Adsorption of ciprofloxacin on surface-modified carbon materials. *Water Res.* **2011**, *45*, 4583–4591. [CrossRef]
10. Hou, J.; Wang, C.; Mao, D.; Luo, Y. The occurrence and fate of tetracyclines in two pharmaceutical wastewater treatment plants of Northern China. *Environ. Sci. Pollut. Res.* **2016**, *23*, 1722–1731. [CrossRef]
11. Kuchta, S.L.; Cessna, A.J. Lincomycin and Spectinomycin Concentrations in Liquid Swine Manure and Their Persistence During Simulated Manure Storage. *Arch. Environ. Contam. Toxicol.* **2008**, *57*, 1–10. [CrossRef]
12. Yamaguchi, T.; Okihashi, M.; Harada, K.; Konishi, Y.; Uchida, K.; Do, M.H.N.; Bui, H.D.T.; Nguyen, T.D.; Nguyen, P.D.; Chau, V.V.; et al. Antibiotic Residue Monitoring Results for Pork, Chicken, and Beef Samples in Vietnam in 2012–2013. *J. Agric. Food Chem.* **2015**, *63*, 5141–5145. [CrossRef]
13. Bergeron, S.; Raj, B.; Nathaniel, R.; Corbin, A.; LaFleur, G. Presence of antibiotic resistance genes in raw source water of a drinking water treatment plant in a rural community of USA. *Int. Biodeterior. Biodegrad.* **2017**, *124*, 3–9. [CrossRef]
14. Lundborg, C.S.; Tamhankar, A.J. Antibiotic residues in the environment of South East Asia. *BMJ* **2017**, *358*, j2440. [CrossRef]

15. Shimizu, A.; Takada, H.; Koike, T.; Takeshita, A.; Saha, M.; Rinawati; Nakada, N.; Murata, A.; Suzuki, T.; Suzuki, S.; et al. Ubiquitous occurrence of sulfonamides in tropical Asian waters. *Sci. Total Environ.* **2013**, *452–453*, 108–115. [CrossRef]
16. Tewari, S.; Jindal, R.; Kho, Y.L.; Eo, S.; Choi, K. Major pharmaceutical residues in wastewater treatment plants and receiving waters in Bangkok, Thailand, and associated ecological risks. *Chemosphere* **2013**, *91*, 697–704. [CrossRef] [PubMed]
17. Sinthuchai, D.; Boontanon, S.K.; Boontanon, N.; Polprasert, C. Evaluation of removal efficiency of human antibiotics in wastewater treatment plants in Bangkok, Thailand. *Water Sci. Technol.* **2016**, *73*, 182–191. [CrossRef]
18. Mutiyar, P.K.; Mittal, A.K. Occurrences and fate of selected human antibiotics in influents and effluents of sewage treatment plant and effluent-receiving river Yamuna in Delhi (India). *Environ. Monit. Assess.* **2014**, *186*, 541–557. [CrossRef]
19. Larsson, D.G.; de Pedro, C.; Paxeus, N. Effluent from drug manufactures contains extremely high levels of pharmaceuticals. *J. Hazard. Mater.* **2007**, *148*, 751–755. [CrossRef]
20. Jutarvutikul, K.; Sakulthaew, C.; Chokejaroenrat, C.; Pattanateeradetch, A.; Imman, S.; Suriyachai, N.; Satapanajaru, T.; Kreetachat, T. Practical use of response surface methodology for optimization of veterinary antibiotic removal using UV/H2O2 process. *Aquac. Eng.* **2021**, *94*, 102174. [CrossRef]
21. Enaime, G.; Baçaoui, A.; Yaacoubi, A.; Lübken, M. Biochar for Wastewater Treatment—Conversion Technologies and Applications. *Appl. Sci.* **2020**, *10*, 3492. [CrossRef]
22. Ganiyu, S.O.; van Hullebusch, E.D.; Cretin, M.; Esposito, G.; Oturan, M.A. Coupling of membrane filtration and advanced oxidation processes for removal of pharmaceutical residues: A critical review. *Sep. Purif. Technol.* **2015**, *156*, 891–914. [CrossRef]
23. Ji, L.; Chen, W.; Duan, L.; Zhu, D. Mechanisms for strong adsorption of tetracycline to carbon nanotubes: A comparative study using activated carbon and graphite as adsorbents. *Environ. Sci. Technol.* **2009**, *43*, 2322–2327. [CrossRef] [PubMed]
24. Rivera-Utrilla, J.; Gómez-Pacheco, C.V.; Sánchez-Polo, M.; López-Peñalver, J.J.; Ocampo-Pérez, R. Tetracycline removal from water by adsorption/bioadsorption on activated carbons and sludge-derived adsorbents. *J. Environ. Manag.* **2013**, *131*, 16–24. [CrossRef]
25. Shimabuku, K.K.; Kearns, J.P.; Martinez, J.E.; Mahoney, R.B.; Moreno-Vasquez, L.; Summers, R.S. Biochar sorbents for sulfamethoxazole removal from surface water, stormwater, and wastewater effluent. *Water Res.* **2016**, *96*, 236–245. [CrossRef]
26. Liao, P.; Zhan, Z.; Dai, J.; Wu, X.; Zhang, W.; Wang, K.; Yuan, S. Adsorption of tetracycline and chloramphenicol in aqueous solutions by bamboo charcoal: A batch and fixed-bed column study. *Chem. Eng. J.* **2013**, *228*, 496–505. [CrossRef]
27. Zeng, Z.-w.; Tan, X.-f.; Liu, Y.-g.; Tian, S.-r.; Zeng, G.-m.; Jiang, L.-h.; Liu, S.-b.; Li, J.; Liu, N.; Yin, Z.-h. Comprehensive Adsorption Studies of Doxycycline and Ciprofloxacin Antibiotics by Biochars Prepared at Different Temperatures. *Front. Chem.* **2018**, *6*, 80. [CrossRef]
28. Stylianou, M.; Christou, A.; Michael, C.; Agapiou, A.; Papanastasiou, P.; Fatta-Kassinos, D. Adsorption and removal of seven antibiotic compounds present in water with the use of biochar derived from the pyrolysis of organic waste feedstocks. *J. Environ. Chem. Eng.* **2021**, *9*, 105868. [CrossRef]
29. Ausavasukhi, A.; Kampoosaen, C.; Kengnok, O. Adsorption characteristics of Congo red on carbonized leonardite. *J. Clean. Prod.* **2016**, *134*, 506–514. [CrossRef]
30. Chammui, Y.; Sooksamiti, P.; Naksata, W.; Thiansem, S.; Arqueropanyo, O.-a. Removal of arsenic from aqueous solution by adsorption on Leonardite. *Chem. Eng. J.* **2014**, *240*, 202–210. [CrossRef]
31. Sakulthaew, C.; Watcharenwong, A.; Chokejaroenrat, C.; Rittirat, A. Leonardite-Derived Biochar Suitability for Effective Sorption of Herbicides. *Water Air Soil Pollut.* **2021**, *232*, 36. [CrossRef]
32. Rico, A.; Phu, T.M.; Satapornvanit, K.; Min, J.; Shahabuddin, A.M.; Henriksson, P.J.G.; Murray, F.J.; Little, D.C.; Dalsgaard, A.; Van den Brink, P.J. Use of veterinary medicines, feed additives and probiotics in four major internationally traded aquaculture species farmed in Asia. *Aquaculture* **2013**, *412–413*, 231–243. [CrossRef]
33. Keiluweit, M.; Nico, P.S.; Johnson, M.G.; Kleber, M. Dynamic Molecular Structure of Plant Biomass-Derived Black Carbon (Biochar). *Environ. Sci. Technol.* **2010**, *44*, 1247–1253. [CrossRef]
34. Sakulthaew, C.; Chokejaroenrat, C.; Poapolathep, A.; Satapanajaru, T.; Poapolathep, S. Hexavalent chromium adsorption from aqueous solution using carbon nano-onions (CNOs). *Chemosphere* **2017**, *184*, 1168–1174. [CrossRef]
35. Chokejaroenrat, C.; Watcharenwong, A.; Sakulthaew, C.; Rittirat, A. Immobilization of Atrazine Using Oxidized Lignite Amendments in Agricultural Soils. *Water Air Soil Pollut.* **2020**, *231*, 249. [CrossRef]
36. Deng, H.; Mao, Z.; Xu, H.; Zhang, L.; Zhong, Y.; Sui, X. Synthesis of fibrous LaFeO3 perovskite oxide for adsorption of Rhodamine B. *Ecotoxicol. Environ. Saf.* **2019**, *168*, 35–44. [CrossRef]
37. Wu, F.-C.; Tseng, R.-L.; Juang, R.-S. Characteristics of Elovich equation used for the analysis of adsorption kinetics in dye-chitosan systems. *Chem. Eng. J.* **2009**, *150*, 366–373. [CrossRef]
38. Weber, W.J.; Morris, J.C. Kinetics of Adsorption on Carbon from Solution. *J. Sanit. Eng. Div.* **1963**, *89*, 31–59. [CrossRef]
39. Wu, F.-C.; Tseng, R.-L.; Juang, R.-S. Initial behavior of intraparticle diffusion model used in the description of adsorption kinetics. *Chem. Eng. J.* **2009**, *153*, 1–8. [CrossRef]
40. Wakkel, M.; Khiari, B.; Zagrouba, F. Textile wastewater treatment by agro-industrial waste: Equilibrium modelling, thermodynamics and mass transfer mechanisms of cationic dyes adsorption onto low-cost lignocellulosic adsorbent. *J. Taiwan Inst. Chem. Eng.* **2019**, *96*, 439–452. [CrossRef]
41. Ayawei, N.; Ebelegi, A.N.; Wankasi, D. Modelling and Interpretation of Adsorption Isotherms. *J. Chem.* **2017**, *2017*, 3039817. [CrossRef]

42. Hamdaoui, O.; Naffrechoux, E. Modeling of adsorption isotherms of phenol and chlorophenols onto granular activated carbon: Part I. Two-parameter models and equations allowing determination of thermodynamic parameters. *J. Hazard. Mater.* **2007**, *147*, 381–394. [CrossRef]

43. Rozada, F.; Otero, M.; García, A.I.; Morán, A. Application in fixed-bed systems of adsorbents obtained from sewage sludge and discarded tyres. *Dye. Pigment.* **2007**, *72*, 47–56. [CrossRef]

44. Jiménez-Lozano, E.; Marqués, I.; Barrón, D.; Beltrán, J.L.; Barbosa, J. Determination of pKa values of quinolones from mobility and spectroscopic data obtained by capillary electrophoresis and a diode array detector. *Anal. Chim. Acta* **2002**, *464*, 37–45. [CrossRef]

45. Wu, M.; Pan, B.; Zhang, D.; Xiao, D.; Li, H.; Wang, C.; Ning, P. The sorption of organic contaminants on biochars derived from sediments with high organic carbon content. *Chemosphere* **2013**, *90*, 782–788. [CrossRef]

46. Martínez-Mejía, M.J.; Sato, I.; Rath, S. Sorption mechanism of enrofloxacin on humic acids extracted from Brazilian soils. *Environ. Sci. Pollut. Res.* **2017**, *24*, 15995–16006. [CrossRef]

47. Xie, H.; Liu, W.; Zhang, J.; Zhang, C.; Ren, L. Sorption of norfloxacin from aqueous solutions by activated carbon developed from Trapa natans husk. *Sci. China Chem.* **2011**, *54*, 835–843. [CrossRef]

48. Zhao, Y.; Liu, X.; Li, W.; Huang, K.; Shao, H.; Qu, C.; Liu, J. One-step synthesis of garlic peel derived biochar by concentrated sulfuric acid: Enhanced adsorption capacities for Enrofloxacin and interfacial interaction mechanisms. *Chemosphere* **2022**, *290*, 133263. [CrossRef]

49. Bajpai, S.; Bajpai, M.; Rai, N. Sorptive removal of ciprofoxacin hydrochloride from simulated wastewater using sawdust: Kinetic study and effect of pH. *Water SA* **2011**, *38*, 673–682. [CrossRef]

50. Reguyal, F.; Sarmah, A.K. Adsorption of sulfamethoxazole by magnetic biochar: Effects of pH, ionic strength, natural organic matter and 17α-ethinylestradiol. *Sci. Total Environ.* **2018**, *628–629*, 722–730. [CrossRef]

51. Zhang, R.; Zheng, X.; Chen, B.; Ma, J.; Niu, X.; Zhang, D.; Lin, Z.; Fu, M.; Zhou, S. Enhanced adsorption of sulfamethoxazole from aqueous solution by Fe-impregnated graphited biochar. *J. Clean. Prod.* **2020**, *256*, 120662. [CrossRef]

52. Wang, W.; Ma, X.; Sun, J.; Chen, J.; Zhang, J.; Wang, Y.; Wang, J.; Zhang, H. Adsorption of enrofloxacin on acid/alkali-modified corn stalk biochar. *Spectrosc. Lett.* **2019**, *52*, 367–375. [CrossRef]

53. Rajapaksha, A.U.; Vithanage, M.; Lee, S.S.; Seo, D.-C.; Tsang, D.C.W.; Ok, Y.S. Steam activation of biochars facilitates kinetics and pH-resilience of sulfamethazine sorption. *J. Soils Sediments* **2016**, *16*, 889–895. [CrossRef]

54. Xie, M.; Chen, W.; Xu, Z.; Zheng, S.; Zhu, D. Adsorption of sulfonamides to demineralized pine wood biochars prepared under different thermochemical conditions. *Environ. Pollut.* **2014**, *186*, 187–194. [CrossRef]

55. Wang, H.; Dong, Y.-n.; Zhu, M.; Li, X.; Keller, A.A.; Wang, T.; Li, F. Heteroaggregation of engineered nanoparticles and kaolin clays in aqueous environments. *Water Res.* **2015**, *80*, 130–138. [CrossRef]

56. Gros, N.; Camões, M.F.; Oliveira, C.; Silva, M.C.R. Ionic composition of seawaters and derived saline solutions determined by ion chromatography and its relation to other water quality parameters. *J. Chromatogr. A* **2008**, *1210*, 92–98. [CrossRef]

57. Wang, Y.; Lu, J.; Wu, J.; Liu, Q.; Zhang, H.; Jin, S. Adsorptive Removal of Fluoroquinolone Antibiotics Using Bamboo Biochar. *Sustainability* **2015**, *7*, 12947–12957. [CrossRef]

58. Ikem, A.; Lin, C.H.; Broz, B.; Kerley, M.; Ho, T.; Le, H. Occurrence of enrofloxacin in overflows from animal lot and residential sewage lagoons and a receiving-stream. *Heliyon* **2017**, *3*, e00409. [CrossRef]

59. Sigiro, M. Natural biowaste of banana peel-derived porous carbon for in-vitro antibacterial activity toward Escherichia coli. *Ain Shams Eng. J.* **2021**, *12*, 4157–4165. [CrossRef]

60. Masrura, S.U.; Jones-Lepp, T.L.; Kajitvichyanukul, P.; Ok, Y.S.; Tsang, D.C.W.; Khan, E. Unintentional release of antibiotics associated with nutrients recovery from source-separated human urine by biochar. *Chemosphere* **2022**, *299*, 134426. [CrossRef]

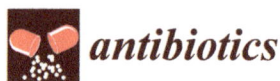

Article

Adsorptive–Photocatalytic Performance for Antibiotic and Personal Care Product Using $Cu_{0.5}Mn_{0.5}Fe_2O_4$

Chanat Chokejaroenrat [1], Chainarong Sakulthaew [2,*], Athaphon Angkaew [1], Apiladda Pattanateeradetch [1], Wuttinun Raksajit [2], Kanokwan Teingtham [3], Piyaporn Phansak [4], Pawee Klongvessa [1], Daniel D. Snow [5], Clifford E. Harris [6] and Steve D. Comfort [7]

[1] Department of Environmental Technology and Management, Faculty of Environment, Kasetsart University, Bangkok 10900, Thailand; eccnc@ku.ac.th (C.C.); athaphon.ak@gmail.com (A.A.); apiladda.pat@ku.th (A.P.); ecpwk@ku.ac.th (P.K.)
[2] Department of Veterinary Technology, Faculty of Veterinary Technology, Kasetsart University, Bangkok 10900, Thailand; cvtwnr@ku.ac.th
[3] Department of Agronomy, Faculty of Agriculture at Kamphaeng Saen, Kasetsart University, Nakhon Pathom 73140, Thailand; agrknw@ku.ac.th
[4] Division of Biology, Faculty of Science, Nakhon Phanom University, Nakhon Phanom 48000, Thailand; pphansak@npu.ac.th
[5] Water Sciences Laboratory, University of Nebraska-Lincoln, Lincoln, NE 68583, USA; dsnow1@unl.edu
[6] Department of Chemistry and Biochemistry, Albion College, Albion, MI 49224, USA; charris@albion.edu
[7] School of Natural Resources, University of Nebraska-Lincoln, Lincoln, NE 68583, USA; scomfort1@unl.edu
* Correspondence: cvtcns@ku.ac.th; Tel.: +66-2942-8200 (ext. 616018)

Citation: Chokejaroenrat, C.; Sakulthaew, C.; Angkaew, A.; Pattanateeradetch, A.; Raksajit, W.; Teingtham, K.; Phansak, P.; Klongvessa, P.; Snow, D.D.; Harris, C.E.; et al. Adsorptive–Photocatalytic Performance for Antibiotic and Personal Care Product Using $Cu_{0.5}Mn_{0.5}Fe_2O_4$. *Antibiotics* **2023**, *12*, 1151. https://doi.org/10.3390/antibiotics12071151

Academic Editors: Anusak Kerdsin, Jinquan Li and Jonathan Frye

Received: 27 May 2023
Revised: 19 June 2023
Accepted: 1 July 2023
Published: 5 July 2023

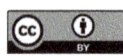
Abstract: The amount of antibiotics and personal care products entering local sewage systems and ultimately natural waters is increasing and raising concerns about long-term human health effects. We developed an adsorptive photocatalyst, $Cu_{0.5}Mn_{0.5}Fe_2O_4$ nanoparticles, utilizing co-precipitation and calcination with melamine, and quantified its efficacy in removing paraben and oxytetracycline (OTC). During melamine calcination, $Cu_{0.5}Mn_{0.5}Fe_2O_4$ recrystallized, improving material crystallinity and purity for the adsorptive–photocatalytic reaction. Kinetic experiments showed that all four parabens and OTC were removed within 120 and 45 min. We found that contaminant adsorption and reaction with active radicals occurred almost simultaneously with the photocatalyst. OTC adsorption could be adequately described by the Brouers–Sotolongo kinetic and Freundlich isotherm models. OTC photocatalytic degradation started with a series of reactions at different carbon locations (i.e., decarboxamidation, deamination, dehydroxylation, demethylation, and tautomerization). Further toxicity testing showed that *Zea mays* L. and *Vigna radiata* L. shoot indexes were less affected by treated water than root indexes. The *Zea mays* L. endodermis thickness and area decreased considerably after exposure to the 25% (v/v)-treated water. Overall, $Cu_{0.5}Mn_{0.5}Fe_2O_4$ nanoparticles exhibit a remarkable adsorptive–photocatalytic performance for the degradation of tested antibiotics and personal care products.

Keywords: adsorption–photocatalysis integration; adsorption isotherms; adsorption kinetics; $Cu_{0.5}Mn_{0.5}Fe_2O_4$ nanoparticles; oxytetracycline removal; paraben removal; root anatomical changes; seed germination

1. Introduction

Pharmaceuticals and personal care products (PPCPs) are substances used for medical, cosmetics, hygiene, and health care. The increased global production of PPCPs and subsequent disposal without environmental controls have negatively impacted some soil–water environments. While newly developed personal care products are continuously entering the environment, older, previously disposed PPCPs may also be a concern. Many PPCPs are non-biodegradable in aerobic environments, especially nitrogen-containing compounds [1]. Because natural PPCP degradation can take several months to years, both parent structure and degradation products can still be found in the environment, long after their initial discharge [2]. Some PPCPs have the capability to be transferred from disposal streams (i.e., manure amendments, wastewater irrigation, and sludge disposal) to agricultural lands, crops, and then humans or animal dietary intake [3]. Because of this, human blood, urine, and breast milk have all recently been found to contain some PPCPs [4,5].

The detection of PPCPs in animals and humans confirms that conventional wastewater treatment approaches are inadequate. Moreover, trace concentrations of PPCPs can produce potential adverse effects on human health, aquatic animals, and aquatic ecosystems [6]. Consequently, there is a need for novel water treatment that can effectively reduce PPCPs while simultaneously removing traditionally encountered organic contaminants. Advanced oxidation processes (AOPs) are primarily recognized for their strong reactivity and harmless by-product production [7]. Heterogeneous photo-Fenton-like processes are considered AOPs and have been previously used in several PPCP treatment [8,9].

The selection of freshly synthesized materials that are reusable and capable of operating across a broad pH range is vital to the success of remedial technologies. By employing manganese ferrite ($MnFe_2O_4$) as heterogeneous catalysts, researchers have found it to be more effective than other catalysts. This is due to the various valences in the nanocomposites, including Mn^{4+}, Mn^{3+}, Mn^{2+}, Fe^{3+}, and Fe^{2+}, which can trigger the synergistic action between the Mn and Fe redox cycles [10,11]. Furthermore, doping manganese ferrite structures with another transition metal (e.g., Cu) can produce ternary transition metal oxides (e.g., $Cu_{0.5}Mn_{0.5}Fe_2O_4$), which have a greater surface area than iron-based transition metal catalysts [12,13]. This is beneficial to photo-Fenton-like AOP treatments by providing larger active sites, an excellent oxygen exchangeability, and an outstanding capability for electron transfer through the Cu^{2+}/Cu^{1+} redox cycle. These characteristics facilitate activating hydrogen peroxide (H_2O_2) and producing hydroxyl radicals that enhance the degradation of recalcitrant organic pollutants [12,13]. As such, $Cu_{0.5}Mn_{0.5}Fe_2O_4$ had higher catalytic activity than other single spinel ferrites (e.g., $CuFe_2O_4$, $MnFe_2O_4$, etc.) in activating H_2O_2 under ultraviolet (UV) light and was unlikely to cause secondary pollution from metal leaching due to its high stability [14,15]. In addition, several researchers reported that $Cu_{0.5}Mn_{0.5}Fe_2O_4$ nanoparticles could be successfully used as an adsorbent to remove several contaminants from wastewater [12,14,16]. However, an evaluation of the cooperative impact between the adsorption and photocatalysis of $Cu_{0.5}Mn_{0.5}Fe_2O_4$ nanoparticles for removing PPCPs has never been reported.

In this study, we selected two representatives for PPCPs: (1) oxytetracycline (OTC), an antibiotic generally used in aquatic veterinary practice, and (2) parabens (e.g., methyl-, ethyl-, propyl-, and butylparaben), an antimicrobial preservative often used in cosmetic and care products. Our objective was to determine the adsorptive–photocatalytic degradation performance of OTC and parabens using $Cu_{0.5}Mn_{0.5}Fe_2O_4$ synthesized using a simple co-precipitation method. The physicochemical properties of $Cu_{0.5}Mn_{0.5}Fe_2O_4$ before and after use were characterized. In the end, we determined any residual toxicity impacts of the treated water on seed germination, seedling growth, and anatomical root changes for *Zea mays* L. and *Vigna radiata* L.

2. Materials and Methods

2.1. Chemicals

Analytical-grade substances from different sources and deionized water (DI) were employed in this research. Loba Chemie Pvt. Ltd. (Mumbai, India) supplied manganese sulfate monohydrate ($MnSO_4 \cdot H_2O$, 99%). QRëC (Auckland, New Zealand) supplied ferric chloride hexahydrate ($FeCl_3 \cdot 6H_2O$, >98%) and acetic acid (CH_3COOH, 99.8%). Merck (Darmstadt, Germany) supplied sodium hydroxide (NaOH), hydrogen peroxide (30%, H_2O_2), copper sulfate ($CuSO_4$, 99%), oxytetracycline dihydrate ($C_{22}H_{24}N_2O_9 \cdot 2H_2O$; OTC, ≥99%), methyl 4-hydroxybenzoate ($C_8H_8O_3$; methylparaben, MP, ≥99%), ethyl 4-hydroxybenzoate ($C_9H_{10}O_3$; ethylparaben, EP, ≥99%), propyl 4-hydroxybenzoate ($C_{10}H_{12}O_3$; propylparaben, PP, ≥99%), and butyl 4-hydroxybenzoate ($C_{11}H_{14}O_3$; butylparaben, BP, ≥99%). RCI Lab-scan (Bangkok, Thailand) supplied acetonitrile (C_2H_3N; ACN) and methanol (CH_3OH; MeOH). Alfa Aesar (Shanghai, China) supplied melamine ($C_3H_6N_6$, 99%).

2.2. Synthesis of $Cu_{0.5}Mn_{0.5}Fe_2O_4$ Nanoparticles

The $Cu_{0.5}Mn_{0.5}Fe_2O_4$ nanoparticles were synthesized via co-precipitation and melamine-assisted calcination. We mixed 125 mL of $CuSO_4$ (0.2 M), 125 mL of $MnSO_4 \cdot H_2O$ (0.2 M), 250 mL of $FeCl_3 \cdot 6H_2O$ (0.4 M), and 500 mL of DI at 80 °C for 1 h. To raise the pH to 10.5, we gently dripped 8 M NaOH solution into the mixture for 1 h. After stirring for another hour, we filtered the precipitates by applying vacuum, washed them with DI water and ethanol multiple times, and dried them at 95 °C for 15 h. The dry particles were blended with melamine in a crucible at a ratio of 2:1. The resulting mixture was subjected to calcination at a temperature of 550 °C for a duration of 3 h, resulting in the production of the final product.

2.3. Chemical and Material Analyses

Temporal changes in OTC and paraben concentrations were analyzed by high-performance liquid chromatography (HPLC) using a photodiode array detector (Waters). With a 20 μL injection volume, an isocratic mobile phase of acetonitrile and 0.1% (v/v) acetic acid (20:80) was used for OTC analysis, whereas a mobile phase of acetonitrile and DI (60:40) was used for paraben analysis. Using a flow rate of 1 mL min^{-1}, samples were separated by a Reversed-Phase 18 (RP-18) Mightysil HPLC column (250 × Ø 4.6 mm) connected with a guard column. Sample peaks were quantified at 354 nm wavelength for OTC and 254 nm for four types of parabens (i.e., methyl-, ethyl-, propyl-, and butylparaben, or MP, EP, PP, and BP) using an external calibration curve.

Morphological structures were analyzed using JEOL (JSM-6010) scanning electron microscopy and Talos (F200X) high-resolution transmission electron microscopy (HRTEM). Material crystallinity characteristics were obtained from a D2 Phaser Bruker X-ray diffractor (XRD), whereas the surface functional groups were acquired from a Bruker (Tensor 27) Fourier transform infrared spectroscopy (FTIR).

Following the photocatalytic degradation experiments, we used ProElut C18 solid-phase extraction cartridges (Dikma) to concentrate the OTC degradates prior to further analyzing them on a liquid chromatography mass spectrophotometer (LC/MS). Initially, the cartridge was preconditioned with 5 mL of methanol followed by 5 mL of ultrapure water at a flow rate of 2 mL min^{-1}. A total of 60 mL of samples was introduced into the cartridge at a flow rate of 5 mL min^{-1}. Then, the samples were eluted with 2 mL of acetonitrile into the glass test tubes prior to filtrating with a 0.45 μm polytetrafluoroethylene (PTFE) syringe filter and transferred to vials for LC/MS analysis (Agilent 6420).

An isocratic mobile phase of freshly prepared acetonitrile and 0.1% (v/v) acetic acid (20:80) was used with a 10 μL injection volume. Using a flow rate of 0.2 mL min^{-1}, samples were separated by a Mightysil C18 column (250 × Ø 4.6 mm). Mass spectral data were obtained by scanning the quadrupole from 200 to 500 m/z with a 1 sec scan and a 30 V cone voltage setting with the following conditions: electrospray ionization source (positive ion mode), 3.7 kV electrospray voltage, 75 psi nebulization gas pressure, 500 °C heater temperature, and 400 °C capillary temperature.

2.4. Varying Dosage of H_2O_2 or Catalysts

Two independent variables that can affect the photo-Fenton catalytic performance are H_2O_2 and catalyst dosage. Here, we varied both parameters (H_2O_2: 0.1–0.6 mg L^{-1}, $Cu_{0.5}Mn_{0.5}Fe_2O_4$: 0–0.5 g L^{-1}) and determined the temporal changes of OTC and paraben concentrations. Initially, 100 mL of 0.1 mM OTC was placed in a 250 mL beaker with a designated catalyst and stirred in the absence of light for 30 min to reach adsorption equilibrium. Then, the beaker was irradiated with a simulated sunlight source using a commercial 75-watt halogen lamp. At a preselected time, 1 mL of sample was filtered through a 0.45 μm PTFE syringe filter. To stop the reaction, 0.7 mL of filtrated sample was transferred to an HPLC vial containing 0.875 mL of methanol. Samples were then stored in a refrigerator at 4 °C until HPLC analysis.

2.5. OTC Adsorption Study

2.5.1. Adsorption Kinetics

The OTC solution was freshly prepared before use in the kinetic and isotherm experiments. A total of 30 mL of 0.1 mM OTC concentrations was placed in a 40 mL amber vial. We selected 6 mg, 12 mg, and 18 mg of $Cu_{0.5}Mn_{0.5}Fe_2O_4$ as adsorbents in this kinetic study (equivalent to 0.2, 0.4, and 0.6 g L^{-1}). The experiments were performed in quadruplicate. The experiment started once the adsorbent had been added. Vials were shaken on a reciprocating shaker at 200 rpm. A total of 0.75 mL of samples was collected at 0.5, 1, 2, 3, 4, 5, and 6 h and filtrated using a 0.45 μM PTFE syringe filter. Samples were kept at 4 °C until HPLC analysis.

The kinetic models used in this study were pseudo first-order, pseudo second-order, Elovich, Brouers–Sotolongo (order 2), and intra-particle diffusion (2 phases) kinetic models (Table 1). The parameters in these models were determined by least squares approximation. In other words, the model used the parameter values that yielded the lowest sum of squared error (*SSE*) between observed and modeled values (Equation (1)).

$$SSE = \sum_{i=1}^{n} (y_i - \hat{y}_i)^2 \tag{1}$$

where n is the count of data, y_i is the value of i the observed data (observed amount of adsorbed OTC), and $\hat{y}_i$ is the value of i modelled data (calculated amount of adsorbed OTC). For each kinetic model, the values of parameters that gave the lowest *SSE* were determined by a generalized reduced gradient (GRG) algorithm [17] with multiple starting points. The GRG algorithm was performed by the Solver add-in in Microsoft Excel.

2.5.2. Adsorption Isotherms

Three amounts of $Cu_{0.5}Mn_{0.5}Fe_2O_4$ (6, 12, and 18 mg) were selected for the adsorption isotherm study (equivalent to 0.2, 0.4, and 0.6 g L^{-1}). The OTC concentrations, which ranged from 0.005, 0.01, 0.025, 0.05, 0.75, 0.1, 0.15, and 0.2 mM, were placed in each vial. The experimental set-up and sample collecting protocol were similar to the adsorption kinetic experiment.

2.5.3. Isotherm Models

This study employed multiple isotherm models (Table 1). However, in this study, the values of parameters cannot be clearly determined for some models. Only the models that give clear values of parameters were selectively reported. These models include Langmuir, Freundlich, and Temkin isotherm models. Since these models can be transformed into linear forms (Equations (2)–(4) for Langmuir, Freundlich, and Temkin isotherm models, respectively), the parameters in these models were determined by least squares linear regression.

$$\frac{1}{q_e} = \frac{1}{q_m b}\left(\frac{1}{C_e}\right) + \frac{1}{q_m} \tag{2}$$

$$\ln q_e = \frac{1}{n}(\ln C_e) + \ln K_f \tag{3}$$

$$q_e = \frac{RT}{B_T}(\ln C_e) + \frac{RT}{B_T}(\ln A_T) \tag{4}$$

From the linearized Langmuir isotherm model (Equation (2)), the value of $1/(q_m b)$ was the slope of the linear relationship between $1/C_e$ (independent variable) and $1/q_e$ (dependent variable), and the value of $1/q_m$ was the y-intercept of that linear relationship. By using a similar approach, the values of K_f and n in the Freundlich isotherm model

(Equation (3)) and the values of A_T and B_T in the Temkin isotherm model (Equation (4)) could be determined.

Table 1. Kinetic and isotherm models used in this study.

Model	Equation	Ref.	Nomenclature
Kinetic Model			A_{KC}: Koble–Corrigan parameter ($\mathrm{L}^{n_{KC}}\mathrm{mg}^{1-n_{KC}}\mathrm{g}^{-1}$)
Pseudo first-order	$q_t = q_e\left(1 - e^{-k_1 t}\right)$	[18]	A_T: Temkin equilibrium binding parameter (L mol^{-1})
			B_{DR}: Dubinin-Radushkevich constant (mol^2 J^{-2})
Pseudo second-order	$q_t = \frac{q_e^2 k_2 t}{q_e k_2 t + 1}$	[18]	B_{KC}: Koble–Corrigan parameter ($(\mathrm{Lmg}^{-1})^{n_{KC}}$)
			B_T: Temkin constant (J mol^{-1})
			b: Langmuir energy constant (L mg^{-1})
Elovich	$q_t = \frac{1}{\beta}\ln(\alpha\beta t)$	[18]	b_K: Khan model constant (L mg^{-1})
			C: constant for intra-particle diffusion kinetic model (mg g^{-1})
			C_e: OTC concentration at equilibrium (mg L^{-1})
Brouers-Sotolongo	$q_t = q_e\left(1 - \left(1 + (n_r - 1)\left(\frac{t}{\tau}\right)^\gamma\right)^{\frac{-1}{n_r - 1}}\right)$	[19]	K_{BS}: Brouers–Sotolongo isotherm constant (L mg^{-1})
			K_d: coefficient for intra–particle diffusion kinetic model (mg g^{-1} h$^{-1/2}$)
Intra-particle diffusion	$q_t = K_d t^{1/2} + C$	[18]	K_f: Freundlich constant (mg g^{-1}(L mg^{-1})$^{1/n}$)
Isotherm model			K_H: Hill constant $\left(\mathrm{mgL}^{-1}\right)^{n_H}$
Langmuir	$q_e = \frac{q_m b C_e}{1 + b C_e}$	[18]	K_j: Jovanovich constant (L mg^{-1})
Freundlich	$q_e = K_f C_e^{1/n}$	[18]	K_{RP}: Redlich–Peterson isotherm constant (L g^{-1})
			K_T: Toth model constant (L mg^{-1})
			k_1: rate constant for pseudo first-order kinetic model (h^{-1})
Temkin	$q_e = \frac{RT}{B_T}\ln(A_T C_e)$	[18]	k_2: rate constant for pseudo second-order kinetic model (g mg^{-1} h^{-1})
			$1/n$: Freundlich adsorption intensity
Dubinin-Radushkevich	$q_e = q_m e^{-(B_{DR}\varepsilon^2)}$ $\varepsilon = RT\ln\left(1 + \frac{1}{C_e}\right)$	[18]	n_{KC}: Koble–Corrigan parameter
			n_H: Hill cooperativity coefficient
			n_r: non-integer reaction order
Jovanovic	$q_e = q_m\left(1 - e^{-K_j C_e}\right)$	[18]	n_T: Toth model exponent
			q_e: amount of OTC adsorbed at equilibrium (mg g^{-1})
Koble-Corrigan	$q_e = \frac{A_{KC} B_{KC} C_e^{n_{KC}}}{1 + B_{KC} C_e^{n_{KC}}}$	[19]	q_m: maximum amount of the adsorbate per unit weight of the adsorbent (mg g^{-1})
Khan	$q_e = \frac{q_m b_K C_e}{(1 + b_K C_e)^{a_K}}$	[19]	q_t: amount of OTC adsorbed at time t (mg g^{-1})
			R: universal gas constant (8.314 J K^{-1} mol^{-1})
			T: temperature (298 K)
Hill	$q_e = \frac{q_m C_e^{n_H}}{K_H + C_e^{n_H}}$	[19]	t: adsorption time (h)
			α: Elovich chemisorption rate (mg g^{-1} h^{-1})
Brouers-Sotolongo	$q_e = q_m\left(1 - e^{-K_{BS} C_e^{a_{bs}}}\right)$	[19]	α_{bs}: Brouers–Sotolongo model exponent
			α_{RP}: Redlich–Peterson isotherm constant ($(\mathrm{Lmg}^{-1})^{\beta_{RP}}$)
Toth	$q_e = \frac{q_m K_T C_e}{\left(1 + (K_T C_e)^{n_T}\right)^{\frac{1}{n_T}}}$	[19]	α_K: Khan model exponent
			β: Elovich desorption rate constant (g mg^{-1})
			β_{RP}: Redlich–Peterson model exponent
Redlich-Peterson	$q_e = \frac{K_{RP} C_e}{1 + \alpha_{RP} C_e^{\beta_{RP}}}$	[19]	γ: fractal time exponent
			τ: characteristic time (h)

2.5.4. Model Evaluation

In this study, the kinetic and isotherm models were evaluated by root mean square error (*RMSE*) and coefficient of determination (R^2) (Equations (5) and (6)).

$$RMSE = \sqrt{\frac{1}{n}\sum_{i=1}^{n}(y_i - \hat{y}_i)^2} \tag{5}$$

$$R^2 = 1 - \frac{\sum_{i=1}^{n}(y_i - \hat{y}_i)^2}{\sum_{i=1}^{n}(y_i - \overline{y})^2} \tag{6}$$

where *RMSE* is the root mean square error, n is the count of data, y_i is the value of i th observed data, $\hat{y}_i$ is the value of i th modelled data, R^2 is the coefficient of determination, and $\overline{y}$ is the average value of the observed data. A low *RMSE* and high R^2 indicate that the model is suitable. Conversely, a high $RMSE$ and low R^2 indicate that the model is not suitable [20].

Since the isotherm models were parameterized by least squares linear regression, the strengths of the linear relationships were also measured using squared Pearson correlation coefficients (r^2) (Equation (7)). Moreover, the adjustment of r^2 according to the count of predictor(s) was also performed (Equation (8)) [21].

$$r^2 = \frac{\left(\sum_{i=1}^{n}(x_i - \overline{x})(y_i - \overline{y})\right)^2}{\sum_{i=1}^{n}(x_i - \overline{x})^2 \sum_{i=1}^{n}(y_i - \overline{y})^2} \tag{7}$$

$$r^2_{adj} = 1 - \frac{(1 - r^2)(n - 1)}{(n - p - 1)} \tag{8}$$

where r^2 is the squared Pearson correlation coefficient, n is the count of data, x_i is the value of i th independent variable, $\overline{x}$ is the average value of the independent variable, y_i is the value of i th dependent variable, $\overline{y}$ is the average value of the dependent variable, r^2_{adj} is the r^2 adjusted according to the count of predictor(s), and p is the count of predictor(s).

2.6. Evaluating Effects of Treated Water on Seed Germination and Root Anatomy

Due to their prevalence in Thai agriculture, *Zea mays* L. and *Vigna radiata* L. were used as representative species (monocotyledon vs. dicotyledon) for assessing the effects of treated water on seedling development and root morphological features. *Zea mays* L. seeds (cv.SW5720, National Corn and Sorghum Research Center, Nakhon Ratchasima, Thailand) and *Vigna radiata* L. seeds (cv.KUML4, Department of Agronomy, Faculty of Agriculture at Kamphaeng Saen, Kasetsart University, Nakhon Pathom, Thailand) were selected for this purpose. The OTC-untreated and treated water were assigned in two separate studies with varying percentages of OTC solution (5 to 15% and 25 to 50%). Fifty seeds from each treatment were planted in a box ($19 \times 28 \times 11$ cm) containing 2.55 kg of sand and 450 mL of three previously described waters and incubated at 25 °C. Each treatment was repeated four times and arranged in a completely random design (CRD). In order to evaluate the vigor and physiological performance of the seeds, the length of the shoots (the length from ground level to the tip of the longest leaf) and roots (the length from the base of the stem to the end of the longest root) were measured 7 d after planting (*Zea mays* L.) or 8 d (*Vigna radiata* L.). Normal seedlings' shoots and roots were weighed in mg (per plant) after drying in a hot-air oven at 80 °C for 24 h. All the obtained data were statistically evaluated. The mean germination time (MGT) and vigor index (VI) were calculated using the following formulas (Equations (9) and (10)):

$$MGT(days) = \frac{\sum(n * d)}{N} \tag{9}$$

$$VI = \text{Final germination}(\%) \times Seedling\ dry\ weight \tag{10}$$

where n is number of seeds germinated on each day, d is number of days from germination, and N is total number of germinated seeds.

Because *Zea mays* L. and *Vigna radiata* L. roots exhibited varying degrees of sensitivity to the constituents present in the treated water, leading to alterations in key anatomical features, their anatomical studies provided valuable insights into the potential physiological and developmental impacts of treated water on root tissues. We investigated the effect of treated water on root anatomy, focusing on parameters such as endodermis thickness, endodermis area, vascular cylinder diameter, metaxylem area, and cortex. These anatomical parameters are responsible for water and nutrient uptake, anchoring the plant, and providing structural support. Three roots per treatment per replication were anatomically analyzed.

The roots were immersed for 2 days in the FAA fixative solution (i.e., formalin (10%)/glacial acetic acid (5%)/ethanol (50%)/DI water (35%)). A table microtome and free-hand sectioning were used to generate cross sections at 4 ± 0.5 cm from the root apex to study *Zea mays* L. and *Vigna radiata* L. root anatomy. The slices were dyed with a 1% safranin-O dye solution for 2 min, mounted on glass slides with 50% glycerin, and then inspected and photographed using a light microscope coupled with Zen 3.5 software (Carl Zeiss, Axio Image 2, Oberkochen, Germany). Tukey's honest significant difference (HSD) was used to compare treatment means at $p = 0.05$.

3. Results and Discussion

3.1. $Cu_{0.5}Mn_{0.5}Fe_2O_4$ Characteristics

The SEM images of $Cu_{0.5}Mn_{0.5}Fe_2O_4$ exhibited a rough, uneven, and porous network structure caused by smaller particles that were well-distributed among larger particles, evidencing the flawless melamine-assisted calcination (Figure 1A,B). The TEM images depict the arrangement of large octahedral shapes surrounded by smaller particle sizes (Figure 1C,D). It is obvious that the morphological characteristics of the material were consistent with those observed through SEM. The HRTEM images also showed lattice fringes of 0.25 nm corresponding to the (311) plane (Figure 1D). In addition, the magnetic properties were more pronounced in comparison to the catalyst that was prepared without melamine addition. This was attributed to the recrystallization process that occurred during the calcination stage with melamine, which served as a coordinating agent. It was confirmed that melamine provided a platform and coordinated with the co-precipitated particles during calcination, resulting in promoting the $Cu_{0.5}Mn_{0.5}Fe_2O_4$ formation without impurity and providing a carbon source for the M-C and C-C/C=C bonds forming a heterojunction structure with $Cu_{0.5}Mn_{0.5}Fe_2O_4$ [12] (Figure 1E–G). Like carbon-based material doping, these carbons could act as an electron acceptor by suppressing photo-excited electron–hole recombination and enhancing the light absorption capability, thereby improving $Cu_{0.5}Mn_{0.5}Fe_2O_4$ photocatalytic activity [22,23]. This ultimately facilitated the formation of a ferrite structure without the α-Fe_2O_3 impurities [12].

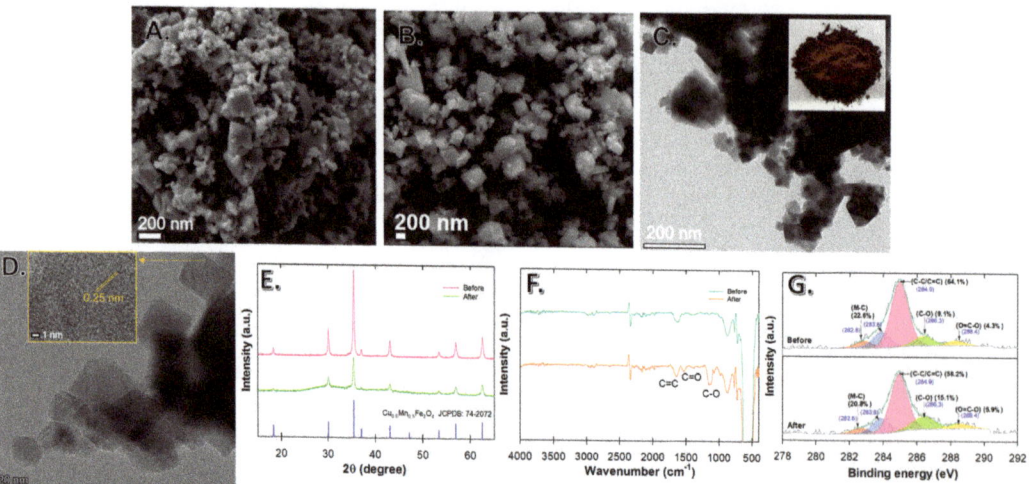

Figure 1. $Cu_{0.5}Mn_{0.5}Fe_2O_4$ nanoparticle characteristics: (**A,B**) SEM images; (**C**) TEM image with a visual observation of particles; (**D**) HRTEM image. The nanoparticle before and after use in photocatalytic reaction: (**E**) XRD patterns; (**F**) FTIR spectra; and (**G**) C 1s XPS spectra.

While the XRD spectra of both materials (before and after use in adsorptive–photocatalytic activity) show similar diffraction peaks at 2θ values of 18.3°, 30.0°, 35.4°, 37.0°, 43.0°,

53.3°, 56.8°, and 62.4° corresponding to the diffraction crystal planes (111), (220), (311), (222), (400), (422), (511), and (440), the unused materials had a slightly higher peak intensity (Figure 1E). This indicates that the occupying of adsorption sites may have occurred, but the crystallinity was still intact, which would still be able to provide a great photocatalytic performance.

The strong vibration spectra in the low wavenumber region (450 to 700 cm^{-1}) were assigned to the M–O band (M=Cu, Mn, and Fe) (Figure 1F). These bands confirmed the formation of M–O bonds at octahedral sites (Cu^{2+}–O^{2-}, and Mn^{2+}–O^{2-} stretching vibration) and tetrahedral sites (Fe^{3+}–O^{2-} stretching vibration) of the Cu$_{0.5}$Mn$_{0.5}$Fe$_2$O$_4$ nanocomposite surface [13,24–26]. These surface metals play an important role in heterogeneous catalytic reactions. The peaks at 1150, 1530, 1640, and ~3000 cm^{-1} can be attributed to C-O, C=O, C=C, and sp2 (–CH) or sp3 (=CH) hybridized carbon atoms (Figure 1F) [25,27,28]. The XPS analysis of the C 1s spectra indicates that the peaks at 282.8 and 283.8 eV corresponded to M-C bonds, while the other peaks at 284.9, 286.3, and 288.4 eV were attributed to C-C/C=C, C-O, and O=C-O (Figure 1G) [25,29]. It also reveals that, after use, C-C and C=C were decreased, while C-O and C=O were increased, indicating that the surface carbons undergo partial oxidation by the active oxygen species or exhibit involvement in the catalytic reaction.

Furthermore, despite the fact that the addition of melamine would result in C–N containing peaks that would aid in the crystal reformation, we did not see such peaks in XRD, FTIR, or XPS analyses. This may be explained by the role of melamine during the calcination stage. Upon heating melamine with the co-precipitated particles, a platform for the distribution of nanoparticles was created. This process was coordinated with the transition metals, leading to the formation of a metal–melamine complex [30,31]. At a high calcination temperature of 550 °C, this compound can undergo further decomposition, resulting in the formation of a spinel ferrite structure and the release of volatile gases (i.e., CO$_X$, NO$_X$, and NH$_3$) [32]. The findings validate the function of melamine as a coordinating agent that effectively enhances the crystalline structure of Cu$_{0.5}$Mn$_{0.5}$Fe$_2$O$_4$ and successfully eliminates the presence of Fe$_2$O$_3$ impurities.

3.2. Photocatalytic Performance

3.2.1. Paraben Degradation Efficiency

A photocatalytic experiment revealed that a >95% paraben degradation efficiency was obtained in 120 min (Figure 2). We did not observe a significant change in the first 30 min in the dark, indicating that the adsorption–desorption equilibrium of catalysts had been reached. The insignificant difference between parabens in the first 30 min of light-irradiation was probably due to the insufficient energy for initiating active oxygen species production. The temporal monitoring of each paraben concentration revealed a rise in the observed pseudo first-order rate constant (k_{obs}), and %removal at 120 min in the order BP > PP > EP > MP (inset of Figure 2), which was due to the generated •OH, photoelectron (e$^-$), and •O$_2^-$, confirmed by our previously proposed radical formation mechanisms in our recent publication by Angkaew et al. [12], which was similarly observed by other works [33,34]. The BP highest degradation efficiency was due to the BP molecular structure with a longer ester chain and the existence of more unsaturated C=C bonds, both of which were preferentially targeted by •OH and •O$_2^-$ [35,36]. These results validate the occurrence of the reaction with •OH in a correlation with the alkyl chain length of the paraben [37].

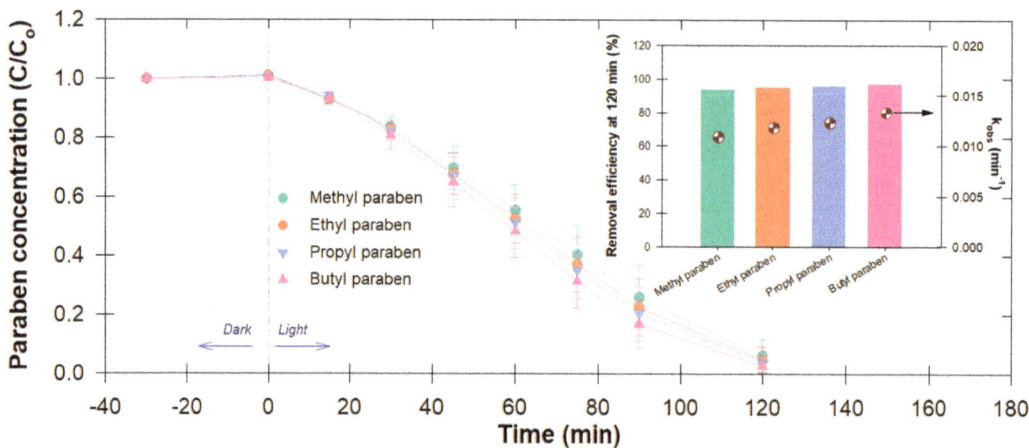

Figure 2. Temporal changes in paraben concentration (i.e., methyl-, ethyl-, propyl-, and butylparaben, or MP, EP, PP, and BP) under the adsorptive–photocatalysis process; (inset graph) removal efficiency (at 120 min) and observed degradation rates of parabens (k_{obs}; min^{-1}).

When the photocatalytic activity was tested by removing parabens individually at different H_2O_2 concentrations and $Cu_{0.5}Mn_{0.5}Fe_2O_4$ dosages, the BP degradation rates were again the fastest, confirming that its molecular structure is more susceptible to oxidative species (Figure 3). The degradation rate exhibited a corresponding increase with the increase in catalyst doses. The degradation rate did not, however, rise by 2.5 times as expected in response to the increase in catalyst dosage, but rather by 1.25 times. Nevertheless, the larger specific area was responsible for this increase because it provided more adsorptive and reactive sites for the H_2O_2 that was present, accelerating the production of reactive species (Figure 3).

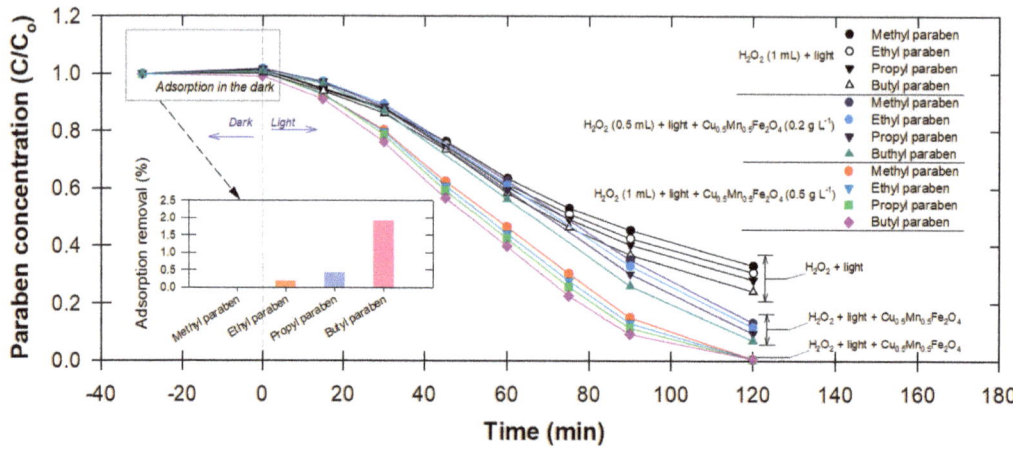

Figure 3. Temporal changes in paraben concentration (i.e., methyl-, ethyl-, propyl-, and butylparaben) under three different oxidative conditions; (inset graph) adsorption removal of each paraben in the absence of light irradiation.

It is noted that, in the dark, BP was also adsorbed, even though there was no photoactivity involved (Figure 3). Up to a 40% increase in paraben removal efficiency was observed following an increase in the $Cu_{0.5}Mn_{0.5}Fe_2O_4$ dose to 0.5 g L^{-1}. This proves that, besides photocatalytic activity, the availability of adsorption sites and a contact surface area also increased. However, Hashemian, et al. [16] reported that, when the quantity of adsorbent exceeds 1.0 g, the increase in removal of pollutants can become negligible due to the occurrence of particle–particle interactions, such as aggregation, which subsequently diminish the available surface area for adsorption sites, and that the adsorption efficiency may play a synergistic important role in this oxidative system.

3.2.2. Oxytetracycline (OTC) Degradation Efficiency

The results of lowering H_2O_2 and catalyst dosages more than the previous experiment show that the increase in these dosages did not necessarily increase the OTC degradation efficiency (Figure 4). The increase in H_2O_2 resulted in a better photocatalytic activity, except for the H_2O_2 doses of 0.4 mL and 0.6 mL, which had a similar degradation efficiency (Figure 4A). This could have been a lack of active sites for the catalyst dose to initiate the reaction. One other possible explanation is that the created $^\bullet OH$ was quenched by the self-scavenging action of the abundant H_2O_2, which itself deteriorated into H_2O and O_2 (Equations (11)–(13)) [10,29].

$$H_2O_2 + H_2O_2 \rightarrow H_2O + O_2 \tag{11}$$

$$H_2O_2 + {}^\bullet OH \rightarrow HO_2{}^\bullet + H_2O \tag{12}$$

$$HO_2{}^\bullet + {}^\bullet OH \rightarrow O_2 + H_2O \tag{13}$$

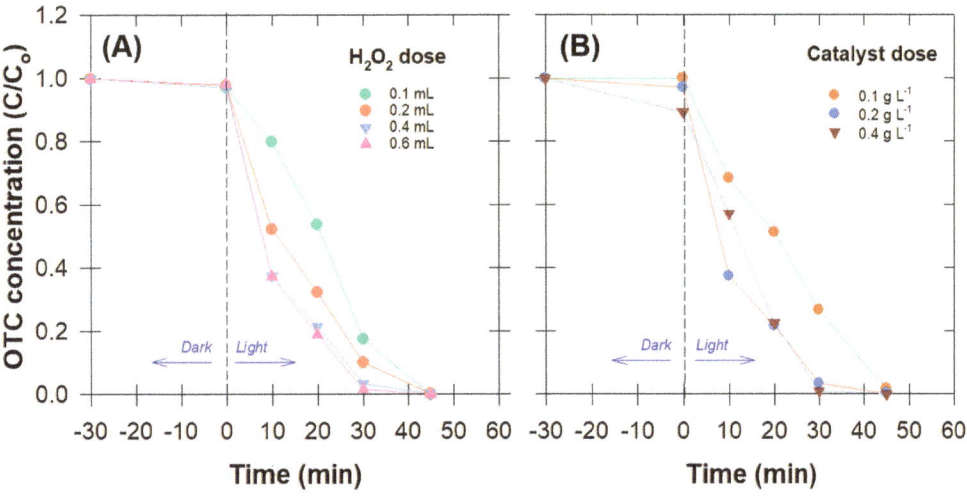

Figure 4. Temporal changes in oxytetracycline concentration (OTC) under the adsorptive–photocatalysis process at varied concentrations of H_2O_2 (**A**) and catalyst dose (**B**).

Increases in the $Cu_{0.5}Mn_{0.5}Fe_2O_4$ dosage had a similar effect on OTC degradation efficiency as increases in the H_2O_2 concentration did (Figure 4B). Besides the lack of H_2O_2 concentration for initiating the reaction, a self-scavenging effect may have occurred from the excessive amounts of Cu^+, Fe^{2+}, and Mn^{2+} in the solution (Equations (14)–(16)) [25,38].

$$Cu^+ + {}^\bullet OH \rightarrow Cu^{2+} + OH^- \tag{14}$$

$$Mn^{2+} + {}^\bullet OH \rightarrow Mn^{3+} + OH^- \tag{15}$$

$$Fe^{2+} + {}^{\bullet}OH \rightarrow Fe^{3+} + OH^{-} \tag{16}$$

Moreover, an excessive amount of suspended catalysts might prevent light from reaching the reaction sites, reducing the amount of ${}^{\bullet}OH$ produced. Notably, the removal efficiency anomaly (>10%) in the dark was observed for the highest catalyst dose (0.4 g L^{-1}) (Figure 4B). This phenomenon indicates the existence of catalyst adsorptivity prior to the generation of active radicals and that some contaminants may have been adsorbed on the catalyst surface. As a result, we ruled out the idea that adsorption was also a key factor in pollution removal. This information is valuable as it pertains to the potential utilization of greater quantities of catalyst in practical applications.

3.3. Adsorptive Performance

At the beginning of the adsorption experiment, a high adsorption rate was seen for all three chosen amounts. This indicates that the catalyst was a viable adsorbent and that there were plenty of adsorption sites accessible, especially as the adsorbent amount increased. This might be attributed to our selected synthesis approaches that used melamine-assisted calcination, which resulted in its octahedral morphology surrounded by tiny spheres. Thus, this is advantageous for both excellent adsorption and excellent photocatalytic properties.

In this study, pseudo first-order, pseudo second-order, Elovich, and Brouers–Sotolongo models were used to explain adsorption, and two-phase intra-particle diffusion was used to explain diffusion (Table 1). $RMSE$ and R^2 values were used to determine the best fit model.

Figure 5A shows the plot of the fitted adsorption models (pseudo first-order, pseudo second-order, Elovich, and Brouers–Sotolongo models). Differences among results from these models can be seen when the $Cu_{0.5}Mn_{0.5}Fe_2O_4$ amount is not very high. Overall, both the Brouers–Sotolongo and the pseudo second-order kinetic models described the OTC-$Cu_{0.5}Mn_{0.5}Fe_2O_4$ adsorption kinetics well, as indicated by the low $RMSE$ and high R^2 (Table 2). Therefore, it can be concluded that the adsorption process between the adsorbent and OTC molecules in the liquid phase was a chemisorption process, and that the efficiency was entirely dependent on the amount of adsorbent used and the concentration of the adsorbate. The OTC-adsorbed mass per $Cu_{0.5}Mn_{0.5}Fe_2O_4$ mass at the equilibrium (q_e) was highest for the lowest $Cu_{0.5}Mn_{0.5}Fe_2O_4$ amount (i.e., 0.006 g) and the decrease at higher $Cu_{0.5}Mn_{0.5}Fe_2O_4$ amounts was due to their more available adsorption sites (Table 2; Figure 5).

At 0.006 g of $Cu_{0.5}Mn_{0.5}Fe_2O_4$, the Brouers–Sotolongo model shows a notably greater q_e than the pseudo second-order model, and the accuracies of these models are low ($RMSE$s are high and R^2s are low), implying that the predicted data may not be as accurate at an extremely low adsorbent amount (Table 2). At higher amounts of $Cu_{0.5}Mn_{0.5}Fe_2O_4$, the predicted adsorbed concentrations from both models were similar (6.04 and 4.06–4.07 mg g^{-1} at 0.012 and 0.018 g of $Cu_{0.5}Mn_{0.5}Fe_2O_4$, respectively) and the accuracies of the models are high ($RMSE$s are low and R^2s are high). By comparing the values of R^2, the OTC adsorption mechanism appeared to be best described by the Brouers–Sotolongo equation. Adsorbate/adsorbent interactions were found to be fractal when the fractal time exponent (γ; also called the global fractal time) was less than 1 [39,40]. This may be attributed to the material's powder-like properties, which may preferentially reside on the edge wall and the inner lid, decreasing the amount of contact with the OTC molecules.

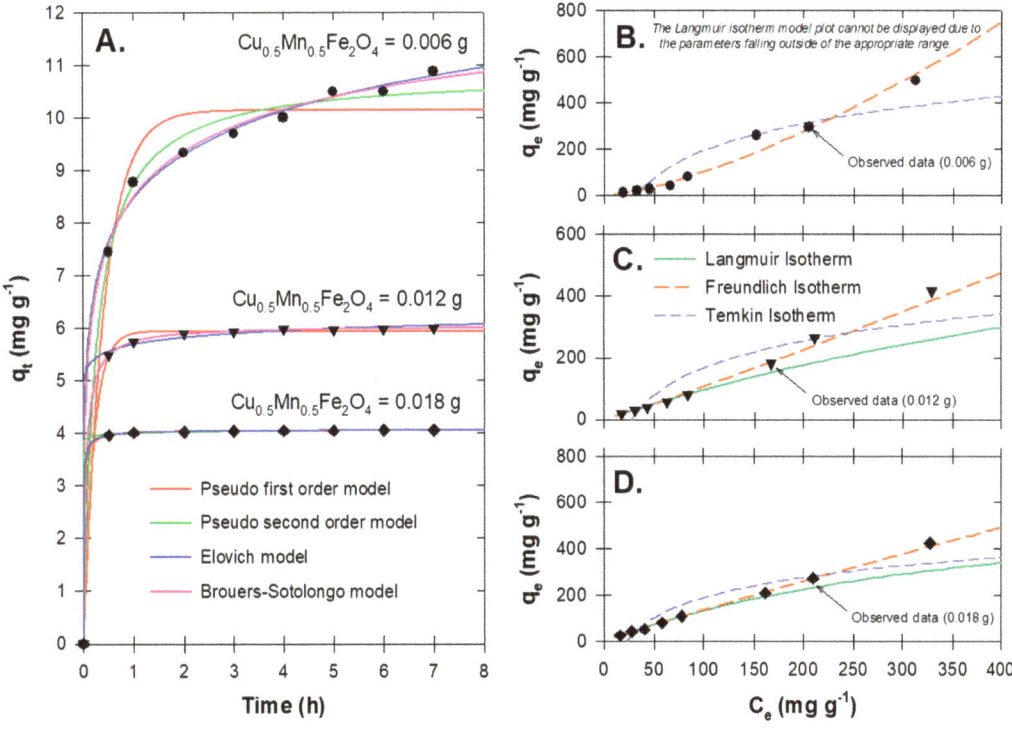

Figure 5. OTC adsorption on $Cu_{0.5}Mn_{0.5}Fe_2O_4$ nanoparticles; (**A**) observed and modeled kinetic profiles; and (**B–D**) observed and modeled equilibrium isotherm profiles.

Table 2. Parameters for the kinetic model determined from least squares approximation and model performance measured by *RMSE* and R^2.

Model	$Cu_{0.5}Mn_{0.5}Fe_2O_4$ (g)	Parameters			RMSE (mg/g)	R^2 (%)
		q_e (mg g^{-1})	k_1 (h^{-1})			
Pseudo first-order	0.006	10.14	2.41		0.48	78.98
	0.012	5.94	5.03		0.07	83.92
	0.018	4.04	7.91		0.01	79.00
		q_e (mg g^{-1})	k_2 (g mg^{-1} h^{-1})			
Pseudo second-order	0.006	10.82	0.38		0.25	94.50
	0.012	6.04	3.26		0.01	99.64
	0.018	4.06	20.72		<0.01	98.35
		α (mg g^{-1} h^{-1})	β (g mg^{-1})			
Elovich	0.006	1.45×10^3	0.84		0.15	97.83
	0.012	6.79×10^{12}	5.49		0.05	90.17
	0.018	2.78×10^{53}	31.63		0.01	92.67
		q_e (mg g^{-1})	τ (h)	γ		
Brouers–Sotolongo (order 2; n_r = 2)	0.006	14.07	0.33	0.38	0.15	97.92
	0.012	6.04	0.05	0.99	0.01	99.64
	0.018	4.07	4.50×10^{-3}	0.78	<0.01	98.73
		K_d (mg g^{-1} h$^{-1/2}$)	C (mg g^{-1})			
Intra-particle diffusion (two phases)	0.006	10.54 if $t \leq 0.58$ h	0.00 if $t \leq 0.58$ h		0.07	99.52
		1.10 if $t > 0.58$ h	8.03 if $t > 0.58$ h			
	0.012	7.75 if $t \leq 0.54$ h	0.00 if $t \leq 0.54$ h		0.03	96.84
		0.13 if $t > 0.54$ h	5.71 if $t > 0.54$ h			
	0.018	5.61 if $t \leq 0.51$ h	0.00 if $t \leq 0.51$ h		<0.01	99.12
		0.02 if $t > 0.51$ h	4.00 if $t > 0.51$ h			

With an increase in adsorbate amount, agglomeration may have started to occur, rendering the adsorbent attachment to the edge wall unlikely. As can be seen, the experiment was contaminant-specific and was conducted in the dark. By using OTC as the target contaminant, the results show that adsorption is playing the main role as OTC was tentatively adsorbed before the start of the photocatalytic performance.

Ho and McKay [41] proposed that the adsorbate diffused through the liquid phase and the film surrounding the adsorbent surface before interacting with the functional groups of the adsorbent–adsorbate (Table 2). Consequently, the kinetic data previously acquired were utilized to selectively examine the intra-particle diffusion stages.

Based on our findings, the adsorption phases (i.e., double-linearity characterization) were divided at 0.51–0.58 h, indicating that the external mass transfer followed by intraparticle diffusion may occur at even lower amounts of adsorbent. This allows OTC molecules to transport to different phases prior to reaching equilibrium. As the adsorbent dosage increased, the first-phase slopes (K_d) decreased, suggesting that self-agglomeration had slightly occurred and that the adsorbent boundary layers had thickened. The rapid disruption in the K_d indicated prompt adsorption on the adsorbent surface, while the subsequent slower rates of adsorption (i.e., a lower K_d) confirmed the occurrence of diffusional phenomena within the adsorbent particles [42,43].

By comparing the values of $RMSE$ and R^2 among three isotherm models (Tables 1 and 3; Figure 5), the Freundlich model better described the adsorption isotherm data, indicating that multilayer adsorption was dominant and that the Cu secondary doping facilitated the uniformly distributed surface for OTC molecules. The n value increased to >1 at 0.018 g of adsorbent, indicating the system's unfavorability [44]. This was probably due to the agglomeration occurring at a higher adsorbent dose, which coincided with the previously described kinetic experiments. Overall, the results provide proof that, during the adsorption/desorption equilibrium, adsorption can occur prior to the photocatalytic reaction that serves as the main oxidation mechanism for degrading unadsorbed OTC molecules.

Table 3. Parameters for the isotherm model determined from least squares linear regression, strength of the linear relationship (between the independent and dependent variables in the linear form of the model) measured by r^2 and r^2_{adj}, and model performance measured by $RMSE$ and R^2.

Model	$Cu_{0.5}Mn_{0.5}Fe_2O_4$ (g)	Parameters		r^2 (%)	r^2_{adj} (%)	$RMSE$ (mg/g)	R^2
		q_m (mg g^{-1})	b (L mg^{-1})				
Langmuir	0.006	-*	-*	-*	-*	-*	-*
	0.012	994.94	1.08×10^{-3}	98.82	98.63	63.08	77.42
	0.018	686.72	2.45×10^{-3}	99.08	98.92	44.64	88.24
		n	K_f (mg g^{-1}(L mg^{-1})$^{1/n}$)				
Freundlich	0.006	0.70	0.14	97.68	97.29	28.30	97.09
	0.012	0.93	0.74	99.06	98.90	14.65	98.78
	0.018	1.09	1.97	99.70	99.65	6.23	99.77
		B_T (J mol^{-1})	A_T (L mol^{-1})				
Temkin	0.006	14.68	14.47	82.87	80.01	68.60	82.87
	0.012	19.48	17.17	82.15	79.17	56.09	82.15
	0.018	19.98	21.34	86.60	84.37	47.66	86.60

* For Langmuir isotherm model applied to 0.006 g of $Cu_{0.5}Mn_{0.5}Fe_2O_4$, the values of parameters are out of appropriate range.

3.4. OTC Degradation Products

Almost certainly, multiple mechanisms for the oxidative degradation of OTC ($m/z = 460$) are occurring simultaneously in this system. The identified intermediates allow us to suggest the reactions that occur, but only a very limited sequence ordering is possible. An inspection of 6,10,12 a-trihydroxy-1,3,11,12-tetraoxo-2,5,6,12a-tetrahydronaphthacene (TC1; $m/z = 340$) allows us to note that the following steps must have occurred, but in any number of different sequences: decarboxamidation at C2; deamination at C4; dehydroxylation at C5, demethylation at C6, and tautomerization at C3 and C12 [45] (Figure 6).

Similarly, OTC was converted to 3,4,4a,10-tetrahydro-1 2,8,10-tetrahydroxy-10-methyl-9-(2H)-anthracenone (TC2; $m/z = 277$) by ring-cleavage at both the C4aC4 and C12a-C1 bonds [46]. This step occurred either before or after dihydroxylation at C5. The observation of degradation intermediates TC1 and TC2 supports the idea of multiple oxidative pathways because TC2 cannot be produced by the degradation of TC1. This is because the methyl group at C6 in TC2 has already been removed in TC1. Finally, either of these compounds or many others could lead to the production of 2,3-dioxosuccinic acid by oxidative cleavage of any ring or sequence of carbon giving a four-carbon chain. Subsequent oxidation of each carbon of that chain would lead to succinic acid ($m/z = 146$) [47].

Further oxidation of that compound would probably lead to oxalic and carbonic acids, and then shortly thereafter to carbon dioxide and water. Thus, the oxidative fate of these compounds is likely to be complete mineralization under the reported conditions. Moreover, our LC/MS results also reveal that the adsorption process was the dominant process throughout the OTC reaction; however, the degradation products may be unstable and may have been adsorbed onto the catalyst surface.

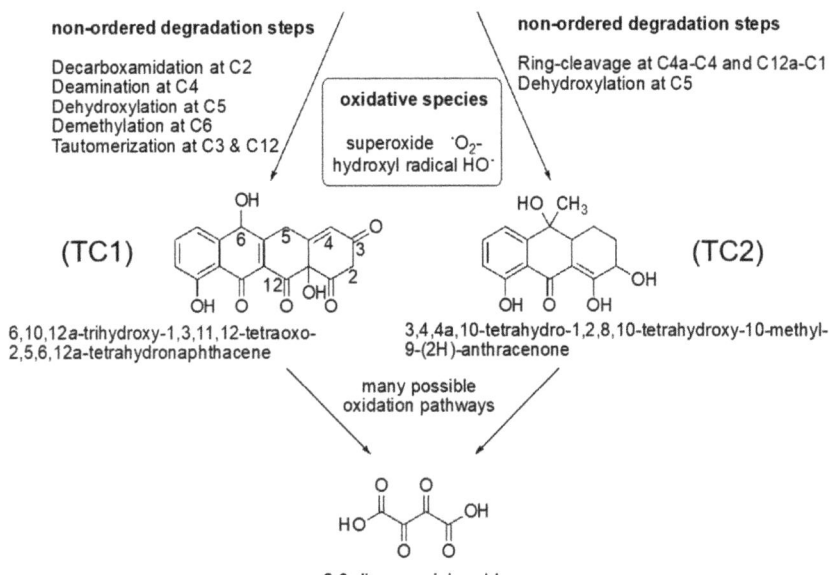

Figure 6. OTC degradation mechanism following the photo-Fenton catalytic activity of $Cu_{0.5}Mn_{0.5}Fe_2O_4$ nanoparticles.

3.5. Effect to Seedling Growth and Root Anatomy

Up to a 50% composition of treated and untreated water, both species had no significant effect on shoot lengths or root lengths for *Vigna radiata* L. (Figure 7). This implies that all of the active radicals had already disappeared and that OTC degradates were not able to trigger *Vigna radiata* L. irregular plant growth nor cause any oxidative stress. This result is consistent with previous works indicating that *Vigna radiata* L. had an inherent ability for growth in chemically contaminated soils [48,49]. For *Zea mays* L. root traits, however, 50% of both tested waters revealed a significantly negative impact on the germination index, vigor index, and root length, while, at a lower composition of tested water (i.e., 25%), there were differences between untreated and treated water, indicating that our treated water was safer for root growth at this lower composition (Figure 7).

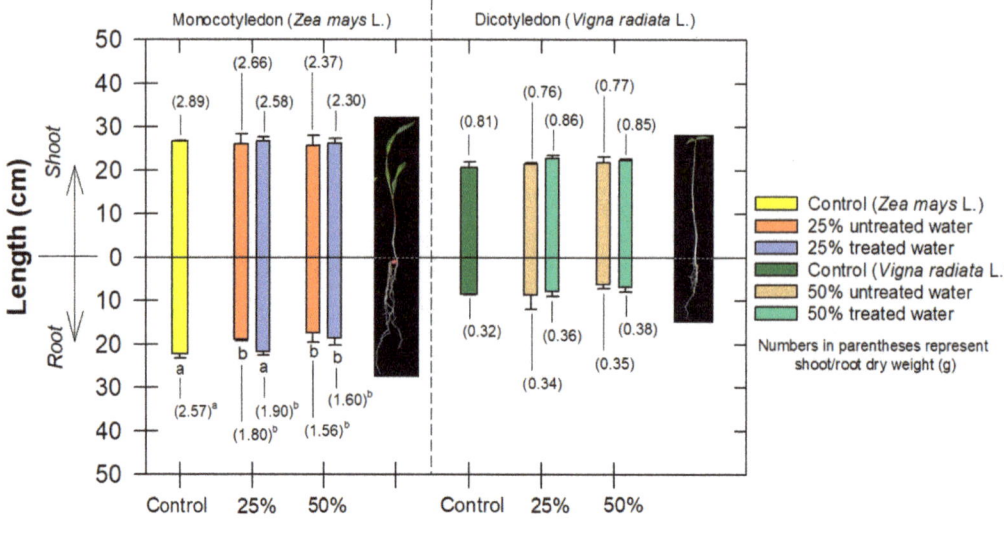

Figure 7. Comparison of shoot and root lengths and their dry weights (g; in parentheses) of *Zea mays* L. and *Vigna radiata* L. following exposure to different compositions of treated water. Values followed by the same letter in each species are not significantly different at $p \leq 0.05$ according to the Tukey's honest significant difference (HSD).

Water plays a crucial role in the germination process since it is necessary for the activation of enzymes that break down the seed's stored nutrients and initiate the growth processes. Therefore, treated water at a high composition, which included OTC-degradates, a minimal amount of inorganic metal, and an abnormal pH, presumably initially interfered with the physiological and metabolic capacity of seeds to germinate and establish themselves as healthy seedlings. OTC-contaminated water at high concentrations has been confirmed to cause disruption in shoot and root growth by inhibiting the photosynthesis and enzyme activity of lettuce [50]. In addition, Bao et al. [51] showed that, when tested at higher concentrations of OTC (i.e., 50–150 mg L^{-1}), the untreated OTC had significant phytotoxic effects on wheat seed germination, root elongation, sprout length, and vitality index. These investigations show the importance of removing as much antibiotic residues as possible before utilizing contaminated water for irrigation.

Following the seedling growth experiment, root samples were analyzed for changes in the anatomical parameters. Our findings reveal significant changes in root anatomy in response to the composition of treated water, where it showed a shrinking of the endodermis thickness and endodermis area, which could be due to the decrease in the size of the parenchyma of the cortex and vascular bundles (Figure 8).

For *Zea Mays* L., changes in endodermis area were observed at 50% of treated water, while changes in the vascular cylinder diameter, metaxylem area, and cortex were observed at only 25% of both treated and untreated water (Figure 8). However, the anatomical results for *Vigna radiata* L. are slightly different. In brief, only metaxylem and cortex were impacted by the tested water, but only 50% of the treated water started to negatively impact the endodermis area and vascular diameter, indicating that *Vigna radiata* L. could tolerate extreme conditions better than *Zea mays* L. (Figure 8). The *Vigna radiata* L. cortex obviously showed more negative impacts from the tested water. This is probably due to the nature of the larger root diameter (i.e., *Zea Mays* L.), which provided a longer radial distance containing more cortexes protecting the absorbed aqueous solution from penetrating into the endodermis area. At higher compositions of treated water, *Vigna radiata* L. root growth indicated that both OTC and OTC-degradates could disrupt maturation and cell division in the roots and may cause anomalous higher auxin production [52]. Because radical remnants were not the main by-products, we believed that either TC1 or TC2 (refer to Section 3.4; Figure 6) could be responsible for the reduction in parenchyma cells (Figure 8).

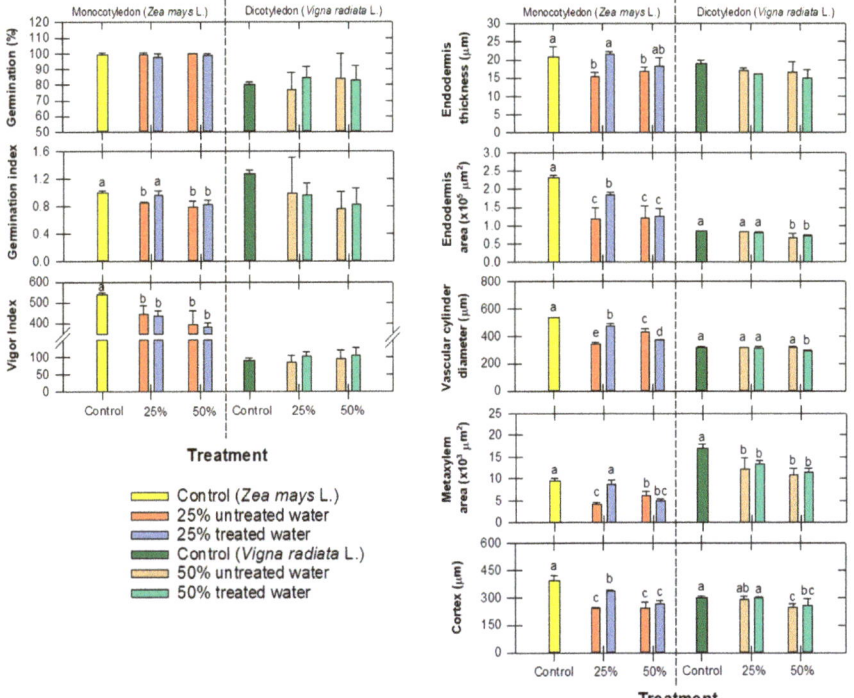

Figure 8. Comparison of seed germination, seedling growth, and anatomical roots of *Zea mays* L. and *Vigna radiata* L. following exposure to different compositions of treated water. Values followed by the same letter (s) in each species are not significantly different at $p \leq 0.05$ according to the Tukey's honest significant difference (HSD).

The reduction in root development is a compelling indication of plant oxidative stress, which results from a reduction in cell division, a decrease in cell elongation, and a reduction in the extension of the root meristem [53]. This decrease in cell size could also cause a reduction in cell wall elasticity, which can eventually lead to overall root contraction [54]. Gomes et al. [52] reported that this cell division impairment was due to the disruption of hormones that may have been associated with auxin production after exposure to treated water, and that any disturbances in auxin signaling can have profound effects on root anatomy and function.

Comparing the germination indices and the anatomical roots of both tested plants, it is clear that *Zea mays* L. was more sensitive than *Vigna radiata* L. Because of the root parameter reductions, it is plausible that the shoot would also suffer the same consequence. Because the plant's root water potential was greater than its shoot water potential, the plant was able to absorb more water through its distorted xylem. Because of this, the plant's capacity to absorb nutrients would have been compromised, and the OTC degrades would still be available for uptake by the roots. If the experiment had been set up for a longer time period (>8 d), we might have seen a different variation in shoot anatomy. In practical applications, a greater concentration of organic matter and other ion constituents can be found in water. Existing antibiotics may be present at much lower concentrations, and they would be naturally absorbed in soils before affecting root development. Most importantly, the dilution would be significantly lower than the mixture that was tested (<25%).

Past research has shown that a decrease in both cell division and cell size and a decrease in xylem vessel size are closely associated with the exposure to heavy-metal-contaminated water that causes the interference of the plant's uptake of several mineral elements by heavy metals [55]. Although metal leaching was not an issue of concern in our study, some micronutrients were found to disrupt the plant mineral nutrient uptake, which consequently reduced enzyme activity, interfered with physiological processes, damaged cell membranes, and limited the biosynthesis of metabolites [56].

These changes in root anatomy can ultimately hinder the overall plant growth and development, can also highlight the sensitivity of root tissues to the composition of treated water, and can have cascading effects on nutrient uptake, water transport, and overall plant growth. Therefore, it is crucial to consider the potential impacts of treated water on root anatomy when assessing the suitability of water sources for irrigation and agricultural practices. Therefore, unless the amount of catalyst is increased to overcome the high loading of organic constituents, there should be no concern that these residuals will interfere with plant growth and yield. Therefore, our $H_2O_2/Cu_{0.5}Mn_{0.5}Fe_2O_4$ oxidative treatment was shown to be successful in removing antibiotics from water while having minimal to no negative effects on plant growth.

4. Conclusions

In this study, we developed $Cu_{0.5}Mn_{0.5}Fe_2O_4$ nanoparticles using the co-precipitation method, calcination with melamine, and tested their adsorptive–photocatalytic performance on four parabens and the oxytetracycline (OTC) removal efficiency. The material showed more crystallinity after melamine calcination and showed no Fe_2O_3 impurity, enhancing the larger adsorption sites as well as the electrons' excellent oxygen exchangeability, which, in turn, can enhance oxidative reactivity for contaminant removal. All four parabens were removed within 120 min and OTC within 45 min, respectively. The optimum condition for pollutant removal was 0.2 g L^{-1} of $Cu_{0.5}Mn_{0.5}Fe_2O_4$ and 40 mM of H_2O_2. In the aqueous phase, both adsorptive and photocatalytic reactions can occur. The OTC diffused through the liquid phase and the film surrounding the adsorbent surface before interacting with the functional groups of the adsorbent–adsorbate. Then, also in the liquid phase, OTC rapidly reacted and generated reactive oxygen species. By fitting the kinetics and isotherm models, the OTC adsorption kinetics fitted well with the Brouers–Sotolongo model, and the OTC adsorption behavior was well described using the Freundlich isotherm. The shoot length of *Zea mays* L. and *Vigna radiata* L. in 25% treated water had less negative impact compared to the root length. The overall results show that $Cu_{0.5}Mn_{0.5}Fe_2O_4$ nanoparticles have provided a relatively good adsorptive–photocatalytic performance for the degradation of tested antibiotics and personal care products.

Author Contributions: Conceptualization, C.C. and C.S.; methodology, C.C., C.S., A.A., A.P., P.P., and K.T.; validation, C.C., C.S. and P.K.; formal analysis, P.K.; investigation, A.A., W.R., A.P.,

P.P., C.E.H. and K.T.; resources, C.C., C.S., D.D.S. and S.D.C.; data curation, C.C., C.S. and P.K.; writing—original draft preparation, C.C. and C.S.; writing—review and editing, C.C., C.S., A.A., W.R., P.P., K.T., P.K., D.D.S., C.E.H. and S.D.C.; visualization, C.C.; supervision, C.S., D.D.S. and S.D.C.; project administration, C.S.; funding acquisition, C.C. and C.S. All authors have read and agreed to the published version of the manuscript.

Funding: This work was financially supported by the Office of the Ministry of Higher Education, Science, Research and Innovation; and the Thailand Science Research and Innovation through Kasetsart University Reinventing University Program 2021, and Kasetsart University Research and Development (KURDI), (grant number FF(KU)18.66).

Institutional Review Board Statement: Not applicable.

Informed Consent Statement: Not applicable.

Data Availability Statement: The authors confirm that the data supporting the findings of this study are available within the article.

Acknowledgments: This work was financially supported by the Office of the Ministry of Higher Education, Science, Research and Innovation and the Thailand Science Research and Innovation through the Kasetsart University Reinventing University Program 2021, and Kasetsart University Research and Development (KURDI), (grant number FF(KU)18.66). Appreciation is expressed to the Department of Environmental Technology and Management, Faculty of Environment, and the Faculty of Veterinary Technology, Kasetsart University, Bangkok, Thailand, for providing facility support.

Conflicts of Interest: The authors declare no conflict of interest.

References

1. Kumar, S.; Kumar, A.; Kumar, A.; Balaji, R.; Krishnan, V. Highly Efficient Visible Light Active 2D-2D Nanocomposites of N-ZnO-g-C_3N_4 for Photocatalytic Degradation of Diverse Industrial Pollutants. *ChemistrySelect* **2018**, *3*, 1919–1932. [CrossRef]
2. Karthikraj, R.; Vasu, A.K.; Balakrishna, K.; Sinha, R.K.; Kannan, K. Occurrence and fate of parabens and their metabolites in five sewage treatment plants in India. *Sci. Total Environ.* **2017**, *593–594*, 592–598. [CrossRef] [PubMed]
3. De Jesus Gaffney, V.; Almeida, C.M.M.; Rodrigues, A.; Ferreira, E.; Benoliel, M.J.; Cardoso, V.V. Occurrence of pharmaceuticals in a water supply system and related human health risk assessment. *Water Res.* **2015**, *72*, 199–208. [CrossRef] [PubMed]
4. Frederiksen, H.; Nielsen, O.; Skakkebaek, N.E.; Juul, A.; Andersson, A.-M. UV filters analyzed by isotope diluted TurboFlow-LC–MS/MS in urine from Danish children and adolescents. *Int. J. Hyg. Environ. Health* **2017**, *220*, 244–253. [CrossRef] [PubMed]
5. Li, X.; Ying, G.-G.; Zhao, J.-L.; Chen, Z.-F.; Lai, H.-J.; Su, H.-C. 4-Nonylphenol, bisphenol-A and triclosan levels in human urine of children and students in China, and the effects of drinking these bottled materials on the levels. *Environ. Int.* **2013**, *52*, 81–86. [CrossRef]
6. Yang, Y.; Ok, Y.S.; Kim, K.-H.; Kwon, E.E.; Tsang, Y.F. Occurrences and removal of pharmaceuticals and personal care products (PPCPs) in drinking water and water/sewage treatment plants: A review. *Sci. Total Environ.* **2017**, *596–597*, 303–320. [CrossRef]
7. Zhang, M.; Shen, J.; Zhong, Y.; Ding, T.; Dissanayake, P.D.; Yang, Y.; Tsang, Y.F.; Ok, Y.S. Sorption of pharmaceuticals and personal care products (PPCPs) from water and wastewater by carbonaceous materials: A review. *Crit. Rev. Environ. Sci. Technol.* **2022**, *52*, 727–766. [CrossRef]
8. Ioannou-Ttofa, L.; Raj, S.; Prakash, H.; Fatta-Kassinos, D. Solar photo-Fenton oxidation for the removal of ampicillin, total cultivable and resistant *E. coli* and ecotoxicity from secondary-treated wastewater effluents. *Chem. Eng. J.* **2019**, *355*, 91–102. [CrossRef]
9. Qian, H.; Yu, G.; Hou, Q.; Nie, Y.; Bai, C.; Bai, X.; Wang, H.; Ju, M. Ingenious control of adsorbed oxygen species to construct dual reaction centers ZnO@FePc photo-Fenton catalyst with high-speed electron transmission channel for PPCPs degradation. *Appl. Catal. B Environ.* **2021**, *291*, 120064. [CrossRef]
10. Angkaew, A.; Chokejaroenrat, C.; Sakulthaew, C.; Mao, J.; Watcharatharapong, T.; Watcharenwong, A.; Imman, S.; Suriyachai, N.; Kreetachat, T. Two facile synthesis routes for magnetic recoverable $MnFe_2O_4$/g-C_3N_4 nanocomposites to enhance visible light photo-Fenton activity for methylene blue degradation. *J. Environ. Chem. Eng.* **2021**, *9*, 105621. [CrossRef]
11. Huang, G.-X.; Wang, C.-Y.; Yang, C.-W.; Guo, P.-C.; Yu, H.-Q. Degradation of Bisphenol A by Peroxymonosulfate Catalytically Activated with $Mn_{1.8}Fe_{1.2}O_4$ Nanospheres: Synergism between Mn and Fe. *Environ. Sci. Technol.* **2017**, *51*, 12611–12618. [CrossRef] [PubMed]
12. Angkaew, A.; Sakulthaew, C.; Nimtim, M.; Imman, S.; Satapanajaru, T.; Suriyachai, N.; Kreetachat, T.; Comfort, S.; Chokejaroenrat, C. Enhanced Photo-Fenton Activity Using Magnetic $Cu_{0.5}Mn_{0.5}Fe_2O_4$ Nanoparticles as a Recoverable Catalyst for Degrading Organic Contaminants. *Water* **2022**, *14*, 3717. [CrossRef]
13. Yang, J.; Zhang, Y.; Zeng, D.; Zhang, B.; Hassan, M.; Li, P.; Qi, C.; He, Y. Enhanced catalytic activation of photo-Fenton process by $Cu_{0.5}Mn_{0.5}Fe_2O_4$ for effective removal of organic contaminants. *Chemosphere* **2020**, *247*, 125780. [CrossRef]

14. Yang, J.; Zeng, D.; Zheng, H.; Xie, Q.; Huang, J.; Xiao, L.; Peng, D.-L. 3D graphene encapsulated ZnO-NiO-CuO double-shelled hollow microspheres with enhanced lithium storage properties. *J. Alloys Compd.* **2018**, *765*, 1158–1166. [CrossRef]
15. Zhang, X.; Ding, Y.; Tang, H.; Han, X.; Zhu, L.; Wang, N. Degradation of bisphenol A by hydrogen peroxide activated with $CuFeO_2$ microparticles as a heterogeneous Fenton-like catalyst: Efficiency, stability and mechanism. *Chem. Eng. J.* **2014**, *236*, 251–262. [CrossRef]
16. Hashemian, S.; Dehghanpor, A.; Moghahed, M. $Cu_{0.5}Mn_{0.5}Fe_2O_4$ nano spinels as potential sorbent for adsorption of brilliant green. *J. Ind. Eng. Chem.* **2015**, *24*, 308–314. [CrossRef]
17. Lasdon, L.S.; Fox, R.L.; Ratner, M.W. Nonlinear optimization using the generalized reduced gradient method. *RAIRO Oper. Res* **1974**, *8*, 73–103. [CrossRef]
18. Chokejaroenrat, C.; Watcharenwong, A.; Sakulthaew, C.; Rittirat, A. Immobilization of Atrazine Using Oxidized Lignite Amendments in Agricultural Soils. *Water Air Soil Pollut.* **2020**, *231*, 249. [CrossRef]
19. Wakkel, M.; Khiari, B.; Zagrouba, F. Textile wastewater treatment by agro-industrial waste: Equilibrium modelling, thermodynamics and mass transfer mechanisms of cationic dyes adsorption onto low-cost lignocellulosic adsorbent. *J. Taiwan Inst. Chem. Eng.* **2019**, *96*, 439–452. [CrossRef]
20. Chicco, D.; Warrens, M.J.; Jurman, G. The coefficient of determination R-squared is more informative than SMAPE, MAE, MAPE, MSE and RMSE in regression analysis evaluation. *PeerJ Comput. Sci.* **2021**, *7*, e623. [CrossRef]
21. Wang, B.; Zeng, D.; Chen, Y.; Belzile, N.; Bai, Y.; Zhu, J.; Shu, J.; Chen, S. Adsorption behaviors of phenanthrene and bisphenol A in purple paddy soils amended with straw-derived DOM in the West Sichuan Plain of China. *Ecotoxicol. Environ. Saf.* **2019**, *169*, 737–746. [CrossRef] [PubMed]
22. Ansari, S.A.; Ansari, S.G.; Foaud, H.; Cho, M.H. Facile and sustainable synthesis of carbon-doped ZnO nanostructures towards the superior visible light photocatalytic performance. *New J. Chem.* **2017**, *41*, 9314–9320. [CrossRef]
23. Wang, X.; Wang, A.; Ma, J. Visible-light-driven photocatalytic removal of antibiotics by newly designed $C_3N_4@MnFe_2O_4$-graphene nanocomposites. *J. Hazard. Mater.* **2017**, *336*, 81–92. [CrossRef]
24. Jiang, J.; Gao, J.; Niu, S.; Wang, X.; Li, T.; Liu, S.; Lin, Y.; Xie, T.; Dong, S. Comparing dark- and photo-Fenton-like degradation of emerging pollutant over photo-switchable $Bi_2WO_6/CuFe_2O_4$: Investigation on dominant reactive oxidation species. *J. Environ. Sci.* **2021**, *106*, 147–160. [CrossRef] [PubMed]
25. Lai, C.; Huang, F.; Zeng, G.; Huang, D.; Qin, L.; Cheng, M.; Zhang, C.; Li, B.; Yi, H.; Liu, S.; et al. Fabrication of novel magnetic $MnFe_2O_4$/bio-char composite and heterogeneous photo-Fenton degradation of tetracycline in near neutral pH. *Chemosphere* **2019**, *224*, 910–921. [CrossRef]
26. Soufi, A.; Hajjaoui, H.; Elmoubarki, R.; Abdennouri, M.; Qourzal, S.; Barka, N. Heterogeneous Fenton-like degradation of tartrazine using $CuFe_2O_4$ nanoparticles synthesized by sol-gel combustion. *Appl. Surf. Sci. Adv.* **2022**, *9*, 100251. [CrossRef]
27. Ahmad, H.; Haseen, U.; Umar, K.; Ansari, M.S.; Ibrahim, M.N.M. Bioinspired 2D carbon sheets decorated with $MnFe_2O_4$ nanoparticles for preconcentration of inorganic arsenic, and its determination by ICP-OES. *Microchim. Acta* **2019**, *186*, 649. [CrossRef]
28. Ghobadi, M.; Gharabaghi, M.; Abdollahi, H.; Boroumand, Z.; Moradian, M. $MnFe_2O_4$-graphene oxide magnetic nanoparticles as a high-performance adsorbent for rare earth elements: Synthesis, isotherms, kinetics, thermodynamics and desorption. *J. Hazard. Mater.* **2018**, *351*, 308–316. [CrossRef]
29. Wang, Z.; Lai, C.; Qin, L.; Fu, Y.; He, J.; Huang, D.; Li, B.; Zhang, M.; Liu, S.; Li, L.; et al. ZIF-8-modified $MnFe_2O_4$ with high crystallinity and superior photo-Fenton catalytic activity by Zn-O-Fe structure for TC degradation. *Chem. Eng. J.* **2020**, *392*, 124851. [CrossRef]
30. Goodgame, D.M.L.; Hussain, I.; White, A.J.P.; Williams, D.J. Synthesis and structure of a copper(II) melamine complex, $[Cu(C_3H_6N_6)(\mu\text{-}OCH_3)(ONO_2)(HOCH_3)]_2$, with direct Cu–melamine coordination. *J. Chem. Soc. Dalton Trans.* **1999**, *17*, 2899–2900. [CrossRef]
31. Wiles, A.B.; Bozzuto, D.; Cahill, C.L.; Pike, R.D. Copper (I) and (II) complexes of melamine. *Polyhedron* **2006**, *25*, 776–782. [CrossRef]
32. Doddamani, J.S.; Hodlur, R.M.; Rabinal, M.K. Melamine assisted large-scale and rapid synthesis of porous copper oxide nanostructures. *Emergent Mater.* **2022**, *5*, 1089–1096. [CrossRef]
33. Farooq, U.; Ahmed, J.; Alshehri, S.M.; Ahmad, T. High-Surface-Area Sodium Tantalate Nanoparticles with Enhanced Photocatalytic and Electrical Properties Prepared through Polymeric Citrate Precursor Route. *ACS Omega* **2019**, *4*, 19408–19419. [CrossRef] [PubMed]
34. Farooq, U.; Ahmed, J.; Alshehri, S.M.; Mao, Y.; Ahmad, T. Self-Assembled Interwoven Nanohierarchitectures of $NaNbO_3$ and $NaNb_{1-x}Ta_xO_3$ $(0.05 \leq x \leq 0.20)$: Synthesis, Structural Characterization, Photocatalytic Applications, and Dielectric Properties. *ACS Omega* **2022**, *7*, 16952–16967. [CrossRef]
35. Domínguez, J.R.; Muñoz, M.J.; Palo, P.; González, T.; Peres, J.A.; Cuerda-Correa, E.M. Fenton advanced oxidation of emerging pollutants: Parabens. *Int. J. Energy Environ. Eng.* **2014**, *5*, 89. [CrossRef]
36. Pattanateeradetch, A.; Sakulthaew, C.; Angkaew, A.; Sutjarit, S.; Poompoung, T.; Lin, Y.-T.; Harris, C.E.; Comfort, S.; Chokejaroenrat, C. Fabrication of Ternary Nanoparticles for Catalytic Ozonation to Treat Parabens: Mechanisms, Efficiency, and Effects on Ceratophyllum demersum L. and Eker Leiomyoma Tumor-3 Cells. *Nanomaterials* **2022**, *12*, 3573. [CrossRef] [PubMed]

37. Gmurek, M.; Rossi, A.F.; Martins, R.C.; Quinta-Ferreira, R.M.; Ledakowicz, S. Photodegradation of single and mixture of parabens—Kinetic, by-products identification and cost-efficiency analysis. *Chem. Eng. J.* **2015**, *276*, 303–314. [CrossRef]
38. Angı, A.; Sanlı, D.; Erkey, C.; Birer, Ö. Catalytic activity of copper (II) oxide prepared via ultrasound assisted Fenton-like reaction. *Ultrason. Sonochemistry* **2014**, *21*, 854–859. [CrossRef]
39. Al-Musawi, T.J.; Brouers, F.; Zarrabi, M. Kinetic modeling of antibiotic adsorption onto different nanomaterials using the Brouers–Sotolongo fractal equation. *Environ. Sci. Pollut. Res.* **2017**, *24*, 4048–4057. [CrossRef]
40. Selmi, T.; Sanchez-Sanchez, A.; Gadonneix, P.; Jagiello, J.; Seffen, M.; Sammouda, H.; Celzard, A.; Fierro, V. Tetracycline removal with activated carbons produced by hydrothermal carbonisation of *Agave americana* fibres and mimosa tannin. *Ind. Crops Prod.* **2018**, *115*, 146–157. [CrossRef]
41. Ho, Y.S.; McKay, G. Pseudo-second order model for sorption processes. *Process Biochem.* **1999**, *34*, 451–465. [CrossRef]
42. Chokejaroenrat, C.; Sakulthaew, C.; Satchasataporn, K.; Snow, D.D.; Ali, T.E.; Assiri, M.A.; Watcharenwong, A.; Imman, S.; Suriyachai, N.; Kreetachat, T. Enrofloxacin and Sulfamethoxazole Sorption on Carbonized Leonardite: Kinetics, Isotherms, Influential Effects, and Antibacterial Activity toward *S. aureus* ATCC 25923. *Antibiotics* **2022**, *11*, 1261. [CrossRef] [PubMed]
43. Sakulthaew, C.; Chokejaroenrat, C.; Poapolathep, A.; Satapanajaru, T.; Poapolathep, S. Hexavalent chromium adsorption from aqueous solution using carbon nano-onions (CNOs). *Chemosphere* **2017**, *184*, 1168–1174. [CrossRef]
44. Sakulthaew, C.; Watcharenwong, A.; Chokejaroenrat, C.; Rittirat, A. Leonardite-Derived Biochar Suitability for Effective Sorption of Herbicides. *Water Air Soil Pollut.* **2021**, *232*, 36. [CrossRef]
45. Zhang, X.; Xu, B.; Wang, S.; Li, X.; Wang, C.; Liu, B.; Han, F.; Xu, Y.; Yu, P.; Sun, Y. Tetracycline degradation by peroxymonosulfate activated with CoNx active sites: Performance and activation mechanism. *Chem. Eng. J.* **2022**, *431*, 133477. [CrossRef]
46. Bembibre, A.; Benamara, M.; Hjiri, M.; Gómez, E.; Alamri, H.R.; Dhahri, R.; Serrà, A. Visible-light driven sonophotocatalytic removal of tetracycline using Ca-doped ZnO nanoparticles. *Chem. Eng. J.* **2022**, *427*, 132006. [CrossRef]
47. Wang, J.; Zhi, D.; Zhou, H.; He, X.; Zhang, D. Evaluating tetracycline degradation pathway and intermediate toxicity during the electrochemical oxidation over a Ti/Ti$_4$O$_7$ anode. *Water Res.* **2018**, *137*, 324–334. [CrossRef]
48. Chokejaroenrat, C.; Sakulthaew, C.; Chantakulvanich, S.; Angkaew, A.; Teingtham, K.; Phansak, P.; Poompoung, T.; Snow, D.D.; Harris, C.E.; Comfort, S.D. Enhanced degradation of herbicides in groundwater using sulfur-containing reductants and spinel zinc ferrite activated persulfate. *Sci. Total Environ.* **2023**, *892*, 164652. [CrossRef]
49. Chouychai, W.; Paemsom, T.; Pobsuwan, C.; Somtrakoon, K.; Lee, H. Effect of Indole-3-Acetic Acid-Producing Bacteria on Phytoremediation of Soil Contaminated with Phenanthrene and Anthracene by Mungbean. *EnvironmentAsia* **2016**, *9*, 128–133. [CrossRef]
50. Chi, S.L.; Wang, W.Z.; Xu, W.H.; Li, T.; Li, Y.H.; Zhang, C.L. Effects of Tetracycline Antibiotics on Growth and Characteristics of Enrichment and Transformation in Two Vegetables. *Huan Jing Ke Xue* **2018**, *39*, 935–943. [CrossRef]
51. Bao, Y.; Pan, C.; Li, D.; Guo, A.; Dai, F. Stress response to oxytetracycline and microplastic-polyethylene in wheat (*Triticum aestivum* L.) during seed germination and seedling growth stages. *Sci. Total Environ.* **2022**, *806*, 150553. [CrossRef] [PubMed]
52. Gomes, M.P.; Richardi, V.S.; Bicalho, E.M.; da Rocha, D.C.; Navarro-Silva, M.A.; Soffiatti, P.; Garcia, Q.S.; Sant'Anna-Santos, B.F. Effects of Ciprofloxacin and Roundup on seed germination and root development of maize. *Sci. Total Environ.* **2019**, *651*, 2671–2678. [CrossRef] [PubMed]
53. Yuan, H.-M.; Huang, X. Inhibition of root meristem growth by cadmium involves nitric oxide-mediated repression of auxin accumulation and signalling in *Arabidopsis*. *Plant Cell Environ.* **2016**, *39*, 120–135. [CrossRef] [PubMed]
54. Tripthi, D.K.; Varma, R.K.; Singh, S.; Sachan, M.; Guerriero, G.; Kushwaha, B.K.; Bhardwaj, S.; Ramawat, N.; Sharma, S.; Singh, V.P.; et al. Silicon tackles butachlor toxicity in rice seedlings by regulating anatomical characteristics, ascorbate-glutathione cycle, proline metabolism and levels of nutrients. *Sci. Rep.* **2020**, *10*, 14078. [CrossRef]
55. Pandey, A.K.; Zorić, L.; Sun, T.; Karanović, D.; Fang, P.; Borišev, M.; Wu, X.; Luković, J.; Xu, P. The Anatomical Basis of Heavy Metal Responses in Legumes and Their Impact on Plant–Rhizosphere Interactions. *Plants* **2022**, *11*, 2554. [CrossRef]
56. Cole, J.C.; Smith, M.W.; Penn, C.J.; Cheary, B.S.; Conaghan, K.J. Nitrogen, phosphorus, calcium, and magnesium applied individually or as a slow release or controlled release fertilizer increase growth and yield and affect macronutrient and micronutrient concentration and content of field-grown tomato plants. *Sci. Hortic.* **2016**, *211*, 420–430. [CrossRef]

MDPI

St. Alban-Anlage 66

4052 Basel

Switzerland

www.mdpi.com

Antibiotics Editorial Office

E-mail: antibiotics@mdpi.com

www.mdpi.com/journal/antibiotics

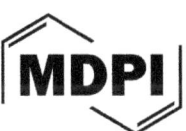